T0133213

AMERICAN STUDIES – A MONOGRAPH SERIES
Volume 236

Edited on behalf
of the German Association
for American Studies by
REINHARD R. DOERRIES
GERHARD HOFFMANN
ALFRED HORNUNG

Communicating Disease:

Cultural Representations of American Medicine

Edited by
CARMEN BIRKLE
JOHANNA HEIL

Universitätsverlag
WINTER
Heidelberg

Bibliografische Information der Deutschen Nationalbibliothek

Die Deutsche Nationalbibliothek verzeichnet diese Publikation
in der Deutschen Nationalbibliografie;
detaillierte bibliografische Daten sind im Internet
über *http://dnb.d-nb.de* abrufbar.

COVER ILLUSTRATION

Student Dissecting a Leg, *Frank Leslie's Illustrated Newspaper*,
April 16, 1870

ISBN 978-3-8253-6215-7

© 2013 Universitätsverlag Winter GmbH Heidelberg
Imprimé en Allemagne · Printed in Germany
Druck: Memminger MedienCentrum, 87700 Memmingen

Gedruckt auf umweltfreundlichem, chlorfrei gebleichtem
und alterungsbeständigem Papier

Den Verlag erreichen Sie im Internet unter:
www.winter-verlag.de

Table of Contents

CARMEN BIRKLE

Communicating Disease: An Introduction

Bridging the Gap

The present volume on cultural representations of American medicine is the outcome of an interest in the intersections of literature and medicine and, more generally, cultural representations and the natural sciences. As the medical historian Dietrich von Engelhardt points out, "[m]edicine needs history and culture because it is not only a natural science but also a humanistic science and art" ("Teaching History of Medicine" 1). Engelhardt goes on to explain the need for teaching the history of medicine from the perspective of the "medical humanities" by foregrounding the intricate entanglement of culture and disease: "Culture is the cause of disease and the product of disease as well. Culture shapes the disease, diagnosis and therapy, situation of the patient, and activity of the physician" (1). Therefore, phenomena of health and illness and their definitions are very much subject to the characteristics of the respective cultures, a phenomenon which Engel-hardt defines as "the cultural, social, and political dimensions of the disease" (2). As he points out, "concepts of health and disease require new definitions, as well as the understanding of culture and the arts. Separation of the sciences and the humanities is inappropriate in medicine. These initiatives aim at bridging the gap between the natural sciences and humanities in medicine. The history of the patient should be as important as the history of the illness" (5). Similarly, the medical psychiatrist Allan Beveridge, after weighing the pros and cons of whether those in his profession should read fiction, comes to the conclusion that "there is a growing acknowledgement of the value of the humanities in medical education, and perhaps this is part of a wider trend that recognises the limitations of a purely biotechnological approach to patient care" (386). It is this exclusive dominance of biotechnology at the expense of the humanities in medicine that our collection of essays seeks to dispute.

However, at first sight, literature and medicine seem to be, as common preconceived notions suggest, incompatible areas of human life. While the one, in Horace's famous and pertinent dictum, is meant to educate and to entertain (*prodesse et delectare*), or, as the idea of art for art's sake and the New Critics many centuries later advocates, has to be seen as an aesthetic object to be appreciated disregarding any historical context, the other is expected to improve and save people's lives and provide means to fight disease and even death. These expectations presuppose literature to be pleasurable but ultimately not really necessary and medicine to be of utmost importance for human survival. By analogy, the same distinction applies to the scholars and practitioners in both fields. While the literary critic finds it hard to produce insights and hard facts relevant for the progress of humanity, the medical researcher and practitioner can easily turn into a proverbial "God in white" who is expected to save the world. Obviously, these distinctions boil down to the frequently discussed dichotomy between the humanities and the natural sciences.

However, in more recent years, as Dietrich von Engelhardt's essay suggests, scholars have moved forward to postulate a mutual recognition of these fields. We no longer have to resort to Hans Robert Jauß who, as early as 1967, declared that literature does not just mimetically reproduce reality or, for that matter, human life, but has to be understood as a medium that shapes human perception and changes human life. Consequently, for Jauß, art for art's sake needed to be replaced by a form of reader-response theory in which not only each reader with his or her specific knowledge and expectations gives meaning to and interprets a literary text, but begins to see the impact of literature as something fluid and forever changing in conjunction with the larger realm of human history. The subsequent theories of a new historicism with its understanding of the textuality of history and the historicity of texts (cf. Montrose; Barry 166) as well as its non-hierarchical reading of all texts as co-texts (cf. Greenblatt; Veeser), and of cultural studies (cf. During; Grossberg, Nelson, and Treichler; Storey), which not only considers literature a cultural practice but also as representing cultural practices, have contributed their share to the rising recognition of the intersections of literature and human life and, in the case at hand, of literature and life sciences.

In his 2004 study *ÜberLebenswissen: Die Aufgabe der Philologie*, the literary and cultural studies scholar Ottmar Ette discusses the idea of literary studies/literary criticism as life sciences (14). As he points out, literature "knows" about life and never ceases to offer this knowledge to its readers. However, as Ette notes with regret, literary scholars do not seem to be aware of the essential questions literature asks or, better, offers about life. He posits that this ignorance is highly dangerous because it excludes literature and literary studies from ways of producing knowledge which are crucial to human life and, therefore, quite popular as an area of investigation. Although scholars of literature think to the contrary, the recognition of literary studies as a life science will open up hitherto untapped areas of knowledge, in particular if accessed jointly and in search of interdisciplinary synergies. For Ette, it is important to protect life and knowledge of life from a purely biologically motivated investigation and to engage in new forms of inter- and transdisciplinary collaboration in the exploration of life (16-18).

As Ette furthermore argues, this knowledge needs to be gained from a look at what he calls, based on Giorgio Agamben, "[d]as 'nackte', das 'bloße' Leben" (19), which is inextricably linked to political, social, and cultural life. Thus, nature and culture need to be seen in their webs of entanglement (19). This interdisciplinarity produces heterotopias of knowledge (19), as Ette explains, which cannot be left for investigation to one or the other discipline but transcend traditional disciplinary boundaries (20), most relevant in the encounter of a multiplicity of different cultures. Literature, as Ette then concludes, offers a form of knowledge that cannot be reduced to simple instructions on how to live but has to be embraced in its entire complexity (21).[1] In this sense, the literary text is no longer seen just as a mimetic mirror of reality but offers an imaginary representation of life, which is, at the same time, an interpretation of and influence on life. Memory, that is, the remembering

---

[1] Ette's pun on the German "ÜberLebenswissen," i.e., knowledge about life and knowledge about how to survive, can, unfortunately, not be reproduced in English.

and making use of a usable past, connects past, present, and future. Narratives can experiment with past and present in order to offer visions for a (potentially different?) future. They can be subversive, pointing to shortcomings, problems, and dangerous developments; they can be utopian or dystopian in tone and mood; they can be liberating or conforming, manipulative or critical. Literature can be all this with regard to the representation of the medical profession.

The volume at hand looks at precisely this complexity of literature, with the particular focus on some of the intersections of literature and medicine, thus on aspects of the representation of what Charles Percy Snow once called *The Two Cultures* in his book of the same title (cf. also Brockman). The present volume shows that literature/literary studies and medicine are not two warring disciplines but that "biology and culture" and their respective disciplines have what Rüdiger Kunow calls "double jurisdiction . . . over human life" (30), with both always cross-fertilizing each other. Admittedly, this attempt here will be undertaken exclusively by scholars of American, English, and Canadian Studies, with the exception of the medical historian Dietrich von Engelhardt. Nevertheless, the present enterprise of exploring the interfaces of literature and medicine can be considered a first step— from a literary and cultural point of view—toward a possible inter- disciplinary collaboration, in which each discipline will first have to clarify and be aware of its own premises, expectations, and aims.

What are some of these premises in literary and cultural studies and how do they offer ground for medical investigation? To argue with Ette, literature and cultural representations are both about life and comprise life and, therefore, take on the qualities of archives and vessels through which medical issues are debated, as can be seen, for example, in Puritan accounts of Native American contact with epidemics, Louisa May Alcott's sketches on Civil War hospitals, or in Siri Hustvedt's autobiographical narrative on psychotherapy. On a more structural level, narratives display techniques of storytelling, the analysis and under- standing of which helps medicine to deal more competently and successfully with their patients' narratives. If trained properly, the doctor becomes a literary critic who knows how to analyze elements such as narrative perspective, imagery, mode of representation, logical structure of representation, choice of words, among other literary devices that all, broadly, contribute to meaning-making practices in general (cf. Brody; Charon; Davis). In the past few decades, a new field of medicine, that is, narrative medicine, has been developed into a field of interdisciplinary expertise in medical training, for example, as established by the physician and philologist Rita Charon and the literary and cultural studies scholar Maura Spiegel at Columbia University in New York City. An analysis of, first, content-related and, second, structural elements of narratives contributes to the formation of practitioners—literary critics as well as doctors—who are well versed in the study of life, that is, the life sciences.

An initial content-related analysis of literature and other cultural representations of medicine offers historians of medicine a substantial corpus of information for the creation of a cultural history of medicine. While the depiction of medical phenomena may not necessarily be adequate or based on historical knowledge of their respective times, narratives may negotiate social norms and values, for example, portraying the interactions of doctors and patients, discussing the social and moral impact of diseases on societies and nations, or revealing the complexities of the concepts of illness and health. Without the need for a scientifically accepted truth, literature can juxtapose and intersect various discourses, as Bettina von Jagow and Florian Steger point out with reference to Rudolf Käser's study *Arzt, Tod und Text* (1998):

> Der medizinische Diskurs stehe demnach immer in Zusammenhang mit anderen Diskursen, die den Anspruch haben, Normen für unser Handeln definieren zu können. Literatur biete einen diskursiven Ort, in dem auch als 'unwissenschaftlich' disqualifizierte Konzepte von Leben, Krankheit und Tod thematisiert, das heißt konfligierende Kompetenzansprüche verschiedener Diskurse namhaft gemacht und diskutiert werden könnten. (11)

Literature may thus offer a whole inventory of depictions of illness and their social, cultural, and historical implications (cf. 12), which can help students of medicine understand the history of medicine in context. After all, illness and its symptoms are never just isolated medical and biological phenomena, but have emerged in the body and the mind of a human being embedded in a social, personal, and cultural environment shaping the individual and his/her identity. Therefore, as Jagow and Steger suggest: "Literarische Texte sind wichtige Quellen für die Medizinhistoriographie und mit ihren ganzheitlichen Beschreibungen

von Gesundheit und Krankheit, Geburt und Tod, Arzt und Patient auch
für die Medizin und den medizinischen Unterricht" (13).

Narrative medicine makes use of both the content and structure of
narratives. It focuses on literature's knowledge of life, its aesthetics and
structures, and aims at an understanding thereof as a tool for the doctor
to approach the patient and to get more profound access to and
understanding of patient narratives. What the doctor needs, as Rita
Charon suggests, is "narrative knowledge" (9). As Gert H. Brieger
explains:

> We constantly tell stories, listen to them, and watch them. Our human
> experiences, including those we tell to our doctors, are the stuff of
> narrative. Narrative, then, is the way we make sense of the world. As the
> clinical narrative tells us much about the patient's illness, so the way we
> tell our history of medical ideas and practices indicates a great deal
> about how we perceive ourselves as an occupational group, as a
> profession, as healers. (406)

While illnesses can be used metaphorically, they are at the same time
very real, and ill persons certainly agree with Susan Sontag that "illness
is *not* a metaphor" (3) although illness is often represented metaphorically. To interpret a patient's metaphoric language is a major step on the
way toward a doctor's diagnosis. Rita Charon highly values this
interpersonal relationship as an element of successful medical treatment:
"Along with their growing scientific expertise, doctors need the
expertise to listen to their patients, to understand as best they can the
ordeals of illness, to honor the meanings of their patients' narratives of
illness, and to be moved by what they behold so that they can act on
their patients' behalf" (3). This narrative knowledge will help the doctor
in understanding the individual and his/her illness "as a singular and
meaningful situation," and it also "attempts to illuminate the universals
of the human condition by revealing the particular" (9). Narrative
medicine thus postulates "the centrality of storytelling" (11) through
which identities are created (cf. 11). Charon takes recourse to
narratology and singles out "five narrative features of medicine—
temporality, singular-ity, causality/contingency, intersubjectivity, and
ethicality" (39). The story told by a patient is always singular, unique,
and non-reproducible so that careful attention has to be paid to its

structure, logic, and context. Charon answers the question of what literature or literary studies contribute to medicine in the following way:

> What literary studies give medicine is the realization that our intimate medical relationships occur in words. Our intimacy with patients is based predominantly on *listening to what they tell us*, and our trustworthiness toward them is demonstrated in the seriousness and duty with which we listen to what they entrust to us. Yes, doctors touch patients and do rather extraordinary physical things to them, but the textuality and not the physicality defines the relation. (53)

Therefore, for narrative medicine the narrativization of the doctor figure is a most crucial point of interest in its analysis of representations, since they reveal more about the profession than any student of medicine may find in medical textbooks. Medical students realize how much their future job is embedded in larger personal, cultural, and social contexts, the impact of which often eludes most practitioners, as Patricia Anne Vertinsky explains: "As agents of society, male and female physicians have demonstrated, in their practices, particular cultural values and orientations, and the importance attributed to their diagnoses and prescriptions has depended upon the active participation and collusion of members of society" (1). The analysis of doctor-patient relationships is crucial to the work of narrative medicine because *both* sides produce narratives, "the patient's story of illness and the doctor's story of diagnosis" (Wells 35) as outcomes of their mutual engagement, which *both* need to be analyzed to understand the mechanisms and structures of their often ritualized communication (cf. Wells 35).[2]

---

[2] As Wells continues: "Patients want to tell stories, to articulate the development and changes of their symptoms, while doctors use the interview to pursue a serial and necessarily disconnected investigation of specific themes:

D: How long have you been drinking that heavily?
P: Since I've been married.
D: How long is that?

Replies are interrupted when the doctor responds to what she feels or sees, opening a new line of questions. The medical interview is inherently discontinuous, since the patient experiences the symptom as a history, while the doctor attempts to localize it within a segmented body" (35).

This interest in the doctor figure inevitably leads to the doctor-author who is both a doctor listening to his/her patients and an author writing about his/her experiences, translating the medical communicative act into a written discourse, often exhibiting narrative features. For doctors who are also authors, literature can serve as a means to reflect on their own positions, acts, and emotions. Writing can become a way of coming to terms with both the joy of healing but, most prominently, with the pain, suffering, and often death that cannot be prevented (cf. Jagow and Steger 87). While some strictly separate their literary and medical lives, such as the nineteenth-century doctor Mary Putnam Jacobi, who ceased to write short stories when she received her medical degree in 1871, a prominent example of the conjunction of both fields is the U.S.-American poet, writer, and doctor William Carlos Williams (1883-1963). As he explains in his *Autobiography*, he could not be one without the other: "[A]s a writer I have never felt that medicine interfered with me but rather that it was my very food and drink, the very thing which made it possible for me to write" (357). Much of what we today know about the medical profession derives from the practitioners themselves, often situating themselves in the contexts of their discipline and historical environment in autobiographies. However, a cautionary note is necessary here. As memory studies have shown, even autobiographical writing is never an exact transposition of life into writing, thus never a one-to-one rendition of reality and as such its interpretation requires expert knowledge in autobiography studies.

Finally, no matter whether we analyze content or structural phenomena, the engagement with narratives is always a communicative act and is itself based on such acts. Literary critics as well as medical practitioners and historians or researchers need to be trained in the reading of interpersonal communication without which "ÜberLebens-wissen" (Ette) would not be productive. If all our lives are stories, these stories will have to be told to affect humanity. Tracing the representation of a communicative act reveals the historical changes in the position of the individual, in power relations, in the use and function of language. Communicative acts are shaped by a sender and a receiver, a medium and a message as well as a code. Additionally, the very manifestations of each shift and change in this framework over the centuries, and processes of encoding and decoding depend on the respective contexts of sender and receiver. Consequently, the more an understanding of the mechanisms of such an act is enhanced, the more successful the act will be. Both patient and doctor become sender and receiver and need to be able to en- and decode each other's messages, thereby jointly producing the diagnostic narrative. Ultimately, communication takes place in two locations: intrinsically between characters, for example, doctors and patients; and extrinsically between texts and readers, between texts and co-texts, between literature and medicine.

Both patient and doctor—whether in cultural representations or actual life—are deeply embedded in the rules and norms, mores and values of their time. By definition they are, therefore, also influenced by the dominant gender roles and norms that have strongly shaped literature and medicine. Gender is loosely defined as social and cultural construction visible in gender roles, which are in turn subject to change but are, however, often considered permanent, natural, and given. Gender roles are—in spite of their quality of construction—often firmly attached to the biological sexes of men and women and define what men or women can or cannot do from the point of view of society. While existing gender conceptions shape literature and medicine, literary and medical discourses also create gender norms. As Vertinsky points out, "medical representation, through its discourse, constituted women in particular ways . . ." (11-12). Binary oppositions, including a hierarchical understanding of these oppositions, characterize gender relations and reveal a socially sanctioned power structure accepted as natural or even, in some contexts, as God-given. Women's desire to write, to embrace the idea of authorship, was for centuries regarded as unfeminine and unnatural so that many women used pen names, did not write, or simply felt guilty and suffered from social disapproval for breaking gender roles. Similarly, women were considered to be too physically weak to get a higher education and to pursue a career, for example, in medicine. This supposedly unnatural desire, as people continued to believe up until the twentieth century, would not only destroy women's physical and mental health, but would also render them unable to fulfill their "natural" and biological duties as wives, mothers, and housewives. Female authors and doctors struggled with these gender norms; female patients suffered from the inflicted and hierarchically coded "healing" methods.

It is the aim of this volume not only "to disclose a surprising past and to reconstruct a usable past" (Wells 145), but to show that literature and other cultural products do not stage gigantic monologues addressed to no one in particular, but rather offer the opportunity for dialogue between the humanities and the natural sciences, between literary studies and medicine as two sides of the same life-science coin. The volume is organized in four sections that prominently explore one major aspect each of the interfaces of literature and medicine while all being infused—explicitly or implicitly—with the notion of gender as a normative category of life. Parts I, II, and III look at literary and cultural narratives as representations of or meta-comments on the medical profession and its debates on possible medical and socio-political treatments of specific illnesses, diseases, and epidemics or on the entrance of women into the field. Part IV reverses this medical gaze by focusing on the patient's gaze and more explicitly discusses the potential healing powers of narratives and some of the implications in the cognitive sciences.

Negotiating Medical Practice

Part I discusses fictional or historiographical representations of medical practice from the early eighteenth to the twenty-first century. While mostly focusing on U.S.-American practices, English and Canadian case studies are instrumental in emphasizing the inter-connectedness of medical practices from a more global perspective as well as the webs of entanglement with ethnic practices that are often considered irreconcilable with dominant epistemologies in North America. Marc Priewe is concerned with the intersections of medicine and religion. He examines the conversion debates in the eighteenth century that reveal the mutual infiltration of these two hardly separable areas of human life. Shifting the medical gaze to the smallpox epidemic in eighteenth-century Boston, Marcel Hartwig sheds light on the first attempts to use inoculation as a form of preventive medicine. Not only does Hartwig discuss the transatlantic notion of medicine at the time, but also the overlap in the professions of the clergy and the physicians with both a rejection and acceptance of inoculation as God's will. Ultimately, the often more than heated dialogue between theology and medicine proved fruitful in the final acceptance of inoculation. Sonja Fielitz ponders cultural representations of age and aging in eighteenth-century

English geriatric discourse as represented in both historio-graphical and fictional texts, above all triggered by Francis Bacon and the Royal Society. Based on major changes in medicine around 1650, Jonathan Swift's *Gulliver's Travels* (1726) satirizes the ambitions of the practitioners of the natural sciences and gives old age a very bleak outlook. Ultimately, Swift illustrates, as the essay argues, that medical advancement is not unlimited and that life cannot be forever prolonged. In general, Age Studies is part of a scholarly discourse which has most recently risen to prominence again (cf. Hartung and Kunow; Kunow). Martin Kuester's Canadian shaman Dr. Hullah gives insights into a medical practice that sees mind and body as a whole and, even more, combines Native North American and traditional Old World ways of healing. Like Swift, Robertson Davies, the author of *The Cunning Man* (1994), doubts that the progress of European medicine is never-ending but, in contrast to Swift, proposes an alternative way of healing in a hybrid and holistic form of medicine that integrates mind and body, Native and European views, and individual and community. From the early American colonies via England and Canada, Stephanie Browner takes us to a postcolonial setting and raises the often neglected questions of literature's engagement with poverty and, more precisely, with the availability of treatment and medication for the poor. Her analysis of the structures of power and inequality in two postcolonial novels literally points to the difficulties of survival in the face of non-existent health care and waste management and mismanagement in the field of medical administration. The resulting violence and disease, no matter whether the setting is New York or Calcutta, serve as vivid reminders of literature's and medicine's social responsibilities.

Subverting the Medical Profession

While the contributions to the first section engage with the debates occurring within the different medical factions in a profession still in the making and about treatments still to be developed, Part II offers illuminating insights into the role that gender plays in shaping the power distribution of the newly emerging medical profession. Susan Wells points out with reference to women physicians: "If science is understood as constructed by, among other things, certain practices of language,

then it is worthwhile to study how women performed those practices"
(12). The mid-nineteenth century saw a decline in respect and power
concerning the medical profession that, ironically, facilitated the
entrance of women into the medical profession. There had always been
female healers, and some women had frequently also worked as doctors
without being considered as such and without having a degree in
medicine. Even though American women entered the profession in the
mid-nineteenth century and fought hard to earn their degrees, the
emerging image of the doctor as a gentleman and "a national icon of
refined masculinity" (Browner 137) as well as "the masculinization of
empiricism" (Browner 137) shaping late nineteenth-century medical
practice prevented many women from successfully practicing medicine.

For a long time, medical training was not standardized. Ruth J.
Abram explains: "Neither the absence of a college education nor the
lack of a medical degree prevented anyone from practicing medicine
. . ." ("Soon" 17). Frequently, young men acquired some knowledge by
training, for a short period of time, with a practicing physician:

> After about three years, the students received certificates attesting to
> their medical abilities and good characters. Thus armed, new 'doctors'
> commenced their practices. Even after medical schools were established
> in the United States (the first, the University of Pennsylvania Medical
> School, was founded in 1765), training at these institutions was regarded
> simply as a supplement to the apprenticeship or preceptor system. (17)[3]

Training at these medical schools, as Elizabeth Blackwell also
experienced at Geneva Medical School, "consisted of a three- to four-
month series of lectures, and students were awarded degrees after
completing only two such terms, the second of which was an exact
repetition of the first" (Abram, "Soon" 18), the length depending on the
respective schools and times. Professors with no salary sold admission
tickets to large lecture classes. Thus, medical training did not have a
high reputation because if medical schools wanted to survive, they had
to take anyone who would pay—any man, that is. It was not until 1869

---

[3] In the early 1850s, Dr. Ann Preston (1813-72) studied at the Woman's
Medical College of Pennsylvania, "the first regular medical college for
women in the world . . ." (Abram, "Will There Be a Monument?" 78).

that Harvard University introduced longer periods of study, fixed salaries for its professors, and minimum standards for medical education.

The second half of the nineteenth century saw the rise of more and more women, for example, Elizabeth (1821-1910) and Emily Blackwell (1826-1910), Harriot K. Hunt (1805-75), Lydia Folger Fowler (1822-79), Marie Zakrzewska (1829-1902), Mary Putnam Jacobi (1842-1906), Ann Preston (1813-72), Rebecca J. Cole (1846-1922), Rebecca Lee Crumpler (1831-95), Susan La Flesche Picotte (1865-1915), Angenette Hunt (1819-1901), and others, working hard to overcome all obstacles imposed by the cult of True Womanhood (cf. Welter) and become doctors, sometimes because they felt they had a talent given to them by God, and sometimes because they listened to the pleas of women who would much rather be treated by women than men because of the decency norms of the time. Elizabeth Blackwell, the first American woman doctor with a medical degree, relates in her autobiography the story of a female friend who is terminally ill and who tells Blackwell: "'If I could have been treated by a lady doctor, my worst sufferings would have been spared me'" (Blackwell 74). Women doctors would also have helped their female patients to more easily tell their stories, as Susan Wells suggests: "If the female patient were treated by a female physician, she would have had a wider scope for telling her story; it is certain that she faced a less constricted speech situation" (54).[4]

Carla Bittel's contribution sets the tone for an in-depth under-standing of the role of pioneering women in American medicine. Her case study of the American doctor Mary Putnam Jacobi's substantial body of fictional, social, and medical writings testifies to these disci-plines' intimate connections. Being the first woman to be admitted to the École de Médecine in Paris, Putnam returned to the U.S. as one of the few American women doctors in the nineteenth century with a medical

---

[4]   For more information on women in the medical profession as well as their literary treatment, cf. Morantz-Sanchez, *Sympathy and Science* and "The Female Student Has Arrived"; More; Bittel, *Mary Putnam Jacobi* and "Mary Putnam Jacobi"; Browner; Furst, "From Speculation to Science" and "Halfway Up the Hill." For examples of "scientific" texts denying women the right to pursue higher education, cf. Clarke; Mitchell.

degree. Her life serves as an example of gender as a powerful exclusionary category in the male-dominated field and of the challenges women had to face in their desire to work in medicine (cf. also Walsh). As early as the late nineteenth century, women who aspired to become doctors had to negotiate whether and how they could integrate professional work and private family life. Antje Dallmann chooses to analyze such "doctor romance" novels, which present female practitioners' struggle to overcome all kinds of social obstacles. While William Dean Howells's protagonist fails in her endeavor, Sarah Orne Jewett, Elizabeth Stuart Phelps, and Annie Nathan Meyer offer more successful women doctors who, however, often practice medicine by actively renouncing marriage. Kirsten Twelbeck's contribution shifts the focus from doctors to nurses during the American Civil War. While nursing as such was a socially accepted yet also little valued profession for women but in times of war more than appreciated, as Louisa May Alcott's *Hospital Sketches* portray, Sarah Emma Edmonds is a very interesting case in point of a Canadian woman nurse (cf. also Dodd and Gorham) and spy—aided by cross-dressing—in the American Civil War. Twelbeck's intertextual analysis of Alcott's short fiction and Edmonds's autobiographical text not only reveals how the nineteenth-century ideal of True Womanhood undergoes a significant trans-formation toward the idea of the New Woman, but also how the emancipation of women and African Americans were intimately connected. Edmonds's frequent, obvious but often also hidden references to Alcott take gender and race one step further to an almost postmodern flexibility and fluidity and ask American women to leave home and hospital and become active shapers of history. Katja Schmieder unfolds a late twentieth- and early twenty-first-century per-spective on individual agency, as asked for by Edmonds, and takes recourse to a different medium, namely television. She offers an in-depth analysis of the American TV series *Bones* and *Crossing Jordan*, which feature an extraordinary female forensic anthropologist and pathologist respectively, crossing the borders of femininity by assuming the empirical medical gaze in the traditionally male-dominated work of criminal investigation and law enforcement and, thus, separating it from the voyeuristic male gaze, as Schmieder points out. As transgressor figures, Dr. Temperance Brennan and Dr. Jordan Cavanaugh, in their very different ways, succeed in solving criminal cases through expertise, persistence, and will power and, therefore, in transforming the scientific laboratory into a feminine space. Ultimately, however, as Schmieder concludes, the pioneering and emancipatory potential for subversion of a male domain, as begun in the late nineteenth century, is constrained by the introduction of male father figures and partners on whom both female scientists seem to increasingly depend in the respective series.

Transmitting Disease

In contrast to Parts I and II, which focus on the medical profession and its internal as well as social, cultural, religious, and political debates as such, Part III turns toward communicable diseases that have affected human beings for centuries, such as the plague, yellow fever, AIDS, and typhoid. The concept of communicating disease is doubly coded in its reference to the acts of representing disease and of passing it on—that is, infecting someone with an illness. As Giovanni Boccaccio's *Il Decamerone* (ca. 1349-53) famously illustrates, seven ladies and three young men survive the plague in Florence in 1348 only because they leave the city, stay for ten days in the country, during which time each one of them has to tell a story about a chosen topic. After ten times ten, thus one hundred stories, they are able to return to Florence. Not only does Boccaccio's text serve as a historical document which offers realistic information on the plague, but it has also become the perfect example of the power of storytelling,[5] thus communicating disease in its double meaning. Yet, although storytelling may spread hope of healing and survival, epidemics, as transgressive and transnational phenomena, ultimately know no borders. Any narrative on epidemics will inevitably include theories about possible origins such as miasma, inadequate sanitation, importation or contagion, ideas that variously blame poor waste management, foreigners, or immoral behavior for the outbreak. While these epidemics, often known to us through their written transmission, have literally brought devastation, destruction, and death to virtually every part of the world at various moments in time, while

---

[5] The 2007 film version *Virgin Territories* by David Leland shows that Boccaccio's impressive narrative has not lost its power, impact, and appeal.

they have been fought with multiple means and treatments respective to the particular times, and while with each medical victory over one disease a new one emerges as the chronological sequence of plague, yellow fever, and AIDS shows, the history of these epidemics has not only often revealed disturbing evidence of human nature, behavior, and relationships, but has also been used metaphorically to explain human life and its connection to possible divine powers. People in dire situations and without effective medical treatment have frequently pointed to disease as God's punishment for sins committed, as debated in Daniel Defoe's *Journal* or Charles Brockden Brown's *Arthur Mervyn*, for example, through so-called immoral and anti-religious behavior. Often it is the patient who is seen as the guilty party. Narratives of the plague, cholera, and other infectious diseases discussed in this section show the almost unnarratable existential fear of contagion and subsequent death, the horror that leads to isolation, the separation of families, friends, neighbors, colleagues, etc., to violence and brutality, to racism, homophobia, and classism, in short, to the worst in human behavior at times of severe crises (cf. Bergdolt 9).

The four contributions in this section discuss narratives that represent different ways of coping with the respective individual and national crises. As Imke Kimpel shows with her discussion of Daniel Defoe's *Journal* (1722), seventeenth-century London was devastatingly affected by the plague, a bacterial disease that is highly contagious and difficult to communicate. Yet, the narrator is in need of communication, and the narrative *Journal* is his only way of doing so in order to survive in spite of witnessing the altered and inhuman burial rites, social isolation, and suffering from the constant fear of contagion. As an observer, however, noting down his insights in the journal, the narrator turns into an outsider; nevertheless, he himself is buried before the end of his narrative. Ingrid Gessner picks up on the idea of communication (and contagion) across borders and prominently focuses on the psychological aspects of fear of infection. Gessner reads yellow fever texts as representations of crises and looks at Charles Brockden Brown's novel *Arthur Mervyn, or, Memoirs of the Year 1793* (1799/1800) and Wesley Bradshaw's lesser known sentimental novella *Angel Agnes or, The Heroine of the Yellow Fever Plague in Shreveport* (1873) and these texts' crisis management and suggestions for integrative solutions. It was not until 1900 that army pathologist Major Walter Reed and James

Carroll confirmed that this disease was spread by the female *Aedes aegypti* mosquito. Astrid Haas's essay on AIDS comedies establishes that infectious diseases are not phenomena of the past but, as medical history (often through fictional representations) shows, have been present throughout the centuries and have found new forms and outlets in new societies, never ceasing to produce personal, social, national, and, even, international crises. Haas discusses the much debated question of whether comedy and humor are adequate means to deal with diseases as devastating as AIDS. She shows how the choice of genre can be essential in the reception of narrative representations of crises. While narratives in general, as the final section of this volume indicates, can have healing powers, comedy or satire, in particular, as Haas emphasizes, can become an outlet and a form of therapy for anxieties that otherwise would not find representation (cf. Berger). As Gessner and Kimpel have also depicted, narratives about epidemics always also negotiate the power of authorities to deal with a medical crisis and the ways in which medical scientists and political officials interact in their common desire to regain control of the crisis and restore socio-political order and health.

As all the contributions show, there is an intimate link between disease, nationhood, and the dehumanization of certain life forms, a connection which Rüdiger Kunow picks up and situates in the triangulation of mobility, governmentality, and disciplinarity. Kunow's essay can serve as an additional theoretical foundation for the discussion of epidemics since he stresses the biological mobility of life forms such as bacteria, germs, microbes, and viruses as a form of transnational mobility. He discusses the case of Mary Mallon a.k.a. Typhoid Mary, an Irish servant and cook who, in the early years of the twentieth century, was said to be spreading typhoid among her employers, carrying the virus herself but never actually being infected, thus serving, as Kunow points out, as a "Trojan stranger." Typhoid Mary's story reveals that governmentality, that is, mechanisms of institutionalized power over human life, has taken charge of the human body, an appropriation and exertion of biopolitics through which the private and the public have increasingly merged in both the ill and the elderly. Biology has moved to the forefront of public life with people suffering from contagious diseases and with the elderly as examples of "failed bodies"[6] that can only be approached through a "biotechnicalization of human life," as Kunow points out. It is here that the natural sciences fully enter the stage of human life. However, it is the task of cultural studies to counter the public dehumanization through biomedical sciences of human suffering and weakness because the human being as body (and in Kunow's essay senescence in particular) "is intensely personal *and* collective, physical *and* cultural" (Hartung and Kunow 16). It is here that the humanities can be true to their name.

Healing Narratives

It is with this understanding of the humanities as contributing knowledge to the improvement of human life that Part IV of this volume negotiates the possible healing functions of literature or narratives in general. What I have delineated so far has addressed the question of what literature as well as other cultural products such as, for example, TV series, have to offer to the medical researcher and practitioner in order to understand his or her own discipline. Moreover, as the essays in Part IV show, literature itself can be a medical tool used for healing purposes. Reading literature with its aesthetic qualities, its interesting topics, and perhaps didactic features can contribute to a person's entertainment, relaxation, and well-being whether as a negotiation of or an escape from societal events. Under-standing one's own positionality in society may also be enhanced through narratives. Even more so, the production, thus the writing of narratives may give expression to one's own physicality and emotion-ality, for example, when dealing with personal illness, and may thus serve as therapy. Bibliotherapy has long recognized the healing potential of reading; narrative medicine adds doctors' recognition of how patient narratives work and attributes to the writing of narratives as the expression of personal feelings and ideas a further medical function.

---

[6]   In his article "Chronologically Gifted?" Rüdiger Kunow draws attention to "a perceived biological normativity" that finds "aged bodies" "to fail to conform to the standards of bionormativity. They thus become 'failed bodies'" (32).

Narratives dealing with personal experiences of illness often emphasize or at least search for the healing power of grief and its narrativization in various sub-genres, such as written testimonies, diaries, blogs, and artists' books as well as fiction, thus in a multiplicity of autobiographical or autoethnographical writings. Some authors inter-weave theoretical discussions or analyses of other people's narratives with their own illness narratives. In doing so, they demonstrate that they share a belief in the illness narrative as a new space of communication between readers and artists and, ultimately, doctors and patients. Translating personal experiences, which have shattered the "reliance on the orderly functioning of [people's] bodies" (Becker 12), into nar-rative—and thus overcoming "the resistance of a collapsing body to verbalization" (Rimmon-Kenan 245)—gives voice to its author by transforming silence into language and action, as Audre Lorde proclaims in her *Cancer Journals* (1980). Moreover, such a narrative gives structure and coherence to often traumatic events in someone's life that help overcome "the multiple difficulties that arise in trying to articulate [trauma]" (Gilmore 6), thus contributing to "narrating the unnarratable" (Rimmon-Kenan 241) and to "the formation and maintenance of our sense of identity" (Eakin 123). Such a narrative also reaches out to its readers and establishes a community or continuum between author and reader. The healing powers of narrative allow the patients to regain (at least partial) control over their bodies.

While all the other contributions concentrate on language and the writing of narratives as means of coming to terms with trauma, be it the gradual loss of one's mental capacities—as in the case of Alice James and Charlotte Perkins Gilman's unnamed narrator—or Siri Hustvedt's therapeutic treatment of her shaking, or Richard Powers's protagonist's suffering from Capgras Syndrome, Christine Marks focuses on the metaphorical language that is used in illness narratives. Communicating pain human beings suffer from is a struggle to come to language and express the inexpressible or unnarratable. While physical pain isolates the individual from a community, metaphors offer a possible sharing and mediation of painful experiences and, thus, transcend the boundaries between the sick and the healthy. Language, after all, can overcome the silence imposed on an individual through illness. Anca-Raluca Radu's contribution shifts the perspective away from the therapeutic illness narrative and the patient-doctor story toward the experiences of witnesses of a disease, that is, of relatives having to come to terms with the loss of a beloved person. Examining one Canadian and one Irish novel, Radu concentrates on people who are affected by a patient's story and subsequent death. Ultimately, as Radu exemplifies, fiction can serve as the stage for figuring out how to deal with the death of beloved people in one's life. Thus, from the metaphors we heal by in Marks's essay we have come to those metaphors which fail to heal. The two male protagonists of the respective novels lose their wives and other relatives to cancer. Radu uses the concepts of "witness involvement" and "responsible narration" to mark the position of the (unreliable) narrators but also the ethicality of their narratives with which they turn toward the past in order to locate themselves in the present. As Christine Marks points out in her essay and Anca-Raluca Radu affirms, those who suffer and those who witness use metaphors in order to overcome the inadequacy of language to express such pain. Moreover, it is the sharing of narratives that seems to have a healing effect.

Giving voice and words to an illness is equally relevant in the case of mental illness. While language can give order and structure to a disintegrating body, it can do even more for the mind. According to Peter Schneck, the emergence of the medical humanities sheds light on the relevance of the interfaces of literature and medicine. The "narrative turn" within the humanities and the social sciences has led to a recognition of illness narratives, which, for Schneck, have to be divided into fictional and autobiographical compositions, each challenging interdisciplinary approaches in their own respective ways. Illness narratives—whether fictional or autobiographical—always unfold the narrative construction of self and, thus, a sense of agency that defies the public and authoritative definition of one's illness. Like Gilman's unnamed narrator, Hustvedt's shaking woman, a narrativized version of her own self, inscribes herself into a discourse that promises self-determination and wholeness. Anna Thiemann shows that while Gilman's narrator's narrative may be that of a victim, Siri Hustvedt's *The Shaking Woman*, in spite of being indebted to the same feminist discourse, also departs from it by engaging in an intertextual dialogue with Gilman's short story both as a critical reflection on feminism and as a pop culture phenomenon, an ambiguity which is the very essence of post-feminism. Hustvedt's psychoanalytical narrative, through which she seeks to come to terms with her own shaking, in contrast to

Gilman's narrator, allows her to acknowledge and accept her divided self in a (post-)feminism that is still very much alive.

Johanna Heil's analysis of Richard Powers's novel *The Echo Maker* and its protagonist's neurological illness, that is, Capgras Syndrome, adds another layer of narrative medicine to Hustvedt's therapeutic narrative reconstruction of her own multiple selves. Powers, as Heil argues, embeds both the patient's and the doctor's narratives into a narrative that seeks to establish a coherent sense of self. While the doctor, as a firm believer in the epistemological power of narrative, wants to consider Capgras Syndrome as merely a psychodynamic response to the trauma of the car accident and almost runs the risk of ignoring the syndrome's physical or biological side, the novel ultimately is a plea for the integration of science and narrative since although narratives are needed for both the reconstruction of the old self and for a diagnosis, they can also be the result of delusion or confabulation. Heil's conclusions clearly advocate the use of narrative medicine in clinical diagnosis, but they also warn of an all too exclusive reliance on narrative; rather, both science and narrative need to be consulted in medical practice. Birgit Däwes extends Johanna Heil's analysis of Powers's novel into the larger political realm of 9/11 fiction and its preoccupation with trauma. She departs from the individual case of Powers's protagonist and moves into what she calls "neurological metafiction." Däwes points out that collective trauma, as in the case of 9/11, only becomes trauma because this very meaning is attributed to the events and then affirms, in this case, welcome national ideologies. Different characters in the novel suffer from traumatic experiences, but, as Däwes argues, the novel goes far beyond the individual toward what she calls a traumorama or global experience and an ethics of empathy. To Heil's conjunction of narrative and science, Däwes adds empathy in the process of possible healing of more than just the individual.

The volume closes with a contribution by the medical historian Dietrich von Engelhardt, who not only sheds light on the complexity of the world of medicine in the medium of literature but also broadens the geographical realm by branching out into some of the many texts pertaining to medicine which literature has to offer from antiquity to the twenty-first century. As a concluding essay, it helps to once more draw into focus the transnational—in the sense of going beyond the individual nation—and multi-level nature of the intersections and reciprocally influential interests of literature and medicine. Not only are narratives an essential part of any form of medicine anywhere and at any time in human history, but medicine or, better, medical phenomena are an indisputable element in human life and, thus, in literature since literature not only reflects but *is* human life.

Acknowledgements

The present volume would never have been published without the help of colleagues, institutions, and students alike. I gratefully acknowledge the support of the University of Marburg, the German Association for American Studies, the Center for Gender Studies and Feminist Research as well as the Ursula-Kuhlmann-Fonds, Novartis Vaccines and Diagnostics GmbH, and the City of Marburg for their kind support of the 2011 international conference on the intersections of literature and medicine, on which this publication is based. Miriam Apell, Carmen Fels, Jan Hölker, Christina Maria Koch, Janina Rojek, and Waltraud Nau lent their helping hands to the organization of the conference. Volker Bischoff's comments on the preparation of both the conference and this volume have greatly contributed to these endeavors' completion. Furthermore, Christina Koch dedicated her expertise in proofreading to the final shape of this volume. It is with particular gratefulness that I acknowledge the help of Sabine Kim, who, as native speaker, not only detected even the minutest linguistic flaws but also errors in content and format in the submitted essays. My most sincere thanks go to my co-editor Johanna Heil, who never tired of reading, discussing, and formatting the present volume and has literally seen it into print.

Works Cited

Abram, Ruth J. "Soon the Baby Died: Medical Training in Nineteenth-Century America." *"Send Us a Lady Physician": Women Doctors in America 1835-1920*. Ed. Abram. New York: Norton, 1985. 17-20. Print.

---. "Will There Be a Monument? Six Pioneer Women Doctors Tell Their Own Stories." *"Send Us a Lady Physician": Women Doctors in America 1835-1920*. Ed. Abram. New York: Norton, 1985. 71-106. Print.

---, ed. *"Send Us a Lady Physician": Women Doctors in America 1835-1920*. New York: Norton, 1985. Print.

Agamben Giorgio. *Homo sacer: Die souveräne Macht und das nackte Leben*. 1995. Trans. Hubert Thüring. Frankfurt am Main: Suhrkamp, 2002. Print.

Barry, Peter. *Beginning Theory: An Introduction to Literary and Cultural Theory*. 1995. 3rd ed. Manchester: Manchester UP, 2009. Print.

Becker, Gay. *Disrupted Lives: How People Create Meaning in a Chaotic World*. Berkeley: U of California P, 1999. Print.

Bergdolt, Klaus. *Die Pest: Geschichte des Schwarzen Todes*. 2006. München: Beck, 2011. Print.

Berger, Peter L. *Redeeming Laughter: The Comic Dimension of Human Experience*. Berlin: de Gruyter, 1997. Print.

Beveridge, Allan. "Should Psychiatrists Read Fiction?" *British Journal of Psychiatry* 182 (2003): 385-87. Web. 4 Apr. 2013.

Bittel, Carla. *Mary Putnam Jacobi and the Politics of Medicine in Nineteenth-Century America*. Chapel Hill: U of North Carolina P, 2009. Print.

---. "Mary Putnam Jacobi and the Nineteenth-Century Politics of Women's Health Research." *Women Physicians and the Cultures of Medicine*. Ed. Ellen S. More, Elizabeth Fee, and Manon Parry. Baltimore: Johns Hopkins UP, 2009. 23-51. Print.

Blackwell, Elizabeth. *Pioneer Work in Opening the Medical Profession to Women*. 1895. Introd. Amy Sue Bix. Amherst: Humanity, 2005. Print.

Brockman, John. *The Third Culture: Beyond the Scientific Revolution*. New York: Simon and Schuster, 1996. Print.

Brieger, Gert H. "Bodies and Borders: A New Cultural History of Medicine." *Perspectives in Biology and Medicine* 47.3 (2004): 402-21. Print.

Brody, Howard. *Stories of Sickness*. New Haven: Yale UP, 1987. Print.

Browner, Stephanie P. *Profound Science and Elegant Literature: Imagining Doctors in Nineteenth-Century America*. Philadelphia: U of Pennsylvania P, 2005. Print.

Charon, Rita. *Narrative Medicine: Honoring the Stories of Illness*. 2006. Oxford: Oxford UP, 2008. Print.

Clarke, Edward Hammond. *Sex in Education, Or, A Fair Chance for Girls*. 1873. N.p.: General, 2009. Print.

Davis, Cynthia J. *Bodily and Narrative Forms: The Influence of Medicine on American Literature 1845-1915*. Stanford: Stanford UP, 2000. Print.

Dodd, Diane, and Deborah Gorham. Introduction. *Caring and Curing: Historical Perspectives on Women and Healing in Canada*. Ed. Dodd and Gorham. Ottawa: U of Ottawa P, 1994. 1-15. Print.

During, Simon. *Cultural Studies: A Critical Introduction*. London: Routledge, 2005. Print.

Eakin, Paul John. *How Our Lives Become Stories: Making Selves*. Ithaca: Cornell UP, 1999. Print.

Engelhardt, Dietrich von. "Teaching History of Medicine in the Perspective of 'Medical Humanities.'" *Croatian Medical Journal* 40.1 (1999): 1-7. Print.

Ette, Ottmar. *ÜberLebenswissen: Die Aufgabe der Philologie*. Berlin: Kadmos, 2004. Print.

Furst, Lilian R. "From Speculation to Science." *Medical Progress and Social Reality: A Reader in Nineteenth-Century Medicine and Literature*. Ed. Furst. Albany: State U of New York P, 2000. 1-21. Print.

---. "Halfway Up the Hill: Doctresses in Late Nineteenth-Century American Fiction." *Women Healers and Physicians: Climbing a Long Hill*. Ed. Furst. Lexington: UP of Kentucky, 1997. 221-38. Print.

Gilmore, Leigh. *The Limits of Autobiography: Trauma and Testimony*. Ithaca: Cornell UP, 2001. Print.

Greenblatt, Stephen. *Marvelous Possessions: The Wonder of the New World*. Chicago: U of Chicago P, 1991. Print.

Grossberg, Lawrence, Cary Nelson, and Paula A. Treichler, eds. *Cultural Studies*. New York: Routledge, 1992. Print.

Hartung, Heike, and Rüdiger Kunow. "Introduction: Age Studies." *Amerikastudien / American Studies* 56.1 (2011): 15-22. Print.

Jagow, Bettina von, and Florian Steger. *Was treibt die Literatur zur Medizin? Ein kulturwissenschaftlicher Dialog*. Göttingen: Vandenhoeck and Ruprecht, 2009. Print.

Jauß, Hans Robert. *Literaturgeschichte als Provokation*. Frankfurt am Main: Suhrkamp, 1970. Print.

Kunow, Rüdiger. "Chronologically Gifted? 'Old Age' in American Culture." *Amerikastudien / American Studies* 56.1 (2011): 23-44. Print.

Lorde, Audre. *The Cancer Journals*. San Francisco: spinsters/aunt lute, 1980. Print.

Mitchell, S. Weir. *Wear and Tear, Or, Hints for the Overworked*. 1871. Introd. Michael S. Kimmel. Walnut Creek: Altamira, 2004. Print.

Montrose, Louis A. "Professing the Renaissance: The Poetics and Politics of Culture." *The New Historicism*. Ed. H. Aram Veeser. New York: Routledge, 1989. 15-36. Print.

Morantz-Sanchez, Regina. *Sympathy and Science: Women Physicians in American Medicine*. 1985. Chapel Hill: U of North Carolina P, 2000. Print.

---. "The Female Student Has Arrived: The Rise of the Women's Medical Movement." *"Send Us a Lady Physician": Women Doctors in America 1835-1920*. Ed. Ruth J. Abram. New York: Norton, 1985. 59-69. Print.

More, Ellen S. *Restoring the Balance: Women Physicians and the Profession of Medicine, 1850-1995*. 1999. Cambridge: Harvard UP, 2000. Print.

Rimmon-Kenan, Shlomith. "What Can Narrative Theory Learn from Illness Narratives?" *Literature and Medicine* 25.2 (2006): 241-54. Print.

Snow, C. P. *The Two Cultures*. 1964. Cambridge: Cambridge UP, 1993. Print.

Sontag, Susan. *Illness as Metaphor/AIDS and Its Metaphors*. New York: Doubleday, 1990. Print.

Storey, John, ed. *What Is Cultural Studies? A Reader*. London: Arnold, 1996. Print.

Veeser, H. Aram, ed. *The New Historicism*. New York: Routledge, 1989. Print.

Vertinsky, Patricia A. *The Eternally Wounded Woman: Women, Doctors, and Exercise in the Late Nineteenth Century*. 1989. Manchester: Manchester UP, 1994. Print.

Wald, Priscilla. *Contagious: Cultures, Carriers and the Outbreak Narrative*. Durham: Duke UP, 2008. Print.

Walsh, Mary Roth. *"Doctors Wanted, No Women Need Apply": Sexual Barriers in the Medical Profession, 1835-1975*. New Haven: Yale UP, 1977. Print.

Wells, Susan. *Out of the Dead House: Nineteenth-Century Women Physicians and the Writing of Medicine*. Madison: U of Wisconsin P, 2001. Print.

Welter, Barbara. "The Cult of True Womanhood: 1820-1860." *American Quarterly* 18.2 (1966): 151-74. Print.

Williams, William Carlos. *The Autobiography of William Carlos Williams*. New York: New Directions, 1967. Print.

PART I:

NEGOTIATING
MEDICAL PRACTICE

Marc Priewe

Staging Final Illnesses: Medicine and Religion in Experience Mayhew's *Indian Converts* (1727)

The first official seal of the Massachusetts Bay Colony featured a Native American dressed in a loincloth, with braided hair, a bow, and an arrow pointing to the ground as a gesture of peace. The ironic caption of the image—"Come over and help us"—reminded readers that one of the initial purposes of settling New England was to "wynn and incite the Natives . . ., to the Knowledg and Obedience of the onlie true God and Savior of Mankinde, and the Christian Fayth" ("Charter" 82). The "help" that the Indians ostensibly desired was English culture, commerce, and Calvinism. Yet, while English settlers were quick to trade with, and on occasion fought against, Native groups after gaining a foothold in the New World, their professed goal of winning Native souls for Christ was tackled only after a decade of settlement. Beginning around 1640, concerted missionaries activities centered primarily on the establishment of "Praying Towns," i.e., English-style villages in which Algonquians, separated from colonists and other Natives, were to learn European manners and Christian virtues. As a means of justifying and funding their acculturative efforts, early New England missionaries— among them John Eliot, Thomas Mayhew, and George Whitfield— wrote letters and reports known to readers of Early American literature as the *Eliot Tracts* (cf. Clark). One decisive feature of these texts is the authors' critique and contestation of traditional Native healing practices or powwowing. Eliot and his colleagues viewed the Algonquian pawwaws' rituals, gestures, and chants as obstacles to proselytizing the Natives because, in their view, these practices constituted anchors of undesirable cultural memory and, even worse, signs of allegiance with the devil (Gookin 14; Wood 83).

Native American conversion narratives recorded by Puritan missionaries constitute proto-ethnographic sources that display indigenous attitudes toward Christianity and illustrate how Natives sought ways of coping with the trauma brought about by the land-clearing epidemics of the first decades of the seventeenth century. Hence, in the following pages I want to examine the writings by Experience Mayhew, grandson of John Eliot's friend and colleague, Thomas Mayhew, Jr., who recorded the missionary work of four generations of family preachers among the Wampanoag people of Martha's Vineyard. Rather than aiming to capture the moment of Native conversion to indicate successful missionary work, Mayhew's *Indian Converts* (1727) stresses how Native subjects conducted themselves during the final moments of their lives. Mayhew "staged" the final illnesses of Native converts in narrative space in order to convince his readers of the efficacy of Calvinist theology, in general, and its configuration of illnesses, in particular. At the same time, his accounts of sick and dying Natives can never fully cover up the missionaries' denial and disavowal of Native otherness in favor of presenting culturally "purified" colonial subjects.

New World Bodies, Old World Pathogens

When English Protestants began to cross the Atlantic in increasing numbers during the seventeenth century, they (as well as their livestock) were an infectious multitude, acutely dangerous to their less immunologically protected neighbors. In New England, at least two major "virgin-soil epidemics" (i.e., communicable diseases which are introduced into a region hitherto unaffected) preceded and accompanied the arrival of European settlers (cf. Crosby, "Virgin-Soil"). The first recorded pandemic induced by colonial exchanges occurred from 1616 to 1619 and killed between seventy-five and ninety percent of the coastal population, while sparing most Native settlements in the interior and west of Narragansett Bay (present-day Rhode Island and Connecticut). The exact nature and scope of the calamitous disease(s) is impossible to determine retrospectively; some early reports call it the "plague," others "a sore consumption," while still others claim that Native people turned yellow before dying. Based on these observations as well as archaeological evidence, historians have speculated that the first lethal epidemic may have been jaundice, influenza, typhoid, yellow fever, chicken pox, viral hepatitis, and/or smallpox.[1]

In 1633, Algonquians living near Windsor, Connecticut, were among the first indigenous groups faced with another wave of epidemics. This time, Native New Englanders were afflicted by smallpox, which had been introduced in the Western hemisphere by Spanish conquistadors in 1518 and continued to spread throughout the Americas in the wake of growing commercial contacts with Europe, Africa, and the Caribbean.[2] Transmitted from one individual to another by droplets of moisture expelled from the upper respiratory tract, by contact with pustules on the skin, or by exposure to contaminated cloth, smallpox proved a most detrimental disease for indigenous communities, reaching epidemic proportion in 1633-1634. Forced to witness helplessly how their villages succumbed to a particularly malignant strain of *variola major*, many Algonquians, most likely in panic, escaped to other settlements and thereby unwittingly fueled the disease, which soon ravaged indigenous communities from New England to the Great Lakes region and the St. Lawrence River valley. Because smallpox was frequently exacerbated by respiratory infections and gastrointestinal disorders, the epidemic had an estimated mortality rate of ninety percent among the already

---

[1] Crosby claims that either typhus or the plague caused Native depopulation before the arrival of the Pilgrims ("'God'"); Spiess and Spiess argue in favor of hepatitis; Snow and Lanphear as well as Bratton consider smallpox as the most likely candidate.

[2] The exact origins of epidemic illnesses and routes of transmission cannot be conclusively traced. Due to the relatively long voyage to America during the seventeenth century, the Atlantic Ocean functioned as a filter for diseases that had already run their course before a ship reached soil. While endemic illnesses (e.g., respiratory ailments, digestive disorders, or venereal diseases) remained non-virulent on ships from Europe and were often transferred to Native Americans after arrival, epidemic diseases such as smallpox and measles were most likely introduced via northern fur-trading regions and the Caribbean (Cronon 86). A useful historical overview of smallpox outbreaks in colonial America is provided by Duffy; Fenn 13-43.

decimated Native New England population, with only a few English casualties (Bragdon 26-28).[3]

Seventeenth-century Algonquians, as well as many other Native Americans previously and thereafter, were utterly unprepared to cope with the imported epidemics—many of which had been childhood diseases in Europe—both physically and culturally: Their medical repositories lacked sufficient treatment methods; their system of caring for the sick, which included familial gatherings at the bedside of the afflicted, fostered contamination and collapsed as the disease took its toll; and survivors were traumatized by the horrors they had to face. As a consequence, Algonquian fields were left untended, hunts canceled, and kinship networks destroyed, causing many hungry survivors to seek food, shelter, and companionship in neighboring villages, which were often equally struck by epidemics. In short, the European diseases were a major factor in the colonization of the Americas. They destroyed the foundations of a subsistence economy, leading to a growing dependence on trade with Europeans (especially fur). This, in turn, increased the transfer of pathogens, created new political alliances and causes for violence, and further destroyed the traditional socio-cultural fabric of indigenous communities (Salisbury, *Manitou* 103-05).

In the course of the disease-induced disorganization of Native communities, the pawwaw's (shamanic healer) elevated social status, which depended significantly on his medical success, was questioned and caused a number of cultural reconfigurations. Some surviving priest-healers attributed the Narragansett's exemption from the first wave of epidemic diseases (1616-1619) to periodic sacrifices and, as a result, transformed and intensified their own healing rituals accordingly. Recent archaeological expeditions indicate that both the quantity and the quality of critical rites (performed during famines, droughts, wars, and collective illnesses) changed after European arrival. Scholars believe

---

[3] Grob asserts that the relative genetic homogeneity of Native Americans contributed to the high mortality rate because once a virus had adapted to the immune response of one person, it became more virulent in other, genetically similar persons. In addition, the lack of knowledge about methods of contagion and the fact that Native dwellings often housed up to twenty people, often genetically related, increased the speed and severity with which viral infections spread (44-45).

that due to a shifting disease ecology, many Native people felt compelled to acquire more goods for sacrificial purposes. Seventeenth-century burial sites exhibit an increase in Indian and European artifacts, suggesting that healing rituals, too, sought to address the new social and medical realities (Bragdon 239-41; McBride; Baker 37-39).

While some Native Americans modified their healing traditions to meet these new realities, others sought medical help from their new English neighbors. Most Indians recognized a causal, yet unspecified, link between the arrival of the colonists and the appearance and dissemination of hitherto unknown diseases. Demoralized by pandemics, many indigenes were convinced that the Christian God was more powerful than their own celestial forces and hence asked English settlers to invoke the help of their God to halt the epidemics. Others decided to convert to Christianity in order to avoid future illnesses. In 1633, John Sagamore, a Pawtucket leader, told Massachusetts Bay Colony leader John Winthrop, before succumbing to smallpox: "[D]iverse of them [the Natives] in their sicknesse, confessed that the Englishe mens God was a good God, & that, if they recovered they would serve him" (Winthrop 105). The severe challenges that epidemics posed to indigenous spirituality and medicine did not result in a complete demise of Algonquian cultural practices. As will be shown below, certain traditional healing methods survived by shifting and adapting over time, while others endured as (suppressed) medical knowledge in colonial and later American culture and society. It is difficult, if not impossible to determine, however, why some belief structures and curative techniques crumbled under the impact of Old World pathogens while others persisted.

Contagious Conversions

Interpreting the loss of family, knowledge, and way of life since the first major epidemic in 1616 as the result of unfavorable supernatural forces, many Algonquians became receptive to the message, meaning, and order which Puritan ministers promised if they converted to the Christian faith and forsook their previous religious rituals and cultural beliefs. In order to do so, Natives were not only coerced into adopting English culture (including dress, speech, and housing) but also had to display the "morphology of conversion" that Puritan settlers had brought to the New World and applied vigorously in their meetinghouses (Morgan 66).[4] The primary spiritual goal of Puritans on both sides of the Atlantic was the conversion from a life of sin to an inward experience of God's saving grace (justification) and its outward manifestation in behavior and speech (sanctification). Conversion, seen by Calvinists as a means of preparing for salvation, could only come about through intense and continual self-examination. Constituting the central spiritual experience for English Protestants, the conversion of the heart through knowledge of the divine and the self was considered not necessarily as a single event of enlightenment, but as a process of personal change and growth over time that was brought about by God's gradual entrance and intervention in the life of the sinner. Conversion, in other words, marked an intricate part of a lifelong spiritual pilgrimage during which a person, guided by Providence and scripture, discovered sin, repented, doubted, prayed, combated temptations, attended sermons, and conversed with ministers and fellow believers in preparation for eternal bliss.[5]

After a decade of setting up shop, New England colonists began to "universalize" their practice of conversion and undertook concerted missionary efforts among the remaining Algonquians, seeking to convert those many souls prior to the imminent return of Jesus Christ. The millenarian impulse for missionizing New England Native Americans was especially evident in the work and life of John Eliot, preacher at Roxbury, Massachusetts, who devoted much of his energy to spreading

---

[4] According to the "morphology of conversion," a sinner's successful conversion could be recognized by a series of signs and stages: conviction in sin, fear of God's judgment, desire for redemption, faith-building through prayer and Bible study, realization of justification, manifestation of piety and devotion in thought and action, and vigilance through continual introspection. Although Puritan theologians devised different sequential stages of conversion, they concurred in their basic outline of a teleological process, one that could potentially be identified and rationalized by individual believers and by the outside world as a successful conversion (Perkins 36-45).

[5] The prospects of preparation were at the center of numerous theological debates in old and New England. For a seminal study on conversion and preparation in the American colonies, cf. Pettit.

the Gospel among the local Natives. Eliot's missionary activities, which began around 1640 and lasted until 1680, were prompted by religious, economic, and political motives. He and other Puritan divines hoped that Native subjects who pronounced their allegiance with the Christian faith would signify to the world the cultural superiority of English ways and manners, facilitate further trade relations between the two groups, and procure alliances that could prove helpful in the disputes over the boundaries between English and French zones of influence in the Western hemisphere (cf. Salisbury, "Red Puritans"; Morrison; Cogley).

In the closing decades of the seventeenth century, after King Philip's War had ended Eliot's concerted missionary experiment, conversion efforts took place mainly on the fringes of English colonial rule. One such place in which sustained missionary efforts were still undertaken was Martha's Vineyard. Over a period of eighty years, four generations of preachers from the Mayhew family taught and examined the indigenous population of the island. Similar to other Algonquian tribes, the Wampanoags living on the island repeatedly expressed their doubts and uncertainties about the power of their deities, power that seemed to have decreased with each passing epidemic and the ensuing trauma of depopulation and social disintegration. By the time the youngest Mayhew missionary, Experience, had completed his account of Native conversions to Christianity, the indigenous adult population of Martha's Vineyard had dwindled from approximately 3,000 in 1642 to about 800 in 1720 (Cook 502). Mayhew's account, entitled *Indian Converts* (1727), covers the missionary work on the island from the beginnings, and, in doing so, captures the profound social, cultural, and political changes among the Aboriginal population shortly before its almost complete demise at the end of the eighteenth century. The text is useful for scholars of Early American literature because it provides insights into how New England Native Americans endowed their illnesses with meaning in accordance with their tribal traditions, on the one hand, and with medico-religious concepts introduced by the missionaries, on the other.

Mayhew's *Indian Converts*

Experience Mayhew's narrative is an assemblage of testimony about the piety and charity of selected Wampanoags at the end of their lives. Mayhew's 128 entries, each describing the Christian life of an individual Native "saint," are modeled on Cotton Mather's *Magnalia Christi Americana* (1702), which approaches New England history through biographical vignettes. Mayhew's third-person narrative differs from similar missionary writings such as the *Eliot Tracts*, which tend to focus on the early stages of the path to conversion and appear to be genuine transcripts of the converts' own words. In contrast to both Mather and Eliot, Mayhew comprises his hagiographies based on life narratives from or about Native people, including women and children. In doing so, he refrains from offering his reader the impression that the converts *speak through* the minister. Rather, the narrative voice in *Indian Converts* claims authenticity and verisimilitude by asserting to have interviewed the Natives or to have gathered the material from trustworthy informants. Turning oral testimony from aged Algonquians and their English neighbors into biographies allows the author to trace divine salvation in his Native subjects until the very resolution of their lives.[6] By spanning the narrative arc of each biographical entry from the moment of accepting Christ until death, Mayhew seeks to avoid the ever-looming danger of hypocritical conversion and false assurance suggested in previous Native (as well as some Puritan) confessions. The closure that Mayhew's life writings achieve can also be seen as "proving" Indian conversion through quasi-scientific experience and repetition, thus showing, among other things, the potential universality of the Protestant faith. With this methodological and narrative approach, *Indian Converts* solidified the linkage between Puritan theology and emerging scientific epistemologies at the outset of the eighteenth century (cf. Cohen; Webster).

---

[6] The translation and transcription of Algonquian oral narratives into English documents was more complex and problematic than I am able to discuss here. For a thorough analysis of the linguistic, cultural, and power issues underlying the writing of Mayhew's *Indian Converts*, cf. Wyss, "'Things.'"

With regard to death, however, science had no role to play in Mayhew's narrative universe. Throughout the early modern world, death was a grim and terrifying reality. For colonists in New England, as well as for other people around the world, the end of life was seen as especially intimidating and anxiety-laden because of the lingering uncertainty about the soul's future estate. Depending on God's inscrutable wisdom and justice, death could be a release from earthly torments or the beginning of even greater ones in hell. Puritans, accordingly, conceptualized death in ambivalent terms, as either a reward or a punishment. Family members, neighbors, and ministers closely monitored behavior and speech on the deathbed because both were seen as providing essential clues about the imminent salvation of the dying person. How an individual carried him- or herself through the "last sickness" was of central importance, since colonists held that, during this moment, God and the devil staged a final battle over the individual's soul. It was therefore imperative that the sick and dying person follow Job and resist the temptation to turn away from God, maintaining his or her faith and piety (Stannard 72-95).

This conceptualization of death and dying was, similar to other aspects of Calvinist theology, extended to Native converts on Martha's Vineyard and elsewhere (cf. Bross). Virtually every hagiography in Mayhew's book includes an account of a death-preceding sickness, which is consistently depicted as a liminal stage between life and death, when the dying person reconfirms his/her covenant with God. In contrast to most lay Puritan conversion narratives, recounted before the congregation in New England meetinghouses, in which the "first sickness" was emphasized as the moment during which the seeker of divinity embarks on the path to salvation, *Indian Converts* stresses the "last sickness" as a confirmation of a conversion that has already been achieved. For example, Mayhew reports on the final days of Abel Wauwompuhque in the following words: "When in his last Sickness I visited him, I heard him express himself in such Language as became a dying Christian. He appeared not to be at all terrified at the Thoughts of his Dissolution, which he daily expected, but manifested a Willingness to leave the World, whenever it should please God to call him out of it" (Mayhew 164). Instead of attempting a mimetic representation of death's agony, this and almost all other Wampanoag orations recorded by Mayhew stage dying as a harmonious order, guided by soothing prayer and edifying grief.

Taken collectively, Mayhew's biographical exposition of Native lives in Christ replicates a number of culturally conditioned signs of successful conversion and future salvation displayed especially on the sickbed: a lack of sustained wavering between the forces of good and evil; devotion expressed through prayer; confession and repentance of sins; religious advice and counsel to family members and visitors; the reception and implementation of final instructions from a minister; and persistent hopes of salvation. What is especially striking about Mayhew's depiction of the dying converts is the relative dominance of optimism over despair with regard to the prospects of salvation. Lacking the perplexing spiritual doubts expressed in many other colonial writings, particularly in Puritan spiritual journals/diaries and funeral sermons, the majority of Wampanoag testimony represents aged, ill, and dying subjects who seem hopeful of, and well-prepared for, eternity and equipped with all the instruments of piety necessary for a tranquil and safe passing. When Mayhew concludes his sketch of Hiaccoomes (the first indigenous minister on Martha's Vineyard, whose life narrative opens Mayhew's text) with the words, "[i]n his last Sickness, he breathed forth many pious Expressions, and gave good Exhortations to all about him, and so went into Eternal Rest," Mayhew is setting the tone and course for the ensuing narratives, which almost unanimously end with a statement on God's likely acceptance of the repentant Native-cum-universal sinner (106).

It seems reasonable to assume that the author's parade of Native after Native "dying well" was designed to have a positive effect on other Natives considering or still resisting conversion and on (prospective) English sponsors of missionary endeavors. In Mayhew's interpretation of Native death and sickbed scenes, Christianity marks the only viable alternative to the miserable and desperate experiences caused by epidemics, the sustaining of Native ways, and alliance with the devil. *Indian Converts* can hence be read as an accumulation of didactic postmortem reports aiming to convey to Algonquians *and* the New England colonists the notion that, while illness may constitute a taste of torment experienced in hell, the prospects of salvation can be increased by piety and devotion. Mayhew's Native subjects furthermore illustrate the English Protestant conviction that the final illness must not be a cause for a "last-minute sacramental reprieve in which the Catholics and some early Christians had believed" (Stannard 87). Instead, believers have to display a continuity of godliness in both health and sickness. Otherwise, the profession of faith shortly before death might be seen as yet another sign of hypocrisy and delusional assurance.

With its rhetorical configuration of illness, Mayhew's text carves out some of the complexities and unresolved tensions underlying seventeenth-century New England conceptions of death and dying. The physical and spiritual agonies experienced by the dying individual could signal either damnation or redemption after death; a rather tranquil passage, or "dying well" did not necessarily entail acceptance into the Kingdom of God; sickness before death could be a blessing, allowing the believer a limited amount of latitude of preparation, or a curse, indicating that the worst pain and suffering was yet to come.

The tensions between the actual experiences of dying and the prospects of life after death are especially evident in some of the biographical sketches of female Native converts. Throughout colonial New England, women seem to have internalized religious doctrines to a greater extent than men and were often seen as being closer to Christ (cf. Porterfield). However, in Mayhew's text, many Wampanoag women, described as especially pious and godly, suffer from lingering spiritual uncertainties and refuse to become full members of the church, fearing that their sins do not qualify them for communion. Such a stance is rarely, if ever, encountered in the narratives related by male converts, who appear more assured of their "correct" spiritual estate. Some of the indigenous women, by contrast, are depicted as having achieved a deeper grasp of the implications of final sicknesses. Reciting the deathbed experiences of Mary Coshomon, Mayhew explains that she

> magnify'd the Mercy of God in preserving her so long, and declared that she looked upon the Evil wherewith God had visited her, as design'd by him for her spiritual Advantage, and prayed that her suffering of it might not be in vain to her; 'For so,' *said she*, 'the Pain which I must afterwards endure will be infinitely greater than that which I here undergo: I therefore intreat the Lord to help me so to improve this, and all other Providences of his towards me, that I may have all my Pain and Sorrow here in this World, and be for ever happy in that which is to come.' (Mayhew 271)

The notion that illness facilitates spiritual progress is of central importance in this passage. The sufferer has internalized the church's emphasis on affliction as a divine test of faith. The convert's words show, moreover, that she is able to align the results of intense introspection with Calvinist doctrine. This cognitive mapping of illness again underlines that the convert has mastered illness with bravado and, in doing so, can serve as a model for other Natives and the English readership.

Aside from configuring the converts' final illnesses as a sign of probable salvation, Mayhew's work also provides insightful ethno-graphic information on how Wampanoag medical practices evolved after the virtual eradication of New England powwowing during the second half of the seventeenth century. Similar to the reports in the *Eliot Tracts*, Mayhew claims that Christ has replaced the shaman as the central healing figure in post-tribal communities (Eliot 8). However, while Eliot provides only scant information on indigenous medical concepts and procedures after contact and conquest, Mayhew is less restricted. He points out that Native women function as tribal healers, in some cases replacing the pawwaw in newly shaped communities. The most detailed information on the practicalities of healing in early eighteenth-century Wampanoag communities is offered in the account of Nattootumau (a.k.a. Hannah Nohnosoo):

> Having very considerable Skill in some of the Distempers to which human Bodies are subject, and in the Nature of many of those Herbs and Plants which were proper Remedies against them, she often did good by her Medicines among her Neighbours, especially the poorer sort of them, whom she readily served without asking them any thing for what she did for them. Nor did she only serve the *Indians* this way, but was, to my knowledge, sometimes imploy'd by the *English* also. And I have sometimes heard her, when she has been asked whether she could help this or the other Person under the Indispositions wherewith they were exercised, make this wise and religious Answer: *I do not know but I*

> *may, if it please God to bless Means for that end, otherwise I can do nothing.* (Mayhew 255)[7]

This excerpt deviates from the bulk of contemporary Puritan texts, which, with few exceptions, omit all references to English settlers seeking the help of Native physicians because of the healers' perceived and claimed proximity to the devil. While virtually all extant records exclude indigenous botanical knowledge for its supposed satanic involvement, Nattootumau's medicinal practices could only be accepted by and included in New England and later American medicine because they were firmly embedded in Christian doctrines, evinced by the convert's "wise and religious Answer" that attributes medical efficacy exclusively to divine will. In doing so, the female healer reveals how traditional means of curing are both changed and maintained: Direct access to the spirit world is still regarded as a vital component of medical practice even though Native deities have been replaced by the Christian Trinity. This indicates that certain cross-cultural similarities in conceptualizing healing were central for the missionary work as such. Only by stressing that the mode of healing through supernatural powers could be maintained, while the means had to be substituted, could English missionaries convince Native Americans to exchange and align their traditional healing practices with those imported by the colonists (Wyss, *Writing Indians* 72-73; Russell 37-38).

Aside from the accounts of female medical practitioners, Mayhew's conversion narratives reveal merely remnants of indigenous illness conceptions. For instance, Wuttinomanomin's final words are related as follows:

> Some of the Persons that tended him in his Sickness, and were with him when he dy'd, have with great Assurance affirme'd, that . . . there appeared in the Room where he lay far brighter Attendants, in human Shape, than any which this lower World could have afforded, even such as those Spirits may be thought to be, who are *sent forth to minister for them that shall be Heirs of Salvation.* (Mayhew 128)

---

[7] Other female medical practitioners mentioned in *Indian Converts* include Hannah Ahhunnut (232-33), Assannooshque (233-36), and Abiah Paaonit (248-51).

This sickbed narrative presents a noteworthy cultural palimpsest. The appearance or vision of a glowing figure of light could have been induced by the traditional Wampanoag belief that the dying were transformed into Hobbamock (alias Abbomocho, one of two central deities according to pre-contact Native New England cosmology); however, Mayhew immediately deconstructs such an ethnographic reading by overriding it with a quote from Hebrews 1:14 about the "Heirs of Salvation." In his attempt to disavow the dying person's regression into traditional belief, Mayhew actually sustains transcultural ambiguities that point to ineradicable residues of Native worldviews after conversion to Christianity. Mayhew's reference can also be interpreted as an indication of significant changes in New England Puritanism in the early decades of the eighteenth century: Whereas an earlier generation of ministers would have vociferously rejected Wuttinomanomin's deathbed apparition as being caused by the devil or Antinomian/Quaker fallacies, Mayhew represents the emerging "New Light" movement in New England Puritanism that constituted one of the pillars of the First Great Awakening (Leibman 3-16).

Conclusion

Mayhew's Natives offer insights into the intersections between religion and medicine in a colonial contact setting. In the attempt to rationalize their spiritual conditions shortly before death, believers, as well as the community that was asked to validate the conversion report, sought signs in illness that would indicate that God had indeed intervened and reshaped the internal landscape of the sinner. Similar to Puritan lay conversion narratives and spiritual autobiographies written mostly by members of the elite, Native accounts emphasize the centrality of corporeal knowledge for assessing the probability of one's salvation. In other words, the transcultural employment of illness configurations in early American conversion narratives illustrates how colonists had devised a system of signs that could represent the inner state of the convert. For the English, these signs were universal. Anyone who convincingly displayed the morphology of conversion could be considered among the elect. However, Mayhew's attempt to prove Native conversion *conclusively* ultimately turns against itself because

Puritans knew that full assurance was impossible, given God's inscrutable will. With this in mind, the accounts gathered in *Indian Converts* threatened the validity and credibility of *all* conversion narratives emanating from self-examined and god-assured individuals. By insisting that the conversion model can successfully "travel" from English to Native communities, Mayhew devises an uncanny illustration of a modernity that becomes contested in the process of transgressing cultural boundaries.

Works Cited

Baker, Brenda J. "Pilgrim's Progress and Praying Indians: The Biocultural Consequences of Contact in Southern New England." *In the Wake of Contact: Biological Responses to Conquest*. Ed. Clark S. Larsen and George R. Milner. New York: Wiley, 1994. 35-45. Print.

Bragdon, Kathleen J. *Native People of Southern New England, 1500-1650*. Norman: U of Oklahoma P, 1996. Print.

Bross, Kristina. "Dying Saints, Vanishing Savages: 'Dying Indian Speeches' in Colonial New England Literature." *Early American Literature* 36.3 (2001): 325-52. Print.

Bratton, Timothy L. "The Identity of the New England Indian Epidemic of 1616-19." *Bulletin of the History of Medicine* 62.3 (1988): 351-83. Print.

"The Charter of the Massachusetts Bay Company, 1629." *American Colonial Documents to 1776*. Ed. Merrill Jensen. London: Eyre and Spottiswoode, 1955. 72-84. Print.

Clark, Michael P. Introduction. *The Eliot Tracts*. Ed. Clark. Westport: Praeger, 2003. 1-52. Print.

Cogley, Richard W. *John Eliot's Mission to the Indians before King Philip's War*. Cambridge: Harvard UP, 1999. Print.

Cohen, I. Bernard, ed. *Puritanism and the Rise of Modern Science: The Merton Thesis*. New Brunswick: Rutgers UP, 1990. Print.

Cook, Sherburne F. "The Significance of Disease in the Extinction of the New England Indians." *Human Biology* 45.3 (1973): 485-508. Print.

Cronon, William. *Changes in the Land: Indians, Colonists, and the Ecology of New England*. New York: Hill and Wang, 1983. Print.

Crosby, Alfred W., Jr. "Virgin-Soil Epidemics as a Factor in the Aboriginal Depopulation in America." *William and Mary Quarterly* 3rd ser. 33.2 (1976): 289-99. Print.

---. "'God . . . Would Destroy Them, and Give Their Country to Another People.'" *American Heritage* 29.6 (1978): 38-43. Print.

Duffy, John. "Smallpox and the Indians in the American Colonies." *Bulletin of the History of Medicine* 25 (1951): 324-41. Print.

Eliot, John. *Tears of Repentance: or, a Further Narrative of the Progress of the Gospel amongst the Indians in New-England.* London, 1653. *Early English Books Online.* E522. Web. 12 May 2009.

Fenn, Elizabeth A. *Pox Americana: The Great Smallpox Epidemic of 1775-82.* New York: Hill and Wang, 2001. Print.

Gookin, Daniel. *Historical Collections of the Indians in New England. Of Their Several Nations, Numbers, Customs, Manners, Religion and Government, before the English Planted There.* 1674. Boston: Belknap and Hall, 1792. Print.

Grob, Gerald N. *The Deadly Truth: A History of Disease in America.* Cambridge: Harvard UP, 2002. Print.

Leibman, Laura Arnold. Introduction. *Experience Mayhew's* Indian Converts. Ed. Leibman. Amherst: U of Massachusetts P, 2008. 1-76. Print.

Mayhew, Experience. *Experience Mayhew's* Indian Converts. 1727. Ed. and introd. Laura Arnold Leibman. Amherst: U of Massachusetts P, 2008. Print.

McBride, Kevin A. "Bundles, Bears, and Bibles: Interpreting Seventeenth-Century Native 'Texts.'" *Early Native Literacies in New England: A Documentary and Critical Anthology.* Ed. Kristina Bross and Hilary E. Wyss. Amherst: U of Massachusetts P, 2008. 132-41. Print.

Morgan, Edmund S. *Visible Saints: The History of a Puritan Idea.* New York: New York UP, 1963. Print.

Morrison, Dane. *A Praying People: Massachusett Acculturation and the Failure of the Puritan Mission, 1600-1690.* New York: Peter Lang, 1995. Print.

Perkins, William. *A Treatise Tending unto a Declaration, Whether a Man be in the Estate of Damnation, or in the Estate of Grace.* London: John Porter, 1597. Print.

Pettit, Norman. *The Heart Prepared: Grace and Conversion in Puritan Spirit Life.* New Haven: Yale UP, 1966. Print.

Porterfield, Amanda. "Women's Attraction to Puritanism." *Church History* 60.2 (1991): 196-209. Print.

Russell, Howard S. *Indian New England before the Mayflower*. Hanover: UP of New England, 1980. Print.

Salisbury, Neal. "Red Puritans: The 'Praying Indians' of Massachusetts Bay and John Eliot." *William and Mary Quarterly* 3rd ser. 31.1 (1974): 27-54. Print.

---. *Manitou and Providence: Indians, Europeans, and the Making of New England, 1500-1643*. New York: Oxford UP, 1982. Print.

Snow, Dean R., and Kim M. Lanphear. "European Contact and Indian Depopulation in the Northeast: The Timing of the First Epidemics." *Ethnohistory* 35.1 (1988): 15-33. Print.

Spiess, Arthur E., and Bruce D. Spiess. "New England Pandemic of 1616-1622: Cause and Archaeological Implication." *Man in the Northeast* 34 (1987): 71-83. Print.

Stannard, David E. *The Puritan Way of Death: A Study in Religion, Culture, and Social Change*. Oxford: Oxford UP, 1979. Print.

Webster, Charles. *From Paracelsus to Newton: Magic and the Making of Modern Science*. Cambridge: Cambridge UP, 1982. Print.

Winthrop, John. *The Journal of John Winthrop: 1630-1649*. Ed. Richard S. Dunn, James Savage, and Laetitia Yeandle. Cambridge: Harvard UP, 1996. Print.

Wood, William. *New England's Prospect: A True, Lively, and Experimentall Description of that Part of America, Commonly Called New England*. London 1634. *Early English Books Online*. STC 25957. Web. 23 June 2009.

Wyss, Hilary E. "'Things That Do Accompany Salvation': Colonialism, Conversion, and Cultural Exchange in Experience Mayhew's *Indian Converts*." *Early American Literature* 33.1 (1998): 39-61. Print.

---. *Writing Indians: Literacy, Christianity, and Native Community in Early America*. Amherst: U of Massachusetts P, 2000. Print.

MARCEL HARTWIG

"Some with their Fear th' Infection bring, And only shun the Doctor's Skill": Medical Practice and the Paper War during Boston's Smallpox Epidemic of 1721

> [V]accination is one of the greatest of medico-social advances, for it was the first attempt to defeat a disease upon the national scale. Further it was the first attempt to protect the community as opposed to the individual.
> (Charles Creighton qtd. in Cartwright and Biddiss 122)

From Red Linen to Live Virus Implantations

Historically, effective therapies for smallpox patients have always been a result of global knowledge transfers:[1] Some of the first special isolation measures, involving red linen for smallpox patients, were applied in Japan (the so-called red treatment method) in the tenth century. Cloths with red pigamon were also used to treat smallpox

---

[1] Smallpox is said to have already plagued ancient Greece and Rome (cf. Cartwright and Biddiss 116). Illness was understood at the time in Galenic terms, as resulting from imbalances of blood, black and yellow bile, and phlegm. Bloodletting or forced vomiting (emesis) were first approaches to curing the infectious disease.

patients in China. In both Western and Eastern cultures, the red treatment method had been in use for more than 500 years, and in Indochina it was still practiced in the 1890s (cf. Hopkins 296). According to the verse productions of the Italian Salerno Medical School, the first inoculations were undertaken in China in the eleventh century.[2] This precursor to Edward Jenner's vaccination induced a genuine form of smallpox in the inoculees and made them as resistant to subsequent smallpox outbreaks as patients who naturally acquired and survived the disease. It is claimed that this form of variolation was first introduced from India. In Europe, where inoculation belonged to the realm of folk medicine, "the first authentic reports were published in Leipzig between 1670 and 1705" (Blake, "Inoculation Controversy" 489). Even though this method of transplanting the smallpox virus had been known and reported about for more than 500 years, inoculation as a first form of preventive medicine only became a permanently established part of the medical code of practice in the mid-eighteenth century. Since then, knowledge transfers between the hemispheres have shaped and constantly redefined a medical understanding of smallpox.

In the end, inoculation proved to be the most effective preventive method until the arrival of Jenner's vaccination. Yet, until 1721 technical explanations and detailed statistical tables reporting the success of this method were non-existent. Inoculation was hence for a long time known only from hearsay and remained a highly risky venture amongst physicians and doctors around the world. While being unaware of cross-infections, doctors who successfully applied inoculation slowly spread the word through highly restricted channels of communication. The first "scientific" paper concerning systematic inoculation appeared in 1714 in the Royal Society of London's journal, *Philosophical Transactions*. This publication triggered "[t]he first large-scale test of the sort in Western medicine" (Shryock 57) in Boston. It is a common belief among historians that the Boston-episode of 1721-22 eventually led to the permanent establishment of smallpox inoculation in England

---

[2]   The term inoculation was introduced by the Greek scholars Timonius and
      Pylarinus in 1714. Focusing on the process of implanting a live virus in a pa-
      tient, the term is borrowed from horticulture (cf. Wetering 48).

(cf. G. Miller 476) and New England, and from there may have found its way into the code of practice of European doctors.

Here, the institutions and cultural circumstances that introduced a preliminary form of preventive medical variolation into Western medical discourse will be the subject of debate. This paper will inquire into the categories that became subject to institutional interventions with regard to the introduction of inoculation and will further study the circumstances under which knowledge about smallpox and inoculation was produced in both medical and public discourses. Therefore, this article argues that it was only due to England's role as a mediator in transatlantic transfers of professional knowledge between England and her North American colonies during the Boston smallpox epidemic of 1721–22 that the institutionalization of transatlantic medical practice and preventive medical care could be established to begin with. Furthermore, the enormous pressure to conform to scientific publication requirements and the belief in compulsory professionalization of the medical practice of educated medical personnel turns the Boston experiment into a prototype case study for the establishment of a transatlantic channel of medical expertise prior to the large-scale "transit of culture"[3] (cf. Shryock 18) starting in 1730.

This essay will therefore undertake a brief survey of the smallpox epidemic in Boston to trace conflicts in Boston's system of knowledge concerning the smallpox virus. To access the channels of a methodical professionalization of medical personnel, this paper will take a closer look at arguments for and against the systematic adoption of inoculation as published in broadsides and newspapers of the time. Lastly, the connection between American and English publication formats and readership will reveal in order to highlight the authoritative channels of medical expertise existing at the time.

---

[3] The term refers to the institutionalized professionalization of American physicians who traveled in large numbers to Edinburgh and London. Once arrived in one of these "medical centers," they set about to study medicine and then (most often) returned to the colonies as "first-class medical men" (cf. Shryock 18-19).

Smallpox and Inoculation until 1721

For several centuries, smallpox was believed to have an affinity with measles and syphilis. The terminology in Europe ("la grosse verole" [the Great Pox] for syphilis and "la petite verole" [the smallpox]) not only echoes this premise but also codifies the disease with the connotations of syphilis. In the sixteenth and seventeenth centuries, syphilis "acquired moral connotations commonly associated with leprosy, connotations that focused on social stability, . . . [but which also] reflected sexual sins" (Grigsby 67). In this way, the disease and its connotations traveled between the hemispheres and repeatedly triggered the attention of the clergy, whose work involved not only matters of the soul but also medical advice.[4]

Such a "calling" ties in with a common belief among historians that during the seventeenth and early eighteenth centuries the causes of diseases and their treatment were still perceived more in terms of unverified doctrines and divine punishment rather than of a professionalized medical practice[5] (this view has to be reconsidered; see Priewe in this publication). Supposedly, smallpox was perceived in a similar vein as a disease that "had supernatural causes and therefore required an appropriately pious response" (Williams 21).[6] But God's

---

[4] In New England, the first medical advice pamphlet concerned with smallpox was published by the first minister of the Old South Church in Boston, Thomas Thacher, under the title *A Brief Rule to Guide the Common-People of New-England How to Order Themselves and Theirs in the Small Pocks, or Measels* (1677). Supposedly, it "was the only publication in this country of any medical importance during this period" (Viets 389).

[5] Thus, the New England Puritan minister Cotton Mather ponders about the origins of illness in his diary: "I must enquire whether a malignant Cold, bee not the very distemper of my Soul; a cold Indisposition to Religion, accompanied with sinful Malignity" (1: 248).

[6] Particularly in the English colonies in the "New World," the disease was first read as a divine sign in favor of the Puritan mission, since it ravaged approximately two thirds of the Native American population during the seventeenth century. In the words of the first governor of the Massachusetts Bay Colony, John Winthrop, the colonist-imported disease attested to the "goodness and providence of God." In 1634, he wrote: As "for the natives,

benevolence had its limits: Smallpox was already an endemic in London and also became an unwelcome but common phenomenon in the colonies during the seventeenth century. There it posed a challenge to both self-proclaimed physicians and the clergy. In 1721, these two interest groups collided, changing the fate of smallpox and preventive medicine for good.

On the following pages, I will introduce the two oppositional parties in the inoculation debate on the 1721–22 Boston smallpox epidemic. A particular focus will rest on the transnational system of knowledge transfer between England and her colonies in order to locate a discursive center for the distribution of knowledge concerning variolation. This will allow a deeper understanding of the existing epistemological system surrounding the medical profession and the clergy.

In New England, clergymen such as Michael Wigglesworth, Thomas Shepard, John Eliot, or Thomas Thacher often acted as self-proclaimed physicians. Cotton Mather was to follow in their footsteps. His belief in rational scientific explanations and his study of natural philosophy made the Puritan minister a controversial public figure. For instance, during the Salem witch trials, in which he served as an advisor, he proclaimed witchcraft as a rational category that could be empirically studied according to the natural sciences. He advocated these views in *The Wonders of the Invisible World* (cf. P. Miller 191-209). Eventually, his advice would lead to the hanging of nineteen "witches" and to the death of one "wizard" by crushing. Mather later distanced himself from his role in the trials of 1692. Nevertheless, his hunger for an understanding of the natural sciences and of the rational impetus of the Enlightenment remained. His greatest interest was in "natural philosophy," and Mather struggled to gain access to the learned body of London's Royal Society, whose publications inspired Mather's study the most. In November 1712, he wrote thirteen letters on New England's "Natural History" to two members of the Royal Society. Finally, the Puritan minister found a new penpal in Dr. John Woodward. Due to a mutually shared interest in paleontology, this Fellow of the Royal Society would eventually become an important spokesman for Mather in England.

---

they are near all dead of the smallpox, so as the Lord hath cleared our title to what we possess" (qtd. in Stannard 109).

In Boston, Cotton Mather gained access to the latest volumes of the *Philosophical Transactions* of the Royal Society through Dr. William Douglass.[7] Other than Mather, this gentleman "was the only physician in Boston who had actually taken a medical degree rather than read and apprenticed with a practitioner who had been trained in the same way" (Williams 61). Douglass studied medicine at the universities of Edinburgh, Leyden, and Paris and can as such be regarded as a professionally trained practitioner. Something must have sparked an interest between the two men as they first met in Boston, something that prompted Douglass to lend his books to Mather. Even though Mather and Douglass would not maintain a close friendship, the former nevertheless had access to Douglass's private library. In other words, by granting Mather direct access to his private collection of material sources of medical knowledge until then restricted—off limits in the sense of consisting of studies from Europe's most prestigious centers of medical training, and publications of the *Transactions* available only to Royal Society members—Douglass by the same token enabled a "professionally" untrained individual to gain access to medical knowledge, thereby transgressing what Michel Foucault would call the "discursive regularities" of the existing formal medical education.[8]

It must have been around the time of Douglass and Mather's intellectual exchange that the Greek physician Dr. Emanuel Timonius of Constantinople reported the circumstances and means of Dr. Jacob Pylarinus's successful systematic inoculation in Turkey in a letter to the Royal Society. The letter was received by Mather's correspondent Dr. John Woodward, who in 1714 forwarded Timonius's report for publication in the *Transactions*. It was this account that sparked Mather's interest in the matter. He quickly formulated his own theory of

---

7 At the time, Mather believed himself to be a Fellow of the Royal Society. However, his name did not appear in the official register of members as he was not able to sign in person. In 1713, he was informed by the Society's secretary Richard Waller about his fellowship (cf. Kittredge, Cotton Mather's Election 84-85).

8 Foucault (cf. 37-38) holds that "discursive regularities" govern the "rules of formation"—the concepts, objects, and themes of a discourse (he would later prefer the term episteme)—that serve as the external conditions of existence for any discourse or "discursive formation."

the internal workings of smallpox. As the Bostonian was familiar with the writings of Antoni van Leeuwenhoek, the so-called "father of microbiology," Mather held that the disease resulted from the interplay of "animalcules"[9] and humor theory (cf. fn. 1). While pondering the "natural design" of the disease, Mather must have asked his slave, Onesimus, about his experience with smallpox in Africa. The Puritan minister then wrote a letter to Woodward, dated July 12, 1716, stating that he had inquired of

> [m]y Negro-man *Onesimus*, who is a pretty Intelligent Fellow, Whether he ever had the *Small-Pox*; he answered both, *Yes*, and, *No*. and then told me, that he had undergone an Operation, which had given him something of the *Small-Pox*, & would forever praeserve him from it; adding, That it was often used among the *Guramantese* [Coromantee]. . . . How does it come to pass, that no more is done to bring this operation, into experiment & into fashion—in *England*? When there are so many Thousands of People, that would give many Thousands of Pounds, to have the Danger and Horror of this frightful disease well over with. (Mather qtd. in Kittredge, *Some Lost Works* 422)

It is worth remarking here that Mather's first thought is of the commodification of health; he hints at the economic value of institutionalized inoculation rather than advocating his intention to do good for a greater public. Mather also stresses the intellectual capacities of his slave Onesimus when he introduces him as "a pretty Intelligent Fellow" to make his voice heard beyond a possible racial bias. Thus, the value of money, the economy of health, the commodification of medicine, and intellectual capacities are the selling points of Mather's initial smallpox theory. Further, in his letter, Mather acknowledges England and not her colonies as the medical center in which the institutionalization of inoculation by means of a general acceptance of the method has to happen first. Such an acceptance, he hypothesizes, would then remove inoculation from the realm of folk medicine and

---

[9]   Animalculae is van Leeuwenhoek's umbrella term for infinitesimal bacteria, protozoa, hydra, and spermatozoa (cf. Williams 63). In the "New World," Cotton Mather "was apparently the only American to discuss this 'germ theory' prior to the appearance of Dr. John Crawford's papers in Baltimore nearly a century thereafter" (Shryock 56).

transform the procedure into a professional preventive therapy. Yet the Puritan minister's letter remained unanswered.

Mather must have hoped for the publication of his correspondence in the *Transactions*, but Woodward would never do him this favor. As a result, Mather refrained from making his opinion public in Boston for the five years that followed. During this time, the acknowledgement of Mather's theories by a professional body of knowledge was wanting. The Bostonian thus lacked the authority to use his ideas to alter the discursive regularities of the existing medical profession in the sense of introducing a new concept into the medical debates of both England and New England. Maybe this is why "Mather did not discuss the matter with any of Boston's physicians and apothecaries" (Williams 67).

While Mather was waiting for the right time to make himself heard, inoculation experienced a success of its own in England. In 1717, Lady Mary Wortley Montagu had her infant son inoculated in Turkey and would repeat this measure on her daughter in April 1721 while London was held hostage by a severe smallpox epidemic. Her letters reported the success of inoculation to royal families. In August 1721, six Newgate prisoners would serve as inoculees in a public experiment, as recommended by Lady Mary, and eventually George I had his grandchildren inoculated. In England, the introduction of inoculation was thus enforced by means of social class. The validity and outcome of inoculation were substantiated in specific private bodies that served to perform public functions due to their status in society: On the one hand, there were the children of an English aristocratic wife of the British ambassador to Turkey, and the grandchildren of the Prince and Princess of Wales; and on the other, the disposable bodies of prison inmates in a public inoculation spectacle. In other words, the social status of inoculated individuals did not interfere with the prestige and authority of medical professionals. Instead, these "royal bodies" either sought inoculation of their own accord or were selected by government officials. In England, *the spectacular effect* of inoculation made an impact, not *the authority* of the personnel who conducted the procedure. As a result, "many London physicians seem to have been convinced that a safe and effective way had been found to have the almost inevitable disease [smallpox]" (G. Miller 479). Yet, at the same time, newspapers from New England raised public skepticism about inoculation in Europe.[10]

The English *Weekly Journal* then republished selected articles concerning the smallpox epidemic in New England. The story is as follows: It was in April 1721 that the HMS *Seahorse* set sail for Boston harbor. Soon after the ship's arrival in May of the same year, Captain Wentworth Paxton was the first to report the outbreak of smallpox in his crew to Boston's town authorities. The physician John Clark, whose daughter Elizabeth had been Cotton Mather's second wife,[11] was dispatched by the Selectmen to report about the *Seahorse* crew's state of health. Mather may have known about Clark's report in full detail even as the Selectmen decided to isolate the ship's crew on Spectacle Island. Being convinced that he could prevent many lives from being harmed by smallpox, Cotton Mather was eager to save Boston's sinful flock by means of inoculation. Lacking the practical experience of conducting the transplantation of a live virus on his own, Mather sought collaborators among ten established local physicians. On June 6, Mather sent them his "Address to the Physicians of Boston," in which he both summed up the by then eight-year-old findings of the Greek physicians Timonius and Pylarinus and requested a meeting with the city's medical personnel (cf. Blake, "Inoculation Controversy" 491-92). Dr. Douglass apparently never received this address (cf. P. Miller 346), but neither he nor other physicians would respond to Mather's request. All ignored the said letter but one: Dr. Zabdiel Boylston was convinced by the minister's missive. Since Boylston himself was already immunized against smallpox, he intended "to try the experiment . . . [and] chose to make it upon my own dear child and two of my servants" (Boylston 202).

---

[10] In 1723, Abraham Vater, a pro-inoculation professor from Wittenberg, held that the general introduction of *Blattern-Beltzen*, the German term for the "methodo nova transplantandi variolas per insitionem," was indeed held back by the debate concerning inoculation in New England. He wrote: "Was aber den Credit dieser Cur gar über den Hauffen zu werffen geschienen ist wohl die Zeitung aus Neu-Engelland in America gewesen" (qtd. in G. Miller 478).

[11] Elizabeth Clark and Mather's three youngest children died during the measles epidemic of 1713. Due to the disease's conceptual closeness to smallpox, Mather's personal loss may have initially sparked his personal mission to find a preventive method against the disease (cf. Wetering 62).

In 1721-22, Boylston would remain the only physician in New England to openly support inoculation. At that time, England's positive attitudes toward the method were unheard of in New England. Instead, the only professionally trained representative of the English medical elite, Dr. William Douglass, sought to establish a circle of his own to resist inoculation. In his pamphlets, the anticlerical physician would insist on his empirical preferences, professional propriety, and the exclusive right to treat and debate smallpox by representatives of modern, educated physicians. Hence, the lines between the two opposing parties in the ensuing debate concerning inoculation were drawn. From this predisposition it very soon became clear that in the 'New World' the debate concerning inoculation would rest solely on the "question of prestige and authority" (P. Miller 348). Both anti- and pro-inoculation parties settled their dispute in the pages of the town's leading newspapers, the *Boston Gazette,* the *New England Courant*, and the *Boston News-Letter*.

The Paper War

By September 1721, Dr. Boylston had conducted 35 successful inoculations. His unorthodox operations were met by outrage among the literate and educated Puritan public. In the following paragraphs, selected examples will help to illuminate the major arguments for and against inoculation as presented in the respective broadsides and pamphlets. This should allow a better understanding of the discursive "rules of formation" concerning inoculation and the enunciative functions of the statements in support or refutation of variolation.

From the beginning of his experiments, Boylston sought to make his efforts as transparent as possible and advertised his progress in the local newspapers. One of these advertisements appeared in print in the *Boston Gazette* of July 17, 1721, in which Boylston cited Mather's summary of the Greek physicians' systematic inoculation. Boylston further advocated that the method was recommended by "Gentlemen of Figure and Learning," and that he himself had successfully applied the method in his own household. In his statement, he points out that, in due time, he hoped to give his readers "some further proof of their [Timonius and Pylarinus's] just and reasonable Account." Such an announcement of the further conducting of his experiments outraged Boston intellectuals, and William Douglass became the spearhead of the subsequent anti-inoculation sentiment.

In his response, Douglass, who expressed his love of humanity under the pseudonym W. Philanthropos, personally attacked Boylston in an open letter published in the *Boston News-Letter* on July 24, 1721, referring to him as an uneducated physician famous only as a "certain *Cutter for the Stone*, who this [inoculation] without any serious thought undertakes"[12] ("History of Inoculation" 1). In Douglass's words, Boylston's belief in folk medicine and experience as a surgeon do not qualify him as a professional physician. Thus, Boylston's judgment concerning practical aspects of inoculation cannot be regarded as a sound statement in the professional realm. Obviously, in the eyes of Douglass, Boylston was not intellectually capable of correctly interpreting the inoculation report by the Greek physicians. In fact, Douglass headlined his letter "The History of Inoculation" and presented his reading of Timonius and Pylarinus's account. According to Douglass, inoculation originated among the uneducated, Muslims, and elderly Greek women and thus had an unethical nature, a claim also raised by English doctors as well as religious authorities. In order to comply with the implicit authority of modern medical education, Douglass as an "educated" physician thus may have felt the need to put this (hi)story right. In doing so, by the same token, he emphasizes that the intellectual and theoretical capacities of professional medicine significantly outweigh the manual and practical labor of uneducated medical personnel.

Furthermore, Douglass tried to rank himself on the level of both the English medical elite and religious authorities. Even though he himself neither had a theological degree nor could be considered a ministerial authority, in his letter, Douglass addressed the Puritan faith when he raised the question of how

> [t]he Determination of this as a *Case of Conscience*, I refer to Divines, how the trusting more the extra groundless *Machinations of Men* than to our Preserver in the ordinary course of Nature, may be consistent with

---

[12] Douglass's letter refers to Boylston's successful removal of an egg-sized bladder stone in his pharmacy in the Dock Square of Boston's South End.

the Devotion and Subjection we owe to the *all-wise* Providence of GOD Almighty. ("The History of Inoculation" 1)

Douglass thereby emphasized the unethical character of inoculation on religious grounds. In inoculating themselves, men like Boylston and those who supported his experiments thus would not be acting merely as divine tools but be consciously deciding against God's will.

Reading Douglass's "History" and his theological arguments, Cotton Mather may have felt personally attacked as well. Even though Douglass's view must have been considered reasonable by the Puritan readership of the *Boston News-Letter*, in his statement he himself crossed the professional line between medicine and theology in the same way Mather did when proposing inoculation to Boston's physicians. Mather then gathered some of his pro-inoculation allies (Reverends Benjamin Colman, John Webb, Thomas Prince, and William Cooper) to rebut Douglass's "History" and to ready an open letter "In Defense of Dr. Zabdiel Bolyston" (July 31, 1721) for printing in the *Boston Gazette*. In this letter, the newly allied pro-inoculators in part acknowledge Douglass's argument concerning medical education when they state that

> [t]he Town knows and so does the Country how *long* and with what *Success* Dr. *Boylston* has practis'd both in *Physick* and *Surgery*; and tho' he has not had the honour and advantage of an *Academic* Education, and consequently not the *Letters* of some *Physicians* in the Town, yet he ought by no means to be call'd *Illiterate*, *ignorant* &c. Would the Town hear that Dr. *Cutler* or Dr. *Davis* should be so treated? no more can it endure to see *Boylston* thus spit at. (1)

In other words, Boylston's practical experience and hitherto successful application of the method prove him right. It is not the cause of Boylston's experiments that seem to be of relevance here, but the outcome. Mather et al. conceded Boylston's lack of authority concerning medical professionalization to Douglass. Yet they argued for the practical aspects of Boylston's case study and thus held a counter position to Douglass. For the clergy, intellectual capacities seem to be secondary only to manual labor. That is why Boylston is not necessarily to be considered a man of learning who is making conscious decisions in his experiments but a vessel for divine providence. Thus, they argue:

> As to the *Case of Conscience* referr'd to the *Divines*, we shall only say—
> What *Heathens* must they be, to whom this can be a question. . . . Who
> know not the profanity and impiety of trusting in *Men* or *Means* more
> than in GOD? be it the best learn'd Men, or the most proper Means? But
> we will suppose what in fact is true among us at this Day, that Men of
> Piety . . . accept it with all thankfulness and joy as the gracious
> Discovery of a *Kind Providence* to Mankind for that end.

By such reasoning, the clergymen managed to elevate Boylston's
experiments beyond a purely scientific approach. In their eyes, the
surgeon acted according to his predestined providence. To support him,
then, is to support God's will. Anyone who would argue against
Boylston's experiments would not only discredit the clergy but also
directly oppose God's will. Perry Miller thus argues that both Cotton
and his father Increase Mather "tried to make him [Boylston] serve that
unification of the clergy they had failed to achieve either through their
association or through the *Proposals*" (354). Hence the medical
experiments served as part and parcel of the discursive regularities of the
clergy and thus as a powerful tool to sustain prestige in the clergy.
Along these lines of argumentation further letters and opinion pieces
were published during the summer and autumn of 1721. They would
eventually culminate in personal attacks, taunts, name-calling, and
rivalries. The object of the debate (inoculation) was soon pushed aside
and instead the authoritative question of who was allowed to speak in
favor of the community was debated in the pages of Boston's major
broadsides: The *Boston Gazette* remained the forum for pro-inoculation
arguments whereas the *Boston News-Letter* and the newly published
New England Courant of the Brothers Franklin sided with anti-
inoculation sentiments (cf. Williams; Blake; Wetering).

At the same time, built around similar arguments, the inoculation
debate was held nearby, in the more liberal environment of Harvard
University. During the Leverett era,[13] students and lecturers at Harvard
published the first student paper in 1721, *The Telltale*, which in the
summer of the same year adopted the inoculation issue. It featured a

---

[13] John Leverett succeeded Increase Mather, the father of Cotton Mather, as
president of Harvard. He was the institution's first secular president and
"founded the liberal tradition of Harvard University" (Morison 75).

series of "Argumentative Dialogue[s] concerning Inoculation between
Dr. Hurry [pro-inoculation] and Mr. Waitfort [against]." Therein, both
tutors discussed questions such as: "Is inoculation a sin? Is inoculation
self-induced illness? Is refusing to be inoculated against God's
reasoning? If bleeding is acceptable, why not inoculation?" (Burton 496). By discussing scientific and theological aspects of the
variolation method, the tutors not only made the "paper war" in the city
a topic in Cambridge, they also altered the rules of debating inoculation
by adding new vocabulary from the background of higher education. In
this sense, both intellectuals broached the issue of Galenic traditions and
the Puritan covenant. In *The Telltale*, the public discourse of Boston's
newspapers was thus transformed into a scientific debate. The students
and tutors at the university altered the discursive regularities of
preventive medicine by boosting the issue of inoculation. Eventually,
Boylston also inoculated "thirteen Harvard students, along with
Professor Edward Wigglesworth and tutor William Welsted" (Burton
496). The living examples of the inoculees would convince further
students at Harvard to get inoculated.

At the heart of the debate in both Boston and at Harvard, then, was
the matter of an appropriate language and format to introduce
inoculation to a literate public on the one hand and to make it an object
of science on the other. Therefore, the debate soon continued in the
pages of pamphlets printed in Boston and the publication of open letters
to members of the Royal Society in London. Both Mather and Douglass
started writing to their friends in the Royal Society in order to get
published in a more authoritative context with regard to matters of
science.

Channels of Medical Professionalization

In a letter to Dr. Alexander Stuart of London, William Douglass
formally penned his view of the *Inoculation of the Smallpox as
Practiced in Boston* (1722) as he intended it to be known by the Royal
Society. Again his approach is based on a historical account. In this
pamphlet, Douglass focuses more on presenting a chronology of the
events than on providing arguments based on a more distanced
reasoning concerning the method's therapeutic value. Thus, he does not

seem to be interested in the empirical success of the inoculation as practiced up until then. Rather, in his letter, he aims at vilifying Mather as someone who, "without any weight of Argument ... and [by] reiterated praying, preaching & scribbling" (i), tried to establish inoculation as an institution in Boston and at downgrading Boylston as a beneficiary who "applys to the two Ministers of the Congregation to which he belongs (being himself *illiterate*) to vindicate his Character as an able Practitioner" (2).

Next to warning in great extent about the dangers of furthered infection due to inoculation and trying to establish the claim that the law of neither natural nor divine physics applies to the procedure, Douglass also proposed that the inoculators should be treated according to English law, which states that "*poysioning and spreading infection are by the penal Laws of* England *Felony*" (13). This letter was to be followed by two more anti-inoculation letters. After being published in London, they became a sound argument for anti-inoculators in England and were republished for example in Dr. William Wagstaffe's *Letter to Dr. Friend, Shewing the Danger and Uncertainty of Inoculating the Small Pox* (1722), which became extremely popular and was immediately translated into French (cf. G. Miller 485).

It was also by this reasoning that Boylston, who was regarded as a criminal by Bostonians (according to Viets, parties are reported to have threatened "to hang him to the nearest tree" [400]) and whom the Selectmen had already warned not to proceed with his experiments in July 1721, was formally restricted in his experiments by the Selectmen in May 1722. Hence, due to a publication in the scientific realm of the "mother country," Douglass's rant was turned into a sound argument that not only inspired a similar war of pamphlets in Europe but also paved the way for legal measures against Boylston's experiments.[14]

Cotton Mather in a similar vein made use of his connections to England and readied a letter to the London agent for Massachusetts,

---

[14] Siding with William Douglass and publishing two major anti-inoculation essays, John Williams, then a contemporary tobacconist and medical practitioner, had publicly been advocating the legal argument since the fall of 1721. However, a legal tool to reprimand Boylston was only applied after Douglass's successful publications in London.

Jeremiah Dummer (cf. G. Miller 481). This letter was published and advertised in London's journals in February 1722 as "An Account of the Method and Success of Inoculating the Small-Pox upon Great Numbers of People (who all recovered) in New-England." Mather supposedly further sent his thoughts on "The Way of Proceeding in the Small Pox Inoculated in New England" to the former librarian at Harvard College, Henry Newman, who in April 1722 forwarded Mather's essays to the Royal Society (cf. G. Miller 482). Therein Mather gave detailed descriptions of how and when to apply inoculation. His account sparked interest and was immediately published in the *Transactions*. In addition to Mather's letters, the pro-inoculation writings of the Puritan reverends William Cooper and Benjamin Colman, extended by "An Historical Introduction," were published in England as *A Narrative of the Method and Success of Inoculating the Small-Pox in New England* by Reverend Daniel Neal. Neal's book probably convinced the Princess of Wales to undergo the procedure in April 1722. Her example again proved to be an instrument of popular promotion for variolation. However, it was adumbrated by the death of the Earl of Sunderland's son, who did not survive inoculation. Reacting immediately, London's *Weekly Journal* republished excerpts from Boston's newspapers and detailed how Boylston was constrained in his procedure by the Selectmen in April and May 1722 (cf. G. Miller 483). This series of examples traces Mather's attempts to establish his position in England. In order to make himself heard in the scientific realm, he opted for a factual and technical description of the method and toned down the religious sentiment that dominated his opinion pieces in the Boston newspapers.

In Boston, both Mather's and Douglass's letters became the subject of Harvard graduate Isaac Greenwood's *A Friendly Debate, or A Dialogue, between Academicus; and Sawney & Mundungus* (1722). The required focus on the right use of language to discuss the inoculation matter was at the heart of this satire. In this intellectual attack predominantly directed at William Douglass, Greenwood criticizes the writing style and form of presenting the inoculation controversy to the Royal Society, in particular to Dr. Alexander Stuart. Douglass is accused of having "published a Libel, which is all *Broad English*" (1) and Mather for his use of Latin, a language "his neighbours don't understand" (4). Hence, Greenwood's satire identified both marked and coded elements inside Mather's and Douglass's arguments as improper or highly restricted to a greater readership. Greenwood's is a timely comment on both authors' struggles to be accepted and acknowledged by the scientific body of the Royal Society in order to add authoritative support to their public debates in Boston.

Zabdiel Boylston well understood these channels of knowledge transfer to England and continued his experiments. His successes were repeatedly accompanied by the letters and pamphlets Mather penned for his contacts at the Royal Society. In February 1722, with the smallpox epidemic virtually at an end, Boylston nevertheless carried on with his experiments, to great success:

> Altogether, 5,759 people had had natural smallpox since April [1721], of whom 842 died. During this same period Boylston inoculated 242 persons in Boston and nearby towns, with 6 deaths, and two other physicians inoculated 39 persons with no fatalities. Except for a few recurrences in April and May the epidemic was over in the capital. (Blake, *Public Health* 61)

The numbers spoke for him. Boylston carefully took note of all his patients, the procedure, and the period of latency. In addition to this, his list of patients featured notable VIPs of the time, amongst whom were reverends Thomas Walter and Ebenezer Pierpont, Samuel Hirst (Justice Samuel Sewall's grandson), and Dr. Elijah Danforth (cf. Blake, "Inoculation Controversy" 494). Through them, his practice was blessed by several high-ranking officials in the community. Within a smaller circle his experiment was thus regarded and authorized as an established practice. As he had inoculated more persons than any European physician, Boylston eventually went to London in 1724. "In a letter to the [Royal] Society, Cotton Mather introduced Boylston with effusive praise . . . [as] 'a person so distinguished by an operation of so much consequence'" (Williams 202). In London Boylston lectured about his experiences before the Royal Society and the Royal College of Physicians. There he became a beneficiary and finally a Fellow of the Royal Society (cf. Viets 401). In 1726, his supporters financed the publication of *An Historical Account of the Small-Pox Inoculated in New England* in London (published in Boston in 1730). His historical account featured detailed statistics that dealt with the inoculations he had conducted and also offered highly detailed technical explanations. His "clinical records," as we would call them now, created a certain distance towards the individual patients and the overall success of the practical method. This would eventually establish him as "the Great Inoculator" (Rutkow 11).

Conclusion

As this paper has shown, Mather and Douglass both tried to determine a set of codified relations in order to establish a truth value for inoculation vis-à-vis the English medical and religious authorities. In their writings, however, it was neither religious sentiment nor arguments concerning literacy or professionalization that eventually established a truth value for inoculation in medical science. Rather, the use of formal Standard English and Latin descriptors as well as both the technical documentation and clinical records governed the formation of inoculation as a professional medical concept. This reasoning and its acknowledgement in established circles of knowledge production (the Royal Society) turned the variolation method formerly used in folk medicine into a superior and more professional tool.

By the same token, both Douglass and Mather abandoned the truths of their hitherto professions. The guiding principles of history, natural philosophy, and theology were disregarded in their reasoning. On the one hand, in Cotton Mather's arguments, arithmetic, horticultural studies (the term inoculation was borrowed from this discipline), and technical documentation replaced the moral and ethical doctrines of the clergy. Mather's reasoning in the letters to London ultimately assigned a minor position to his social duties. Moreover, by desperately trying to establish a truth value through the use of a restricted code of communication (Latin) and references to other scientific disciplines, Mather sought to govern the Bostonians' conduct as individual members of their community by propagating inoculation not as an experiment but as an already established practice. He mistook this deed as the right of his profession to work as a religious adviser and as such to control the life of the community. Thus, according to him, every argument against inoculation was by the same turn an "antiministerial sentiment" (P. Miller 357).

For his part, Douglass was more interested in putting right the historical background of inoculation. He downgraded the method as unfit due to its use in Muslim communities and its introduction to Boston by supposedly untrained and medically unskilled personnel. While ignoring the success of the method and overriding any argument in favor of inoculation by applying the established ideology of his professional education, he also violated his code of practice. The Hippocratic oath asks physicians to act for the benefit of the sick. This principle was disregarded in Douglass's writings, which were more focused on the merits of the inoculators than the merits of inoculation. Eventually, he came to his senses in 1730, when he "was the first to urge inoculation" (P. Miller 362) during another smallpox epidemic.

In the end, it was the untrained surgeon Zabdiel Boylston who established a truth value for inoculation because he lacked both ministerial authority and professional training. As such he served as a vessel for mediating Mather's authoritative influence in Boston, and through Mather's knowledge of the institutional structures of the professional medical apparatus, Boylston was authorized to make himself heard in the medical discourse. He was thus enabled to present a set of established statistical values and to publish his *Historical Account* (1726), in which he formulated the guiding principles of the inoculation method. In his publication, he presented precisely detailed descriptions of the procedure and defined medical personnel as the desired agents to conduct inoculations. In this manner, he introduced vocabulary into the medical discourse that in turn could become subject to the discourse's own regulations and institutional interventions in the form of handbooks, medical advice, and training. As such, inoculation could already serve as an established practice in the Boston smallpox epidemic of 1730.

This paper suggests a close connection between European medical discourses and the establishment of a regulated medical profession in the New World. Boston's smallpox epidemic and the introduction of inoculation into a medical professional discourse involved a steady and simultaneous transfer of knowledge between the so-called Old and New Worlds. This opens a new transnational perspective on the origins of the medical profession in the New World and raises questions about authorities and knowledge structures in transnational medical discourse. The specific arguments, codes, and practices that were used to establish inoculation as a scientifically acknowledged standard of practice have been located in this paper by looking at letters and pamphlets as carriers and possible channels of professionalization. A closer study of these "channels" still remains to be done. Such a venture may open a new perspective on the history of medicine in America.

Works Cited

Blake, John B. *Public Health in the Town of Boston, 1630-1822*. Cambridge: Harvard UP, 1959. Print.

---. "The Inoculation Controversy in Boston: 1721-1722." *New England Quarterly* 25.4 (1952): 489-506. Print.

Boylston, Zabdiel. "An Historical Account of the Small-Pox Inoculated in New England." 1726. *The Monthly Anthology, and Boston Review*. Ed. David P. Adams and William Emerson. Boston: Munroe and Francis, 1804. 201-04. Print.

Burton, John D. "'The Awful Judgements of God upon the Land': Smallpox in Colonial Cambridge, Massachusetts." *New England Quarterly* 74.3 (2001): 495-506. Print.

Cartwright, Frederick F., and Michael Biddiss. *Disease and History*. New York: Barnes and Nobles, 1972. Print.

Douglass, William. "The History of Inoculation." *Boston News-Letter* 24 July 1721: 1. Print.

---. *Inoculation of the Smallpox as Practiced in Boston: Consider'd in a Letter to A--S--M.D. & F.R.S. in London*. Boston: Printed and Sold by J. Franklin, at His Printing-House in Queen-Street, over against Mr. Sheaf's School, 1722. Print.

Foucault, Michel. *The Archaeology of Knowledge*. Trans. Alan Sheridan. New York: Pantheon, 1972. Print.

Grigsby, Bryon Lee. *Pestilence in Medieval and Early Modern English Literature*. New York: Routledge, 2003. Print.

Hopkins, Donald R. *The Greatest Killer: Smallpox in History*. Chicago: U of Chicago P, 2002. Print.

Kittredge, George Lyman. *Some Lost Works of Cotton Mather*. Cambridge: J. Wilson and Son, 1912. Print.

---. *Cotton Mather's Election into the Royal Society*. Cambridge: J. Wilson and Son, 1912. Print.

Mather, Cotton. *Diary of Cotton Mather, 1681-1724*. Vol. 1. Cambridge: Massachusetts Historical Society, 1911. Print.

Miller, Genevieve. "Smallpox Inoculation in England and America: A Reappraisal." *William and Mary Quarterly* 3rd ser. 13.4 (1956): 476-92. Print.

Miller, Perry. *The New England Mind: From Colony to Province*. Cambridge: Harvard UP, 1953. Print.

Morison, Samuel Eliot. *Three Centuries of Harvard, 1636-1936*. Cambridge: Harvard UP, 1936. Print.

Rutkow, Ira. *Seeking the Cure: A History of Medicine in America*. New York: Scribner, 2010. Print.

Shryock, Richard Harrison. *Medicine and Society in America, 1660–1860*. Ithaca: Cornell UP, 1960. Print.

Stannard, David E. *American Holocaust: The Conquest of the New World*. Oxford: Oxford UP, 1992. Print.

Viets, Henry R. "Some Features of the History of Medicine in Massachusetts during the Colonial Period (1620-1770)." *Isis* 23.2 (1935): 389-405. Print.

Wetering Van De, Maxine. "A Reconsideration of the Inoculation Controversy." *New England Quarterly* 58.1 (1985): 46-67. Print.

Williams, Tony. *The Pox and the Covenant: Mather, Franklin, and the Epidemic that Changed America's Destiny*. Naperville: Sourcebooks, 2010. Print.

SONJA FIELITZ

Live and Let Die: Viewpoints on Aging in Eighteenth-Century Britain

Introduction

In our contemporary society, electronic media—among others—have brought about a completely new awareness in the perception of space and time, and with regard to the latter, various processes have clearly reshaped the meaning of (old) age. The phenomenon of aging is part of all human societies, and it implies physical processes as well as cultural and societal[1] dimensions. From a historical perspective, as Donald Olen

---

[1] Social critics have approached the phenomenon of aging from various angles, but no single theory has prevailed yet. The "disengagement theory" of aging looks at old age as a time when both the older person and society engage in mutual separation, as in the case of retirement from work. Disengagement thus depends on having some sense of personal meaning that is distinct from the office one holds. The "activity theory" of aging argues that the more active people are, the more likely they are to be satisfied with life. Activity theory assumes that how we think of ourselves is based on the roles or activities in which we engage and thus recognizes that most people in old age continue with roles and life activities established earlier because they have the same needs and values. The third, that is, the "continuity theory" of aging, argues in a similar way by noting that people who grow older are inclined to maintain as much as they can the same habits, personality, and style of life they developed in earlier years. According to both activity theory and continuity theory, any decreases in social interaction are explained in a better way by poor health or disability than by some functional need of society to disengage older people from their previous roles. The ideal of

Cowgill has reminded us, "the status of old age was low in hunting-and-gathering societies, but it rose dramatically in stable agricultural societies, in which older people controlled the land. With the coming of industrialization, it is said, modern societies have tended to devalue . . . the wisdom or life experience of elders, leading to a loss of status and power" (qtd. in Moody 7). In the twentieth and twenty-first centuries, aging in humans has become a most diversified field of multidimensional perspectives, approaches, and aspects of investigation.

This essay (by a literary historian) will not be so much concerned with aspects of chronological, social, or biological aging but rather with cultural representations of age and aging in the early days of the natural sciences in Britain. Taking a look back in history may even result in unexpected realizations for the present.

Historical Background

It is common knowledge that the seventeenth and eighteenth centuries were a period of great scientists and their experiments, inventions, and discoveries. Mathematicians (such as John Wallis), scientists (such as Robert Boyle and William Petty), educational reformers (such as Samuel Hartlib), scientists such as Isaac Newton and Boyle, Johannes Kepler and William Gilbert (Sir Walter Raleigh's half-brother), Gabriel Harvey and Galileo Galilei, Blaise Pascal, Christopher Wren, Robert Hooke, Edmund Halley, and many others changed the world in a hitherto unknown dimension. In the field of the humanities (cf., for instance, David Allan and Thomas Abbott), the most distinguished writers (such as John Dryden,[2] Henry Fielding, William Goldsmith, Dr. Samuel Johnson, and Samuel Richardson) and artists (such as William Hogarth, Joshua Reynolds, and William Gainsborough) gave it excellence. Georg Friedrich Handel's music fascinated the court while David Garrick and Sarah Siddons won

---

active aging seems more a prolongation of middle age rather than something special or positive about the last stage of life (cf. Moody 7-10).

[2]   For Dryden's responses to the intellectual impulses aroused by the scientific moment, cf., for instance, Bredvold.

immortality on the stage, especially in productions of Shakespeare's dramas. In the field of politics, French writers and philosophers such as Voltaire, Montesquieu, Denis Diderot, and Jacques Rousseau spread their ideas of liberty and reform far beyond the borders of France and thus stimulated new political thinking in Europe. Needless to say, with René Descartes, the Enlightenment as one of the most significant movements in the history of Western thought was on the horizon.

The early seventeenth century, and here specifically the years between the death of Queen Elizabeth I (1603) and the beheading of Charles I (1649), witnessed notable winds of cultural change. While the Thirty Years War was still ravaging the continent, in England, numerous forces were at work, be it in the fields of politics, agriculture or religion. The kings of the House of Hanover were not only involved in British but also in Continental European matters as well as in colonial rivalries (the loss of the American colonies occurred under George III). As to foreign affairs, Britain and France were engaged in fierce opposition (with a few short intermissions between the War of the Spanish Succession and the Napoleonic Wars). Explorers and traders brought goods such as tobacco and coffee home and stimulated curiosity to see and learn more about the (new) world. In domestic politics, the divine right of kings was called into question by the increasing influence of Parliament, and the authority of the bishops was contested in church. In the eighteenth century, an increase in population, a further expansion of trade, the practice of enclosures, the Agrarian Revolution, and, from the 1780s on, industrialization gradually transformed English society. Among the lower classes, poverty and smallpox swept away large parts of the population, and many people were debased by gin-drinking. For many human beings, the art of living thus mostly consisted in the skill of surviving the perils of infancy, youth, and middle age. Given the fact that throughout the sixteenth and seventeenth centuries average life expectancy was about forty years, the medical sciences were to address the problem of dying young.

Francis Bacon

English science in the seventeenth and eighteenth centuries acknowledged a great debt to the work of Sir Francis Bacon (1561-

1626), who, despite a busy career in politics and law (he was Lord Chancellor under James I), developed a new program for science. If knowledge were to grow and develop, he maintained, a new method of cognition and a different approach from that of classical antiquity would be needed. Bacon thus went beyond Aristotle's verbal science

> passed down in texts and commentaries, relying on a verbal discipline, logic, which can manipulate received ideas but not find out new sciences. . . . The remedy, according to Bacon, was to start from a fresh examination of reality in all its detail, not rejecting, as earlier theorists had done, certain topics as trivial or sordid, and on the basis of observation and experiment gradually build up axioms or scientific laws of increasing generality and universality. From this level one could return to works, or specific man-made transformations of nature. (Vickers 1-2)

For centuries before Bacon, learned men had used the form of syllogistic or deductive reasoning and had worked out their ideas according to a specific method, moving step by step from major principles to conclusions. No doubt, this reasoning of deduction worked well for the re-statement and confirmation of what was already known. According to Bacon, however, it was not extremely fruitful for the discovery of new knowledge. Thus, he developed an opposing strategy, i.e., to assemble facts by observation and experiment, consider their similarities and dissimilarities, and then conjecture on the basis of the evidence before one's eyes.

> Where traditional logic operated deductively, from first principles down to ever more minute descriptions, Bacon would reverse the process by using induction, ascending from a host of specific instances to general propositions. At this stage experiments would be used, but not in a hasty way, nor designed for a swift material application. (Vickers 3)

In short, proceeding from facts and details to generalizations and principles would lead on to further discoveries, and knowledge would thus expand.

> Some of his [Bacon's] ideas, such as the attack on medieval scholasticism and its purely philological practice of science, had been expressed by others in the European Renaissance, but he was the first to develop a coherent critique of outmoded science and to suggest practical

remedies, while no one else expressed these ideas so forcibly and so eloquently. Yet in the seventeenth century Bacon was actually revered as one of the pioneers in the new philosophy, both as a theorist and an experimenter, his fame spreading throughout Europe. (Vickers 1)

Bacon proclaimed his breach with the old philosophical tradition and the importance of inductive reasoning in his *Novum Organum* (1605), the title itself signaling a clear reference to Aristotle's *Organon*, the standard work on syllogistic reasoning that had dominated Western thinking for about fifteen centuries. In his *Advancement of Learning*, Bacon presented the fields of knowledge as he knew them, pointing out the regions awaiting exploration but also indicating some of the difficulties humans might meet in making those explorations. Unlike other great individuals in the sciences such as Galileo, Kepler, Descartes, and Newton, Bacon thought in terms of institutions that would channel scientific research and then apply it to society at large.

Bacon not only excelled in the field of science, he also gave voice to the advancements of the age in literary texts. In 1627, a few months after his death, his utopia *New Atlantis* was published. It depicts an imaginary country where people live under the government and the institutions Bacon thought to be wisest. The most important one of these is Solomon's House (cf. Colie), a scientific research institute with all the equipment a scientist could dream of and a fully worked out division of specialized responsibilities. This institute, "the noblest foundation ... that ever was upon the earth" (Bacon 229), comprises every imaginable aid for observation and experiment in natural phenomena to uncover their possible utility for mankind. Its end is "the finding out of the true nature of all things" (Bacon 230), that is, the knowledge of causes, and the secret motions of things. For this end, Solomon's House enclosed observatories on high towers, underground laboratories, engines for the enforcing of winds, dissection rooms, breeding stations; in short: all the equipment imaginable for an interrogation of nature.

And in the field of medicine and old age, it was Sir Francis Bacon as well who would be the inspiring presence.

From the early *Essays of Counsels* (1597), the preservation of health became a leitmotif of his writings. Shortly afterwards, in *The Advancement of Learning* of 1605, he provided, for the first time, preliminary advice on diets, exercises, and medicines, thus paving the

way for the prolongation of life. Later, . . . his *New Atlantis* showed the
same medical bias as did the *Magnalia Naturae*. . . . It was *The History
of Life and Death*, however, which was first published under its Latin
title, *Historia Vitae et Mortis*, in 1623 and which formed part of Book
Three of the projected *Great Instauration*, that publicized more than any
other treatise Bacon's determination to make the prolongation of life the
first objective of medical art. . . . In particular, its long list of
recommendations on the various ways and means how to maintain and
prolong life, including advice on medicine and herbs, food and drink,
diet and regimen, sleep and exercises, habitation and air, temperature
and climate, baths and hygiene, established the format for the numerous
treatises of a healthy and long life that were to succeed Bacon
throughout the seventeenth century. (Real 126-28)

The Royal Society

Beside individuals such as Bacon, the *institution* that played a major
part in bringing about an effective scientific revolution in eighteenth-
century Britain was the Royal Society of London as the oldest leading
learned society for science in the world still in existence in the UK.

The first attempts to organize the new developments in England were
undertaken by devotees of science who met informally in casual meeting
places such as clubs in London and Oxford. Those who paved the way
for the development of modern science were enthusiasts in the time of
Elisabeth I (1564-1603) and her successor James I (1603-1624). They
believed that neither of the universities, i.e., Oxford and Cambridge,
prepared young men adequately for their later life either in the king's
councils or in the vastly expanding world of trade and business. In 1645,
the so-called invisible college was founded, and in 1660, these amateurs
formally constituted themselves into an academy for the advancement of
various parts of learning. Charles II, who took considerable interest in
the new organization, granted the society's petition, and the charter
passed the Great Seal on 15 July 1662. As the official *Record of the
Royal Society* states, their Horatian motto "nullius in verba" ("on the
words of no one") "was an expression of their (the Society's)
determination to withstand the domination of authority and to verify all
statements by an appeal to facts" (qtd. in Stimson 64). It thus explicitly
signifies the society's commitment to establishing the truth of scientific

matters through experiment rather than recourse to (classical) authorities.

When the Royal Society was officially granted its Royal Charter in 1662, it united several strands of scientific activities that would change the world to a hitherto unknown extent:

> William Gilbert, Queen Elizabeth's physician, had published his epochal study of terrestrial magnetism (*De Magnete*) in 1600, . . . Kepler's formulation of the laws of planetary motion, together with Galileo's brilliant work in astronomy and mechanics was combined by Newton with the Copernican hypothesis in his fundamental theory of the universe. The laws of attraction and of motion, mathematically demonstrated, governed earth, planets and stars alike in one magnificently ordered system.
>
> Other astronomers like Edmond Halley and Flamstead in England by their studies supplied supporting evidence. . . .
>
> Robert Boyle, the finest virtuoso of them all, for the first time distinguished between element, compound, and mixture and used his improved air-pump to work out the law of the gases that students know today as Boyle's Law. Robert Hooke was his right-hand man in his work . . . . (Stimson 43)

With particular reference to the focus of this collection of essays, that is, medicine and literature, it is safe to say that medicine greatly improved during the seventeenth and eighteenth centuries. Since major discoveries were also made in physics, chemistry, and biology, the sciences formed a basis for various branches of clinical medicine. In the course of the eighteenth century, William Harvey determined how blood circulated through the body, Anton van Leeuwenhoek discovered red blood cells, and Edward Jenner invented vaccination after having investigated the relationship between cowpox and smallpox. Thomas Sydenham developed a treatment procedure which included careful observation and record-keeping in clinical practice. William Smellie, the leading obstetrician of his time in London, was the first to make a scientific study of the physical process of childbirth, published in the three-volume *Treatises on the Theory and Practice of Midwifery* (1752-64). Giovanni Battista Morgangni's *De Sedibus et Causis Morborum per Anatomen Indagatis* (*On the Seats and Causes of Diseases, investigated by Anatomy* [1761]) set the standards in the field of anatomy by describing about 700 cases in which he attempted to correlate the findings after death with the related clinical records. Scientists shared their research in journals, the best-known one being the Royal Society's *Transactions* as the first scientific journal in the English-speaking world. Medical education was also increasingly incorporated into the universities of Europe.

Aging

Historians have long been interested in the history of aging. In classical antiquity, Cicero (106-43 BC) in his *De Senectute* (*On Old Age*) was inspired by the hope that the mind can prevail over the body. "Thus, he viewed old age not exclusively as a time of decline or loss but also as an opportunity for cultivating compensatory wisdom. Cicero, in fact, was one of the first and most eloquent proponents of the ideal of 'successful aging'" (Moody 14). About 200 years later, however, Juvenal's *Satire X* (and Dr. Johnson's eighteenth-century imitation of it in *The Vanity of Human Wishes*) are sharp satires on the idea that long life is a source of happiness.

As Daniel Schäfer has reminded us in his comprehensive study on the relationship between age and illness in the early modern period, up to 1650, the vast majority of medical writings still adhered to Galenic physiology and dietetics. Due to the anatomical and physiological discoveries as well as the growing interest in clinical observation in the seventeenth century, a shift in how medical writers perceived the process of aging occurred in the 1650s. According to Schäfer, the reason for this change lay in the gradual replacement of the older basis of gerocomy, that is, dietetics, by the "new" disciplines of physiology, pathology, and pharmacology.

Opponents

Despite overall enthusiasm, the new science's success saw a number of difficulties. To many, the activities of the members of the Royal Society, for instance, not only seemed futile, useless, and unproductive in themselves but also dangerous to the state and the established church. The earliest critics were academics from Oxford and Cambridge who were highly skeptical about the growth of the new science and also concerned that their own prestige was at stake. In the field of medicine, it was mostly the members and patrons of the Royal College of Physicians, that is, the first medical institution in England to receive a Royal Charter after having been founded in 1518 by Henry VIII (it acquired the "royal" honour in 1674), who censured the institutions. In his manuscript "Life," Dr. Hamey became seriously disturbed at its growing fame and viewed the Royal Society as "a rival society trading close upon ye heels of the Aesculapians, whose vortex would be so great as to comprehend everything . . . whereas all matters within ye sphaere of Medicine, Anatomy and Surgery most properly should belong to ye Royal College of Physicians" (qtd. in Sprat 69). The members of the Royal Society were also accused of disregarding ancient learning and classical authority, foremost of all Aristotelian philosophy. One of the Royal Society's severest critics was Dr. Henry Stubbs, perhaps the most famous classical scholar of his time. In 1670, he attacked Sprat's *History of the Royal Society* in no less than seven books and pamphlets censuring the society from its moral principles to its grammatical competence (cf., for instance, Jones).

In the fine arts, some of the best-known writers of their time heavily criticized the Royal Society, among them Samuel Butler, Thomas Shadwell, and Aphra Behn. Butler's poem "Elephant in the Moon"[3] must suffice as one example:

> In the poem a group of virtuosi observe the moon one night through a long telescope. They discover that the moon's inhabitants are evidently at war and one claims to see an elephant striding across its surface. They fall into eager discussion about this, and a footman standing by decides to look for himself. He reports that he can see nothing because there is something in the tube near the eye-piece. A less credulous virtuoso looks and discovers a mouse caught in the tube. . . . There they discover gnats, flies and other insects caught in it, and they realize that these were their great "armies battling" on the moon. (Stimson 91)

---

[3] Though written sometime in the 1660s or 1670s, it was not printed until 1759, together with a fragment, "On the Royal Society," that was even more scornful.

Furthermore, Shadwell's satirical play *The Virtuoso* (1673) is particularly critical of the scientific discoveries of the age. Shadwell's play became very popular due to the character of Sir Nicholas Gimcrack, who is an untiring and indiscriminate advocate of experimentation. Being superstitious, gullible, and only interested in the monstrous, however, he does not distinguish between the true scientist and the credulous enthusiast: "'Tis below a Virtuoso, to trouble himself with men and manners. I study insects, and I have observed the tarantula does infinitely delight in music, which is the reason of its poison being drawn out by it" (3.3.88-91). In his play, Shadwell ridicules the Royal Society's experiments in blood transfusion by recounting the transfusion of "the blood of a sheep into a madman" (2.2.180). And when his character Longvil laughs at knowledge as an ultimate end, we may assume that Shadwell had in mind the failure of the virtuoso to use his learning for immediate utility:

Longvil: But to what end do you weigh this Air, Sir?

Sir Nicholas: To what end shou'd I—to know what it weighs. O knowledge is a fine thing. Why I can tell to a grain what a gallon of any air in England weighs. (5.2.19-21)

With respect to language, Sir Nicholas uses expressions like "diffusive" (2.2.62), "precelling in physico-mechanical investigations" (2.2.96), "follicular impulsion" (2.2.103-04), "testaceous" (2.2.291), "cacochymious" (2.2.217) and thus ridicules the Royal Society's Latinisms. The most extended parody, however, is the description of how a plum turns blue:

Sir Nicholas: Then for the blue upon plums, it is nothing but many living creatures: I have observ'd upon a wall plum (with my most exquisite glasses, which cost me several thousands of pounds) at first beginning to turn blue, it comes first to fluidity, then to orbiculation, then fixation, so to angulization, then crystallization, from thence to germination or ebullition, then vegetation, then plantamination, perfect animation, sensation, local motion and the like. (4.3.221-28)

Sir Nicholas Gimcrack was such a success that he has lived on in literature. For instance, in the *Tatler* No. 221 (supposedly written by Joseph Addison), the widow Gimcrack writes a letter telling of her husband's becoming a virtuoso. Here, we learn that his death from a fever resulted from chasing an odd-colored butterfly for some five miles. On his deathbed he had made his will, saying that he wanted to relieve his slaves as the Romans had done. In his case, however, the slave is a fly which he had kept in chains for several months.

Jonathan Swift, *Gulliver's Travels*

The best-known satire[4] on the sciences in eighteenth-century Britain is Jonathan Swift's *Gulliver's Travels* (1726), and here the voyage to Laputa and its famous Grand Academy of Lagado in Book Three, in which Swift ridicules the experiments of the Royal Society most clearly. For instance, a scholar in the Academy of Lagado "has eight years upon a project for extracting sunbeams out of cucumbers which were to be put into vials hermetically sealed, and let out to warm the air in raw inclement summers" (223). The most ancient student of the Academy "reduces human excrement to its original food, by separating the several parts, removing the tincture which it receives from the gull, making the odour exhale, and scumming off the saliva" (224). Another is at work to turn ice into gunpowder, and a blind man is "to mix colours for painters, which their master taught them to distinguish by feeling and smelling" (224). In all episodes, Swift's overall satirical technique is to isolate the eccentricity and strangeness of the scientific discourse of his time and play with the intellectual hopes and longings that are, however, far from becoming physical realities. In his depictions, almost any experiment attempts to supersede the inevitabilities of natural processes. Without denying the association between the academy's experiments and the actual experiments reported in the *Transactions of the Royal Society*, of the fourteen projects displayed in Chapter 5 of the third book, many are recognizable derivations from actual experiments published in

---

[4] Aphra Behn's farce *The Emperor in the Moon* (1687) also parodied the Royal Society's fantasies, in this case with reference to people inhabiting the moon.

Transactions (cf. Nicholson and Mohler). For instance, the innovation of the microscope enabled the scientist Robert Hooke in his *Micrographia; or, Some Physiological Descriptions of Minute Bodies* to describe the magnified drawing of a blue fly as follows:

> Sixthly, at the under part of the face FF, were several of the former sort of bended Bristles; and below all, the mouth, out of the middle of which, grew the *proboscis* GHI, which, by means of several joints, whereof it seems to consist, the Fly was able to move to and fro, and thrust it in and out as it pleas'd. . . . This kind of Fly seems by the steams or taste of fermenting and putrifying meat (which it often kisses, as 'twere, with its *proboscis* as it trips over it) to be stimulated or excited to eject its Eggs or Seed on it. (qtd. in Smith 140-41; ellipsis in original)

Gulliver describes the flies that attack him in Brobdingnag in terms that clearly remind us of this newfound objectivity:

> The Kingdom is much pestered with Flies in Summer; and these odious insects, each of them as big as a *Dunstable* Lark, hardly gave me any Rest while I sat at Dinner, with their continual Humming and Buzzing about mine Ears. They would sometimes alight upon my Victuals and leave their loathsome Excrement or Spawn behind, which to me was very visible, although not to the natives of that Country, whose large Opticks were not so acute as mine in the viewing of smaller Objects. Sometimes they would fix upon my Nose or Forehead, where they stung me to the Quick, smelling very offensively. (Swift 129)

When Gulliver returns from the land of the Brobdingnags to England, he proudly presents his cabinet comprising, among others, "a collection of needles and pins from a foot to half a yard long. Four wasp-stings, like joiners' tacks: some combings of the Queen's hair. . ." (188). In Gulliver's Brobdingnag, man is the poor victim of his own invention of the microscope. Gulliver's observation of a louse in Book Two is an obvious allusion to Hooke's *Micrographia* (see above), where Observation 54 is "Of a Louse." In Part 2, Glumdalclitch takes Gulliver into the city, where beggars crowd to the side of the coach providing him with "the most hateful site," that is, "Lice crawling on their clothes"

(Swift 164).[5] All in all, in *Gulliver's Travels*, scientific fact is distorted practically on every page. On the one hand, Swift's satire testifies to the author's fascination with contemporary science; on the other hand, however, it ultimately lays bare its limitations.

The Aging Struldbruggs

Swift had ridiculed the methods and objectives of the new sciences as early as *The Battle of the Books* (1704) and *A Tale of a Tub* (1705), and in the third book of *Gulliver's Travels*, he would resume his attack most memorably. During his stay in the land of Luggnagg, Gulliver learns that a few of the natives, the so-called Struldbruggs,[6] are born into a state of perpetual life but not perpetual youth (Swift 252). On first hearing about them, Gulliver is fascinated and

> cries out as in a rapture: Happy nation where every child hath at least a chance for being immortal! Happy people who enjoy so many living examples of ancient virtue and have masters ready to instruct them in the wisdom of all former ages! But happiest beyond all comparison are those excellent Struldbruggs, who, being exempt from that universal calamity of human nature have their minds free and disengaged without the weight and depression of spirits caused by the continual apprehension of death. (Swift 252-53)

As a Struldbrugg, Gulliver believes, he would have anything he could hope for. As he then learns from the natives, the Struldbruggs (their word for *immortal*) live a normal life until they are thirty, a time when one is expected to have chosen a career and to have made some progress in it, that is, the time when a candidate for fame begins to worry about his talent and his reputation. From this until the age of eighty they become increasingly "melancholic" and "dejected," and as a

---

[5] In Book Four, Gulliver is the sole representative of his species on the island, that is, a human being who is seen by the hybrids around him as suspect.

[6] For the varieties of reading the Struldbrugg episode, cf., for instance, Freedman 457-58. For the three "schools" in the critical history of the episode that have so far established themselves, cf. Real.

group they are "opinionative, peevish, covetous, morose, vain, talkative, but incapable of friendship and dead to all natural affection. . . . Envy and impotent desires are their prevailing passions" (Swift 257). In their later years, they are chiefly moved by envy of the passions of the young and the deaths of the old. At the age of eighty, they are "looked on as dead in law, and their heirs immediately succeed to their estates. . . . At ninety, they lose their teeth and hair," "have no distinction of taste," and "their memory will not serve to carry them from the beginning of a sentence to the end" (258). Their memories fail, they become senile and the walking dead, alive in body but dead in mind, and "they are despised and hated by all sorts of people" (259). Gulliver ultimately comes to the conclusion that "[t]hey were the most mortifying sight I ever beheld. . . . I grew heartily ashamed of the pleasing visions I had formed and thought no tyrant could invent a death into which I would not run with pleasure from such a life" (259). When Gulliver later indeed meets some of the Struldbruggs, he is repelled by their deformity and senility, and his appetite for perpetuity of life is abated immediately.

Swift's Struldbruggs reduce scientific "progress" to nothing but senility and physical as well as moral decay. They thus extend human desire for immortality *ad absurdum* and are a systematic assault on the idea of continuous scientific progress. These creatures rather communicate the message that the only real progress in human history is the progressive degeneration of human beings.

Critics have read the Struldbrugg episode as a lecture in religious morality[7] and as an assault on humanity's intellectual inadequacies and unearned pride as such. With reference to the topic of aging, one of the most highly acknowledged Swift scholars worldwide, Hermann Josef Real, has demonstrated that by the time Swift was finishing *Gulliver's Travels*, longevity had become a pre-eminent preoccupation of the age in many areas and disciplines (cf. Real 126). As sketched at the beginning of my essay, Bacon had paved the way for the belief that it is possible and desirable to significantly extend the length of life by a

---

[7] For instance: "The Struldbruggs represent 'a sermon on the foolishness or fearing death,' and their fate 'is in itself a sermon on the vanity of human wishes,' for which we do not need to 'look beyond Swift's own writings to find its obvious theological explanation'" (Real 120).

reformation of medicine. In sharp contrast to Bacon's positive attitude, the encounter with the Struldbruggs in Swift's novel teaches us that humans are denied the right to enjoy the advantages of old age without experiencing its miseries. In the words of Real, the Struldbrugg episode

> appears to be a vision, as bleak as it is nightmarish through which Swift anticipates, and thinks out, the implications inherent in the "scientific" endeavours of an art which, for him, seemed to be acting without, or beyond, a divinely sanctioned objective. Shorn of such a purpose, medical "science" to Swift was not only conductive to the prolonging of lives that were "barren, wasted, and futile," it also ignored the "rationale" of dying in the divine scheme of things. (133)

Against medicine's belief that it is possible (and desirable) to significantly extend the length of life by human action the Struldbrugg episode in *Gulliver's Travels* signals that Swift was

> entirely sympathetic towards the *methods and means* recommended by the prolongevitivists, [but] he was thoroughly hostile to their proposed *end*, their objective—the prolongation of life. For Swift, prolongevity, the belief that it was possible, *and* desirable, to extend significantly the length of life by human action was an intellectual attitude that inevitably led to interference with the decrees of Divine Providence. . . . If, as Gulliver's encounter with the Struldbruggs teaches him, man is denied the right to enjoy the advantages of old age without experiencing its miseries, any prolongation of life is but a prolongation of misery and a continuation of disease. (Real 132-33)

Conclusion

This essay set out to sketch the complexity of attitudes and actions towards the new science, and here, the discourse of aging, in eighteenth-century England. Even at the beginning of the twenty-first century, the process of aging has remained one of the major fields of investigation in the natural sciences. Aging and death remain a biological inevitability, and so far, we have not learned how to overcome the physiological limits that we know as aging. As Simone de Beauvoir writes in *The Coming of Age*: "Die early or grow old: there is no other alternative.

And yet, as Goethe said, 'Age takes us by surprise'. . . . A limited future and a frozen past: such is the situation that the elderly have to face up to" (qtd. in Moody 119).

In the seventeenth century, Bacon's new method of proceeding from facts and details to generalizations and principles had paved the way for further discoveries in the sciences and the hope of improving human life. Medical advancement in the eighteenth century communicated a widespread optimism for the future. In the field of the arts, however, the possibility that Cartesian rationalism and Baconian science would remedy the ills of the age was indeed denied. The scientific belief in progress, which would imply that mankind naturally improves as it ages, is confuted by what Gulliver learns in Glubbdubdrib. "The medical programme originally envisaged by the New Science as a contribution to the relief of man's estate, the Struldbruggs demonstrate, could end in the burden of life-in-death" (Real 134). Thomas Shadwell's drama *The Virtuoso* in the seventeenth and Swift's *Gulliver's Travels* in the eighteenth century may be the most prominent literary texts that testify to their authors' fascination with contemporary science but which also lay bare its limitations. Most memorably, Swift's Struldbruggs send out a clear signal that medical advancement is not unlimited. The conviction of the age that the human lifespan could be extended by medical advancement finds its (artistic) limits in the Struldbruggs and their implicit message—whose topicality might surprise us in our medical practice in the twenty-first century—live, but also let die.

Works Cited

Allan, D. G. C., and John L. Abbott, eds. *"The Virtuoso Tribe of Arts and Sciences": Studies in the Eighteenth-Century Work and Membership of the London Society of Arts.* Athens: U of Georgia P, 1992. Print.

Bacon, Francis. *The Advancement of Learning and New Atlantis.* Ed. Arthur Johnston. Oxford: Oxford UP, 1974. Print.

Bredvold, Louis I. "Dryden, Hobbes, and the Royal Society." *Modern Philology* 25.4 (1928): 417-38. Print.

Colie, Rosalie L. "Cornelis Drebbel and Salomon de Caus: Two Jacobean Models for Salomon's House." *Huntington Library Quarterly* 18.3 (1955): 245-60. Print.

Erickson, Marianne, "Geriatric Canons: A Look at Aging through Literature." *Gerontology and Geriatrics Education* 11.3 (1991): 67-76. Print.

Freedman, William. "Swift's Struldbruggs, Progress, and the Analogy of History." *SEL* 35.3 (1995): 457-72. Print.

Hooke, Robert. *Micrographia*. New York: Dover, 1961. Print.

Jones, Harold Whitmore. "Mid-Seventeenth Century Science: Some Polemics." *Osiris* 9 (1950): 254-74. Print.

Moody, Harry R. *Aging Concepts and Controversies*. 5th ed. Thousand Oaks: Sage, 2006. Print.

Nicholson, Majorie. *Science and the Imagination*. Hamden: Archon, 1976. Print.

Nicholson, Majorie, and Nora M. Mohler. "The Scientific Background of Swift's Voyage to Laputa." *Annals of Science* 2.3 (1937): 299-334. Print.

Nuessel, Frank, and Arthur Van Stewart. "Literary Examples of Illness: A Strategy for Personalizing Geriatrics Case Histories in Clinical Settings." *Physical & Occupational Therapy in Geriatrics* 16.1-2 (1999): 33-53. Print.

Real, Hermann Josef. "The 'keen Appetite for Perpetuity of Life' Abated: The Struldbruggs, Again." *Fiktion und Geschichte in der anglo-amerikanischen Literatur: Festschrift für Heinz-Joachim Müllenbrock zum 60. Geburtstag.* Ed. Rüdiger Ahrens and Fritz-Wilhelm Neumann. Heidelberg: Winter, 1998. 117-35. Print.

Schäfer, Daniel. *Alter und Krankheit in der Frühen Neuzeit: Der ärztliche Blick auf die letzte Lebensphase*. Frankfurt: Campus, 2004. Print.

Shadwell, Thomas. *The Virtuoso*. Ed. Majorie Hope Nicholson and David Stuart Rodes. Lincoln: U of Nebraska P, 1966. Print.

Smith, Frederik N., ed. *The Genres of Gulliver's Travels*. Newark: U of Delaware P, 1992. Print.

Spiegel, Maura, and Rita Charon. "Editing and Interdisciplinarity: Literature, Medicine, and Narrative Medicine." *Profession* (2009): 132-37. Print.

Sprat, Thomas. *History of the Royal Society*. Ed. Jackson I. Cope and Harold Whitmore Jones. London: Routledge & Kegan Paul, 1966. Print.

Stimson, Dorothy. *Scientists and Amateurs: A History of the Royal Society*. New York: Greenwood, 1968. Print.

Swift, Jonathan. *Gulliver's Travels*. 1726. Ed. Peter Dixon and John Chalker. Introd. Michael Foot. 1967. Harmondsworth: Penguin, 1985. Print.

Vickers, Brian. Introduction. *English Science: Bacon to Newton*. Ed. Vickers. Cambridge: Cambridge UP, 1987. 1-22. Print.

MARTIN KUESTER

Cunning Man and/or Shaman?
Robertson Davies's Dr. Hullah

The Canadian novelist, dramatist, journalist, and scholar Robertson Davies (1913-1995) is one of the relatively small group of Canadian writers who had already established themselves on the international writing scene even before the so-called renaissance of Canadian letters in the 1970s. He was an intellectual who always looked back to Europe as one of the sources of his inspiration, whether it was as Shakespeare scholar and actor in Britain in the late 1930s or as novelist in Canada drawing upon Jungian psychology in his later life.

European inspiration also lies behind Davies's last novel, *The Cunning Man* (1994), which—together with *Murther and Walking Spirits* (1991)—may have been planned as the first two volumes, introducing readers to some of its main characters and their personal histories and involvements, of what Douglas Gibson has referred to as "The Toronto Trilogy" (ix). Surprising for a writer who mostly looked and sounded rather Old World, here, European inspiration is combined with the knowledge, spirit, and culture of Canada's First Nations. Davies's character Dr. Jonathan Hullah in *The Cunning Man* is somewhat of an outsider in his profession. His approach of seeing mind and body as a whole and of empathically listening to the narratives his patients tell him turns out to be successful where traditional Western medicine—dependent on pharmaceutical and medical machinery, if not gadgetry—is not. And Hullah and his creator Robertson Davies are also listened to—in and beyond the field of literature—so that we find references to the novel not only in literary journals but also, and surprisingly, in renowned medical publications such as *The Lancet* or *The British Journal of General Practice.*

My essay will have a look at the ways in which Dr. Hullah's approaches combine the academic and scientific methods used in twentieth-century medicine with Native North American ways of healing and their Old World counterpart: alternative European traditions of "cunning" men and women. That Robertson Davies always approved of holistic rather than purely "scientific" approaches to medicine becomes obvious as early as the late 1940s, when he includes the following entry in his regular newspaper column in the *Peterborough Examiner* that is written in the voice of his curmudgeonly alter ego, Samuel Marchbanks, and later included in the hilarious collections of Marchbanks's musings entitled *The Diary of Samuel Marchbanks*:

> Was talking to a most unusual physician tonight—a man who scorns vitamins and laughs uproariously at talk of allergies. Medicine, he said, was an art and not a science, and could only be usefully practiced after deep study of human nature and of each individual patient. This attitude, he said, was commonplace among the great physicians of the past, but was out of favour with the modern school of pill-peddlers, who like to do their diagnosis by machine as much as possible, and prefer not to see the patient if they can possibly manage with a piece of him. Too many doctors are deeply interested in disease, but don't care much for people, he said. (163)

Davies (or Hullah), I will argue, brings together classical European and Native North American approaches to sickness, thus holistically integrating approaches of the Old World and the New, but his Old World approaches are very different from those of the European Enlightenment which we would normally associate with progress in the field of medicine, as he refers to the cunning men of medieval Europe and Britain in the excerpt from Robert Burton's *Anatomy of Melancholy* that he uses as an epigraph to the novel:

> Cunning men, wizards, and white witches, as they call them, in every village, which, if they be sought unto, will help almost all infirmities of body and mind. . . .
>   The body's mischiefs, as Plato proves, proceed from the soul: and if the mind be not first satisfied, the body can never be cured. (qtd. in Davies, *Cunning Man* 3)

This epigraph, by the way, joins two passages from Burton which do not occur on the same page. Both quotations are from the second partition of the *Anatomy*, but while the first appears under the heading of *"Unlawfull Cures rejected"* (Burton 3), the second is part of the subsection *"Perturbations of the Mind Rectified. From himself, by resisting to the utmost, confessing his griefe to a friend, etc."* (Burton 100).

This is the way Davies's first-person narrator, Dr. Jonathan Hullah, introduces himself to his readers in a "bifurcated" way that already plays upon the rather ambiguous reputation he holds among his peers: "Jonathan Hullah, M.D., F.R.C.P., with a wide reputation in the treatment of stubborn and chronic diseases, and a somewhat murky reputation among some of my colleagues because of the methods I use in such treatment" (*Cunning Man* 19). Hullah comes to the city of Toronto, the Canadian centre of sophistication and science, initially in order to attend a prestigious boarding school and then to attend the University of Toronto as well as becoming an active member of the High Anglican parish of St. Aidan's. But his background is not that of a sophisticated city environment: he grew up in the northwestern Ontario town of Sioux Lookout, which had provided him with a profound exposure to Canada's Native population and also to Native traditions of healing. His own attitude to Native healing traditions is a very positive one, since the local Natives' "treatment" in the case of his own infection with scarlet fever proves to be more efficient than the methods of the bootlegging Toronto-educated Dr. Ogg, who cannot exactly be described as "an ornament of the medical profession" (26). Rather than Dr. Ogg, Elsie Smoke, an Indian "wise woman" (28), saves Hullah by performing the ritual of a "shaking tent" in front of the home in which he is quarantined (29-30). As "the village doctor was not promising as an approach to the white man's medicine" (44), the future doctor decides to learn from Mrs. Smoke, which he undoubtedly does, even though she tells him that he has the "wrong colour" and the "wrong brains" (41) for the Native approach to medicine. Still, she confronts him with a basket containing two Massassaugas ground rattlesnakes which are to be his totem and his "helpers" (43).

Another step toward becoming a "special" physician occurs some years later when Hullah supports his close friend and fellow university student Charlie Iredale during painful medical treatment that is undertaken without anaesthesia. As Charlie is a strong believer, Hullah supports him during surgery by reading the latter's favorite Christian work, Jacobus de Voragine's *Legenda aurea*, another decidedly pre-

Enlightenment work. "Without my being in the least aware of it, this illness of Charlie's was the strong influence that led me to become a physician, and the rather special kind of physician I am" (86). Hullah's friendship with Charlie, he is sure, was a stronger motivation in his becoming a physician than "the murky lessons of Mrs. Smoke, or the shallow certainties of Doc Ogg" (86).

Although he is a gifted student of medicine at the University of Toronto, Jonathan Hullah remembers the holistic Native ways of healing that he had been exposed to in his youth, and he is thus repelled by the purely scientific, taxonomic, and consequently somewhat soul-less approach taken by his university professors (ironically referred to as "Saved Souls"), who condescendingly reject any deviation from the methods of treatment that they deem acceptable and efficient. They have closed their minds to any alternative ways of thinking and of treating diseases:

> The spirit of the medical school was firmly hierarchical; you crept upward, begging acceptance of the greater ones above you, questioning only when questioning seemed to be asked for, and if you had the makings of a True Believer, a Saved Soul, in you, you acquired a detestation of patent medicines, of osteopaths and chiropractors, of homeopaths and herbalists, . . . which was the property of your brotherhood, and you knew with whatever modesty lay in you, that you were a creature apart. The world, for you, was becoming a world divided between patients and healers. (164)

Hullah's medical career includes such stations as that of an army doctor, police surgeon, and, finally, general practitioner. He becomes a "heretic about health" (245) who is propelled by humanism (246) and to whom other, more orthodox doctors send the difficult patients of whom they have grown tired. As a conversation with his patients may explain their health problems, and especially their mental state, much more easily than a judgment based on sheer physical facts, he calls himself a "Talking Doctor" (216). As an army doctor, he comes to understand that in the modern and more and more agnostic society "the physician is the priest of our modern, secular world. The Medical Corps insignia on my sleeve promised a magic that the chaplain's Cross had lost" (217). Among his therapies—besides an intuitive rather than scientific approach to his patients and their suffering—there is also, surprisingly, the exposure of his patients to literature—not necessarily high-brow, but efficient nevertheless—during "Reading Hour" (225). In the army, he makes his fellow soldiers read not only Rudyard Kipling, whose contents and style one might expect to be of a certain appeal to soldiers, but also Geoffrey Chaucer (at least the more bawdy scenes). His medical kit includes a copy of Sir Thomas Browne's *Religio Medici*, Burton's *Anatomy of Melancholy*, and *The Oxford Book of English Verse* (224). Later in Toronto, his patients include persons such as a Mrs. Fothergill, whose illness "Old Burton would have described . . . as Maids', Nuns', and Widows' Melancholy" (278). His uncommon practices, which involve making house calls that will expose the patients' attitudes and living conditions, listening to patients' bowel movements, and sniffing their bodies, become so suspicious to some of his fellow practitioners that they even call in a snoop on the scene from the Canadian Medical Association as part of their program to "chase out quacks. Put chiropractors in the pillory. Geld osteopaths. Brand a huge H on the cheek of the homeopath" (308). As part of his strategy of "pulling the wool over the eyes of a snoop," Hullah tells him about his association with Mrs. Smoke and invents a story about an Indian boy who "'wanted to be a shaman'" (309) and is confronted with a *Windigo*, a cannibal monster in Native mythology. His message, typical of his holistic approach, is thus a "'combination of modern science, intimate and revealing conversation, and intuition'" (312): "'Hear the voice; open the closed place; confront the monster; reason with him; reach a compromise'" (312).

Hullah's insistence on ways of healing that go beyond technology-based Western medicine leads to his being referred to as the "cunning man" among his Toronto friends, and he explains the significance of that nickname to Esme:

> "It was the sort of person that used to be found in a lot of English villages. There was a Wise Woman or else a Cunning Man. Never both at the same place. He could set bones, after a fashion, and knew a bit of horse-doctoring, and if somebody had overlooked your cattle, he could take off the spell, and maybe track down the overlooker, and then there would be a contest of wizards. A Cunning Man was a sort of village know-all." (465; cf. also 232)

Hullah's methods would nowadays be supported by many scholars. Borys Surawicz and Beverly Jacobson, for example, state in their study of *Doctors in Fiction* that

> [m]ost intelligent physicians learn to realize that there are illnesses curable by scientific means, that some are incurable, that many discomforts will disappear without treatment and that the majority of non-life-threatening ills of the body either originate in the mind or are strongly affected by the patient's state of mind. (130-31)

The symbol of Hullah's medical practice is the caduceus representing two snakes. Although the caduceus is mythologically associated with Hermes and the fields of trade and alchemy, it has been linked, especially in North America—somewhat arguably, according to one view, but all the more fittingly in the context of Davies's novel— with the medical profession. Following another tradition, the medical profession is generally associated with the rod of Asclepius, which features only one snake (and also represents the "one-sided" Canadian Medical Association so hated by Dr. Hullah). As Walter J. Friedlander points out in *The Golden Wand of Medicine*, "the ancient writers who referred to the caduceus made no connection between it and the staff which is more often associated with the demigod, Aesculapius" (6).

Fittingly in the context of *The Cunning Man*, the caduceus with two snakes reminds us of the two rattlesnakes to which Mrs. Smoke had exposed young Jonathan. As Hullah puts it, the snakes are his "totem animals":

> ". . . I shall have on my wall a constant reminder of the Warring Serpents of Hermes—Knowledge and Wisdom, balanced in an eternal tension."
> "Knowledge being science and all the accumulated lore you have pumped into you at medical school; science which keeps changing and shifting all through your lifetime, like a snake shedding its old skin—"
> "And Wisdom, with which you have to apply and temper the whole business, and fit it to the patient who sits before you, so that it too has a serpentine sinuosity and of course the wisdom which snakes are—quite mistakenly—supposed to possess." (306)

In his study of Davies's novels, Victor J. Lams points out that the parallel between Mrs. Smoke's rattlesnakes and the snakes of the caduceus "interweaves Greek mythology with the flora and fauna of

Sioux Lookout" (263). Here we are presented with a fusion, whether we want to call it *bricolage* or a hybrid or synergetic creation, which—one might claim—heals the rift that Canadian Métis scholar Jo-Ann Episkenew alludes to in her recent book on indigenous literature, public policy, and healing. Episkenew points out "that Indigenous communities had created a body of knowledge that enabled our ancestors to survive for millennia before the Johnny-come-lately new nation-state of Canada established itself on top of Indigenous peoples' lands" (1).

Jonathan Hullah's references to the caduceus are in fact not so different from points Robertson Davies himself had made during a much-quoted talk given to Johns Hopkins University medical students in 1984 and entitled "Can a Doctor Be a Humanist?" Both novel and talk are referred to by Brendan Sweeney, chairman of the Royal College of General Practitioners' Committee on Medical Ethics, in a lecture in which he insists, like Davies and Hullah, on the interconnectedness and cross-fertilization of science-based and arts-based therapeutic approaches for the general practitioner and on the importance of narrative in the diagnostic process (Sweeney 1001).

Toward the end of the novel, however, the holistically oriented doctor seems to be losing his grasp on reality. He falls in love with Esme, the widow of his godson—or even son, as he sometimes fancies (201)—Conor Gilmartin, the entertainment editor of the *Colonial Advocate*. Esme is a young, attractive journalist who is working on a professional assignment focusing on the death of a possible Canadian saint, Father Ninian Hobbes of St. Aidan's in Toronto. St. Aidan's, we remember, is Dr. Hullah's parish, and Hobbes was in fact murdered by Charlie Iredale.

Another task that the medic puts to himself in his final years, certainly a "delusion of grandeur" (376), is his own anatomy, not of melancholy (as for Burton) this time, but of fiction. His project "will change literature forever, and make necessary new developments and commentaries on the literature of the past. It will keep the whole critical trade hard at work for at least a couple of centuries" (376). In other words:

> I'm going to apply modern medical theory to the notable characters of literature. Why did Micawber lose his hair? Want of keratin? What were his nails like? What did Jane Eyre, as a governess in a gentleman's house, get to eat? . . . We know that Jane Austen was fond of port; does

it show up in any of her heroines? . . . What was the truth behind the
marriage of Dorothea Brooke and Mr. Casaubon? . . . What conclusions
can we draw about the menstrual cycle of Emma Bovary? . . . And . . .
the day will come when no writer will dare to offer a novel or a play to
the public until he has investigated the medical history of all his
characters. Very likely the great writers of the future will all be doctors.
(377-78)

This anatomy seems to be based on a rather naive conflation of "the role
of the critic and author" (Sugars 83) and on a sophomoric
misunderstanding of the literary mode of realism, and is inspired, as
Cynthia Sugars shows, by yet another friend Hullah made while a
student in Toronto, Browchel (Brocky) Gilmartin, the future "honoured
senior professor at Waverley" (201), the fictive University at Salterton
(which is often seen to be based on Kingston, Ontario). Jonathan
Hullah's anatomy has not appeared in bookstores yet, and it never will, I
hope, but his creator, Robertson Davies, himself made sure that most of
his medical statements were based on solid information. For example,
there is an author's note by Davies in the novel thanking Dr. Richard
Davis "for advice on certain medical matters" (6), and there is an
entertaining essay by Rick Davis and Peter Brigg which shows the
writer Robertson Davies checking with the physician Richard Davis
whether all kinds of medical detail in his novel are acceptable not only
to the non-specialized reader but also to Davis's fellow members of the
medical and scientific professions.

Regarding Hullah's literary inspiration, Burton's *Anatomy of
Melancholy*, as Northrop Frye reminds us in his *Anatomy of Criticism*, is
"the greatest Menippean satire in English before Swift," and it is a work
based on a "creative treatment of exhaustive erudition" (311). According
to Cynthia Sugars, Frye's *Anatomy* is in turn Davies's "primary but
unacknowledged intertext" (73). Frye himself famously admitted that
Burton's *Anatomy* had been one of his favorite books (Cayley 69).
According to Frye, "the word 'anatomy' in Burton's title means a
dissection or analysis, and expresses very accurately the intellectualized
approach of his form" (311). Frye even goes so far as to suggest that
"we may as well adopt it as a convenient name to replace the
cumbersome and in modern times rather misleading term 'Menippean
satire'" (311-12). Jonathan Hullah's envisaged *Anatomy of Fiction*
would of course fit in here without any problem.

So how can and should we read Robertson Davies's *Cunning* Man from the point of view of medicine and literature? On the one hand, it is a crime novel about Charlie Iredale trying to create a twentieth-century Anglican saint by murdering an innocuous priest in Toronto. But more than that it presents the views of a twentieth-century doctor who is not willing to sacrifice his holistic view of human beings on the altar of science; he would rather go for the all-encompassing perspective of "narrative medicine" (Charon), of an approach that follows Paracelsus and many others who have not accepted the split between mind and body, between wisdom and knowledge, art and science. It is rather fitting that this integrative approach also combines—pretty much in the way Claude Lévi-Strauss described mythical thinking in *La pensée sauvage* (29)—different myths and concepts, European as well as Native Canadian, in a new (and old) concept that we may call *bricolage*, hybridity or (Frygian or Burtonian) anatomy. And it might hint on the level of Hullah's alternative Canadian medicine toward what John Ralston Saul has claimed of Canada as a whole: that it is a "métis civilization" informed by the influence of the First Nations (Saul 3). Robertson Davies's novel thus gives us an example of holistic medicine based on what Jo-Ann Episkenew describes as "indigenous views on health." These views are, and I would like to close with this description,

> holistic in that they do not separate body from mind, emotions, and spirit. Holism also defines Indigenous communities in which a person is never a singular, isolated individual. Instead, Indigenous people are part of a complex network of relationships that, when healthy, respect the autonomy of the individual within the supportive environment of the group. (Episkenew 194)

Works Cited

Burton, Robert. *The Anatomy of Melancholy*. 1621. Vol. 2. Text. Ed. Thomas C. Faulkner, Nicolas Kiessling, and Rhonda L. Blair. Oxford: Oxford UP-Clarendon, 1994. Print.

Cayley, David. *Northrop Frye in Conversation*. Concord, ON: Anansi, 1992. Print.

Charon, Rita. *Narrative Medicine: Honoring the Stories of Illness*. New York: Oxford UP, 2006. Print.

Davies, Robertson. "Can a Doctor Be a Humanist?" *The Merry Heart: Reflections on Reading, Writing and the World of Books*. 1996. New York: Penguin, 1997. 90-110. Print.

---. *The Cunning Man: A Novel*. Toronto: McClelland, 1994. Print.

---. *The Diary of Samuel Marchbanks*. 1947. *The Papers of Samuel Marchbanks*. 1986. London: Penguin, 1989. Print.

---. *Murther and Walking Spirits*. Toronto: McClelland, 1991. Print.

Davis, Rick, and Peter Brigg. "'Medical Consultation' for *Murther and Walking Spirits* and *The Cunning Man*." *Robertson Davies: A Mingling of Contrarieties*. Ed. Camille R. La Bossière and Linda M. Morra. Ottawa: U of Ottawa P, 2001. 157-74. Print.

Episkenew, Jo-Ann. *Taking Back Our Spirits: Indigenous Literature, Public Policy, and Healing*. Winnipeg: U of Manitoba P, 2009. Print.

Friedlander, Walter J. *The Golden Wand of Medicine: A History of the Caduceus Symbol in Medicine*. Westport: Greenwood, 1992. Print.

Frye, Northrop. *Anatomy of Criticism: Four Essays*. 1957. Princeton: Princeton UP, 1971. Print.

Gibson, Douglas. Introduction. *The Merry Heart: Reflections on Reading, Writing and the World of Books*. By Robertson Davies. 1996. New York: Penguin, 1997. ix-xii. Print.

Lams, Victor J. *Aspects of Robertson Davies' Novels*. New York: Peter Lang, 2009. Print.

Lévi-Strauss, Claude. *Das wilde Denken* [*La pensée sauvage*]. Trans. Hans Naumann. Frankfurt am Main: Suhrkamp, 1989. Print.

Saul, John Ralston. *A Fair Country: Telling Truths about Canada*. 2008. Toronto: Penguin, 2009. Print.

Sugars, Cynthia. "The Anatomy of Influence: Robertson Davies's Psychosomatic Medicine." *Mosaic* 33.4 (2000): 73-89. Print.

Surawicz, Borys, and Beverly Jacobson. *Doctors in Fiction: Lessons from Literature*. Oxford: Radcliffe, 2009. Print.

Sweeney, Brendan. "The Place of the Humanities in the Education of a Doctor." *British Journal of General Practice* 48 (1998): 998-1002. Web. 13 Aug. 2011.

STEPHANIE P. BROWNER

Resocializing Literature and Medicine: Poverty, Health, and Medical Science in Postcolonial Literature

This essay begins with a broad question: In what ways does contemporary literature engage the question of the preventable suffering of those who live in extreme poverty? The answer I can offer in a brief essay is specific but I hope useful as the field of literature and medicine increasingly takes up this larger and important question about poverty, health, medicine, and power. This essay suggests that two novels— Aravind Adiga's *The White Tiger* (2008) and Amitav Ghosh's *The Calcutta Chromosome: A Novel of Fevers, Delirium and Discovery* (1995)—are particularly powerful interrogations of two core issues. Adiga's Booker Prize-winning novel offers a stinging rebuttal to those who are confident that economic development can address public health crises; and Ghosh's novel offers a view of transmission—biological and cultural—that challenges the will-to-power that animates Western medical science.

Poverty, Medicine, and Literature

When literary criticism considers literature's politics, its emphasis is typically on race, gender, ethnicity, and sometimes class, but rarely poverty. As Gavin Jones notes in his study *American Hungers: The Problem of Poverty in U.S. Literature, 1840-1945* (2007), despite "its prominence as a subject in the social sciences, poverty has remained unfocused in literary studies that privilege the cultural identity of the marginalized" (xiii). This is lamentable, Jones argues, since literature has a unique ability to represent poverty:

> Surely poverty is a material condition, a position in the social structure. And literary texts: are they not aesthetic artifacts, retreating by their nature into the privacy of the imagination? Only in this retreat from the tactile and the statistical, I contend, can we approach the complexity of poverty as an ideological formation, or understand the inner life of being poor—the tangled web of emotion and behavior that gets brushed too easily from social study. ("The Truths of Poverty in Fiction")

Jones observes that U.S. literary engagement with poverty is "unrelentingly multicultural," and he also notes a transhistorical and transcultural consistency: "There is something in the nature of literary language, its openness to contradiction and paradox, that attunes it to the difficulty of poverty as a category that hovers on the edge of social thought, that undercuts dominant ideologies of success" ("Truths"). In texts ranging from "Bartleby" to *Native Son*, Jones unearths ideological entanglements, concluding that literature that takes up poverty struggles with the very act of representation. "Bartleby" is an exemplary text for Jones: The scrivener's indigence denies summary and explanation, and leaves the narrator, and by implication the reader, grasping for meaning and understanding. In *Pierre*, Melville's treatment of poverty ends in a similar dead end of nihilism. But it is these very ideological troubles and representational struggles that Jones finds worthy of study. In short, Jones turns to literary texts precisely because they "open up the complexities and contradictions of poverty" (*American Hungers* 3).

Notably, *Lancet* editor-in-chief Richard Horton also believes that literature is particularly effective at helping us think about poverty. Like Jones, he suggests that to understand the "crisis of existence lived by so many," literature may be a better tool than statistics, social science, and science, which "erode the density of human life." Writing for *Literature and Medicine*, Horton suggests that in the nineteenth century Elizabeth Gaskell's novels offered a more trenchant analysis of poverty and disease than did medical journals. Medical journals today, he notes, are not much better—more interested in commercial success than the "diseases of poverty" (210). Ultimately, he hopes that narrative, including fiction, will undertake the task of creating "an urgent literature of human survival" that takes up the "vast inequalities" that are the leading causes of worldwide suffering ("Mr. Thornton's Experiments" 211).

Doctor, medical anthropologist, and healthcare activist Paul Farmer also champions narrative in his work *Pathologies of Power: Health, Human Rights and the New War on the Poor* (2005), a book dedicated to using case studies to reveal the socioeconomic structures that generate power and wealth for a few and poverty and preventable suffering for many. As the Indian Nobel Prize-winning economist, philosopher, and humanitarian Amartya Sen notes in his introduction to Farmer's book, it is through stories that Farmer makes visible the economic and political structures that give rise to and shape the distribution of preventable suffering. "A phenomenon can be either characterized by a terse definition or described by examples. It is the latter procedure that Farmer follows" (xiii). Indeed, Farmer uses case studies and descriptive narrative to establish clear links between local instances of deprivation and global systems.

Numbers have, of course, played a role in building an argument for freedom from poverty as a basic human right. According to the World Bank, 2.7 billion people live in moderate poverty (less than \$2/day); 1.37 billion of these live in extreme poverty (less than \$1.25/day); six million children die of hunger each year; and one third of all deaths each year, or 18 million, are due to poverty-related causes. As a result of this statistical work, many, though not all, now understand human rights to include the rights to basic health care and freedom from dire poverty, malnutrition, and dirty water. In the 1948 Universal Declaration of Human Rights, the United Nations asserted that basic human rights included the right "to a standard of living adequate for the health and well being" of self and family, "including food, clothing, housing and medical care" (United Nations, Article 25, *Universal Declaration*). Obviously, the 1948 declaration was only a beginning, but an important one, since it has allowed what Sidonie Smith calls in her 2005 article in *Literature and Medicine* a "dynamic process" in which local conditions are made public by "recourse to the universalizing discourse" of human rights, which in turn allows witnesses and advocates to "re-form, contest, and reframe the notion of what constitutes a human right" (154).

Framing health as a universal human right challenges the neoliberal position, especially as articulated in the 1980s by Margaret Thatcher, Ronald Reagan, and the World Bank, that healthcare is not a state obligation. Confident in the power of the market to deliver goods and services, neoliberalism understands health as a private good best provided by the market, which has often led to an odd division between medicine and public health. In the U.S., where healthcare has not been included in the basket of public goods provided by the state but understood primarily as a private good, resources—financial and intellectual—have flowed towards the medical practices and medical science serving this private interest. Caring for the poor, while obviously still medical practice at the individual level, is understood more generally as a distinct project, that of public health. Public health has been burdened and even tainted by association with state funds, welfare, and charity, and thus has languished as a stepchild in the world of elite professions. More women have earned degrees in public health; and the field has been synonymous with the routine drudgery of caring for sniffling children and the management of uninteresting diseases that science has understood for decades. In short, public health has not been understood as a science, but rather as a matter of policy and implementation, and, of course, as an expense as the states take on the "burden" of providing minimal health care to the poor, which is to say to those who are sometimes seen as being agents of their own indigence. Most significantly, public health has not benefited from capitalism's tendency to direct resources towards commodities and private goods. As Horton points out, this pattern is evident in the pages of medical journals where the diseases of poverty get little attention.

More recently, the field of public health has garnered some prestige and attention by claiming a role in social justice movements. Building upon the 1948 Universal Declaration of Human Rights, in 2000 the UN adopted the Millennium Development Goals that establish eight anti-poverty targets to be achieved by 2015, with four of the eight directly focused on issues that can only be addressed through public health work. In 2008, a report from the World Health Organization Commission on the Social Determinants of Health included such bold statements as "[s]ocial injustice is killing people on a grand scale." Echoing Paul Farmer, the commission calls for tackling "the inequitable distribution of power, money, and resources," noting that it is the maldistribution of resources and power at global, national, and local levels that creates preventable deaths and suffering on a huge scale (World Health Organization 26, 10).

Hospitals, Sewage, and Rage

Adiga's *The White Tiger* offers precisely what Horton calls for—a representation of the "crisis of existence lived by so many"—and it links, as Farmer urges us to do, a particular story of poverty to global pathologies of power, global economic development, and national politics. Set in modern India, Adiga's novel suggests that post-colonialism is no longer a matter of cultural identity (national, caste, racial, or ethnic) but a matter of materiality, of poverty, disease, deprivation, and hunger. In the 2002 edition of *The Empire Writes Back*, an overview of postcolonial studies, Bill Ashcroft, Gareth Griffiths, and Helen Tiffin call for such a turn to the local, noting that the future of the field "hinges on the balance between the articulation of theoretical generalisations and the analysis of *particular* material post-colonial realities" (147).

The novel is the epistolary rant of an Indian man, Balram, who has risen from rural poverty to become owner of a car rental company, a transformation achieved by murdering his master, an act which Adiga suggests is not only an act of resistance but also the ultimate act of entrepreneurial self-making. The novel is a series of letters written by Balram to the prime minister of China, who has declared an interest in India's famous entrepreneurial spirit. Balram claims, not entirely ironically, that he is a fine example of that spirit—of the success and also of the bitterness, rage, and loneliness that result from becoming aware of one's situation and from acting, desperately and even violently, to climb into the middle class. Notably, the particular material post-colonial realities that serve as the backdrop for Balram's rise from poverty are fundamental public health issues: limited access to health care and the failure to manage human and industrial wastes. The first is typically a rural issue, and the latter an urban one. In *The White Tiger*, Adiga renders each with a specificity that insists on coupling aesthetic pleasure with moral outrage.

Eager to underscore the consequences of the entrepreneurial spirit in India for the benefit of China's prime minister, Balram takes pains to note the role of entrepreneurism in his father's death. Although most of his writing is manic, Balram's description of his father's death is marked by resignation and quiet dismay. He explains that there is no hospital in Balram's hometown of Laxmangarh, despite three separate efforts by three different politicians. Each called for a hospital, raised some funding, and held a celebratory ground-breaking event, but the result is three separate foundations and no hospital. Consequently, Balram and his brother must carry their father, who is suffering from tuberculosis, to a hospital in a neighboring town. In Dhandbad, the hospital entrance is dotted with goat turds "spread like a constellation of black stars on the ground," while inside patients lie on the floor waiting for a doctor. The patients are, on the one hand, reduced to their ailing parts: "[T]he line of diseased eyes, raw wounds, and delirious mouths kept growing" (40). On the other, they are a compassionate community as they thoughtfully spread out newspapers for Balram's father when he settles on the floor to wait. When Balram asks why there is no doctor, one patient tells a parable of India's entrepreneurial spirit in which everything is for sale— politicians sell the job of regional medical superintendent to enterprising doctors, who in turn receive payment from junior government doctors, who are then told to "keep the rest of your government salary and go work in some private hospital for the rest of the week. Forget the village. Because according to this ledger you've *been* there. . . . You've *healed* that girl's jaundice" (41). As Balram's father begins to convulse and spew blood, the other patients scoot away as discreetly as possible. Balram concludes, "[a]round six o'clock that day, as the government ledger no doubt accurately reported, my father was permanently cured of his tuberculosis. The ward boys made us clean up after Father before we could move the body. A goat came in and sniffed as we were mopping the blood off the floor" (42).

The death of Balram's father is a representative case of the inequitable distribution of health care and of the failure to put the same kind of financial efforts into diseases of poverty that we put into diseases of affluence. Tuberculosis is well understood, and yet, after decades of declining worldwide TB rates, in the 1980s, rates began to increase rapidly in poor countries. In 1993, the World Health Organization declared tuberculosis a world emergency, and a 2005 World Health Organization report on tuberculosis called for "the promotion of equity and pro-poor policies," including "health service decentralization," i.e., clinics, doctors, testing, and treatment where the poor live. In 2009, an estimated 1.7 million people died from TB. Undoubtedly, each of these deaths is a story that includes systemic managerial failures, dirt and disease, goat turds and phlegm, as well as acts of kindness between strangers and details of family members going to great lengths to sustain life. And most of these deaths are the result of what Farmer calls the pathology of power: the failure of global, national, economic, and political powers to end preventable suffering. And like Farmer's case studies, Adiga's novel provides some sense of the details of how individuals and communities contend with crises of existence that the poor constantly confront, or what Adiga ironically calls the celestial "constellation of goat turds."

Urban poverty, according to Balram, is no less disturbing than rural poverty, although this is not initially his expectation. As an entrepreneurial, modern "everyman" who hopes to climb the ladder of success, he moves to the city, where he expects to make good. To do so is to plan one's life in accord with the paradigm of economic development, which insists that although urban economic development may make the rich richer it also improves the lives of the poor, as rising tides lift all boats. And city life does give Balram the capacity to see and critique oppressive power structures. As a chauffeur, Balram develops a keen understanding of the master-servant complex, and he chronicles in detail the love and hate the servant feels for the master. Balram kindly rubs Ashok's back when his master is on his knees vomiting after a night of drinking, but begins to hate him when Ashok tells the police that Balram was responsible for a fatal accident even though it was Ashok's wife who had been driving. Recognizing the layers of intimacy and power that make the master-servant relationship particularly disturbing, Balram asks himself, "Do we loathe our masters behind a facade of love—or do we love them behind a facade of loathing?" (160).

The city offers bookstalls, and Balram reads about rebellion, but he concludes that books provide only "signs and symbols" for the poor (217). One writer, he notes, describes a conversation between God and a disobedient angel who refuses to serve anymore. "I am powerful. I am huge. Become my servant again," says God. The disobedient angel, whom Balram imagines as a small black man in a khaki uniform (an apt description of Balram himself), answers, "Ha!" and God asks, "Isn't it all wonderful? Isn't it all grand? Aren't you grateful to be my servant?" And the small black man starts "to shake, as if he has gone mad with anger, before delivering to the Almighty a gesture of thanks for having created the world this particular way, instead of all the other ways it could have been created" (75). And the little black man in the khaki uniform spits again and again at God.

Sensing that he is only a small man, Balram is desperate to confess to someone, even his master, the murderous rage he feels and his desire to claim a middle-class life of dignity. But as Balram attempts to initiate his conversation, Ashok, sitting in the back seat of the car Balram drives for him, opens his wallet, takes out a thousand-rupee note; puts it back; takes out a five-hundred-rupee note; puts it back; and then hands Balram a hundred. Notably, the next scene, Balram's visit to a New Delhi tent city for construction workers, is the climax of both the novel's documentation of poverty and of Balram's decision to kill his master:

> Early next morning I walked out of Buckingham B [Ashok's gated apartment complex] onto the main road. Though it was a brand-new building, there was already a leak in the drainage pipe, and a large patch of sewage darkened the earth outside the compound wall; three stray dogs were sleeping on the wet patch. A good way to cool off—summer had started, and even the nights were unpleasant now.
>
> The three mutts seemed so comfortable. I got down on my haunches and watched them.
>
> I put my finger on the dark sewage puddle. So cool, so tempting.
>
> One of the stray dogs woke up; it yawned and showed me all its canines. It sprang to its feet. The other mutts got up too. A growling began, and a scratching of the wet mud, and a showing of teeth—they wanted me off their kingdom.
>
> I surrendered the sewage to the dogs and headed for the malls. None of them had opened yet. I sat down on the pavement.
>
> No idea where to go next.
>
> That's when I saw the small dark marks in the pavement.
>
> Paw prints.
>
> An animal had walked on the concrete before it had set.
>
> I got up and walked after the animal. The space between the prints grew wider—the animal had begun to sprint.
>
> I walked faster.
>
> The paw prints of the accelerating animal went all the way around the malls, and then behind the malls, and at last, where the pavement ended and raw earth began, they vanished.
>
> Here I had to stop, because five feet ahead of me a row of men squatted on the ground in a nearly perfect straight line. They were defecating.
>
> I was at the slum. . . .

> The men were defecating in the open like a defensive wall in front of the slum: making a line that no respectable human should cross. The wind wafted the stench of fresh shit toward me.
>
> I found a gap in the line of the defecators. They squatted there like stone statues.
>
> These people were building homes for the rich, but they lived in tents covered with blue tarpaulin sheets, and partitioned into lanes by lines of sewage. It was even worse than Laxmangarh. I picked my way around the broken glass, wire, and shattered tube lights. The stench of feces was replaced by the stronger stench of industrial sewage. The slum ended in an open sewer—a small river of black water went sluggishly past me, bubbles sparkling in it and little circles spreading on its surface. Two children were splashing about in the black water.
>
> A hundred-rupee note came flying down into the river. The children watched with open mouths, and then ran to catch the note before it floated away. One child caught it, and then the other began hitting him, and they began to tumble about in the black water as they fought.
>
> I went back to the line of crappers. One of them had finished up and left, but his position had been filled. I squatted down with them and grinned. A few immediately turned their eyes away: they were still human beings. Some stared at me blankly as if shame no longer mattered to them. And then I saw one fellow, a thin black fellow, was grinning back at me, as if he were proud of what he was doing. Still crouching, I moved myself over to where he was squatting and faced him. I smiled as wide as I could. So did he. He began to laugh—and I began to laugh—and then all the crappers laughed together. (221-23)

In this moment, Adiga seeks to bridge the gulf between readers and those who live in abject poverty, and he asks us to follow closely as Balram walks back to the mall, washes his hands in the area reserved for servants of the wealthy, and picks up an iron wrench he considers using to kill his master.

Balram may fulfill Frantz Fanon's prediction that violence is the only response to abject poverty and oppression. But Adiga rejects Fanon's suggestion that through violence a new beginning is possible. Balram takes Ashok's money and his name, sets up his taxi company, and ascends to the middle class. He bribes the police but he doesn't beat his young drivers; he observes on the street "the ones left behind" but predicts there will be no revolution, ever (254). In *The White Tiger*, tuberculosis, open sewers, and the voice of the thinking poor man give the lie to promises of economic development. Balram warns the Chinese prime minister that the sacred Ganges, often called the river of emancipation and frequently a destination spot for tourists, is "full of feces, straw, soggy parts of human bodies, buffalo carrion, and seven different kinds of industrial acids" (12). And, by implication, he suggests that the famous Indian entrepreneurial spirit the prime minister is coming to see has fundamentally failed to provide Indians with the basics—access to healthcare for treatable diseases and waste management.

Medical Science and the Global South

Richard Horton's indictment of medicine's failure to address the diseases of poverty is scathing. He observes that medical journals' "claims of dedication to human health are mostly marketing." He continues: "We editors remain elitist, insular, and parochial despite the fact that, at the global level, most of the problems . . . are as acute today as one hundred and fifty years ago" ("Mr Thornton's Experiments" 210). Horton holds public health spending to the same high standard— genuine and effective engagement with the leading causes of ill health worldwide. In his review of Bill Shore's 2010 book on malaria, *The Imaginations of Unreasonable Men: Inspiration, Vision, and Purpose in the Quest to End Malaria*, Horton lambasts public health research that is predicated on the hope that brilliant laboratory scientists with radical visions and entrepreneurial disregard for traditional methods will discover cures, which can then be coupled with market mechanisms to conquer malaria. This approach marries "a top-down effort to parachute in a technology" with an economic development model of improving lives by depending upon the market to distribute services and medicines essential for health. Horton notes that "horizontal programs, by contrast, build capacity to improve health care—including clinics, trained medical workers, and education about disease and infection—from the ground up" ("Stopping Malaria").

Amitav Ghosh takes up the question of who "owns" medical science and whom it serves in his novel *The Calcutta Chromosome*, suggesting that we may need to complement our commitment to a universal science with attention to local science in which local communities and cultures participate not as subjects or recipients but as actors in the creation of medical knowledge and practices. In other words, Ghosh reconceives medical science as a fundamentally horizontal and chaotic activity that includes the vernacular, the past, the uncanny, and the relational.

In the vertical model, medical achievements move in one direction, as a kind of intellectual export, from the West or Global North to the Global South. Funding for medical research typically operates under this assumption. For example, 40 percent of the total giving of the Gates Foundation over the last ten years went to supranationals (e.g., the World Health Organization, the World Bank, and the Global Fund to Fight Tuberculosis, Malaria, and AIDS), and another 50 percent went to recipients based in the United States (cf. McCoy et al.). The approach is reminiscent of colonialism, and critics point out that as missionaries sought to eliminate local religious practices and to convert the natives to Christianity, and colonial public health officers sought to eradicate indigenous medicine, so the postcolonial agenda has "integration as its goal and its dominant metaphor" (King 782). Not surprisingly, some critics were particularly troubled when the World Health Organization briefly dedicated resources to combating the spread of diseases of affluence (high blood pressure, etc.) in poorer countries. Many health ministers in developing countries suggested that such concerns were misplaced and that they would rather focus on such health problems as malaria, tuberculosis, and dysentery. Noting this "talk back," scholars now suggest that in identifying Western dominance in public health discourse, we must understand the non-Western world not as a screen but as a "living space of encounter and exchange" (Driver and Martins 5). Put differently, "the global diffusion of public health knowledge and practice is not a one-way flow" (Brown and Bell 1572).

Ghosh's novel participates not only in this effort to make visible a two-way flow of knowledge and practice, but also in a broader project that uses the liberties of science fiction to imagine a multi-directional, chaotically networked world of cultures and people out of which knowledge and practices are constructed. The traditional story of malaria science focuses on Sir Ronald Ross, his life as the son of a colonial officer in India, his training in England, his return to India where he boldly rejects conventional wisdom about malarial transmission, his Nobel Prize in 1902, and his numerous appointments and awards in England. These accounts make little to no reference to

Indian places, people, or culture, although some accounts note that
Ross's Indian assistant Kishori Mohan Bandyopadhyay was awarded a
gold medal.

Ghosh's retelling embeds stories within stories and weaves jerkily
across time and geography, revising the traditional, linear heroic tale of
medical discovery into a feverish delirium of storytelling. Set in the not
too distant future, the outer frame story features Antar, a melancholy
information technology worker who monitors a wall-sized screen in his
New York City apartment as reams of historical detritus scroll by. He
describes himself as a "Dust-Counter," a term he used as a child in
Egypt when watching an archeologist sift through sand for fragments of
the past. The second frame story is set in 1995 and features Murugan,
Antar's co-worker, who goes to Calcutta in an effort to piece together
Ross's story, which he is convinced has significant missing pieces.
Within this story are additional stories, including ghost stories, folktales,
and accounts of Ross and other colonial scientists. Notably, Ghosh made
extensive use of archives in the British museum and Welcome Institute,
and every line given to Ross comes from Ross's own meticulously and
obsessively kept memoirs. In fact, every character, from Antar to
Mangala—the Indian subaltern working in Ross's lab in pursuit of her
own project focused on the transmigration of human knowledge and
souls through the malaria mosquito—is primarily engaged in archeology
as they gather and sift through bits and pieces of information, ideas,
possibilities, facts, and perspectives in order to develop knowledge.

Trained as an anthropologist, Ghosh believes that it matters whose
voices we hear, which places are featured, and which cultures are
foregrounded in the histories we tell and the stories we honor and
preserve. In 2001, Ghosh asked to be removed from the list of nominees
for the Commonwealth Writers Prize because only fiction written in
English is eligible and thus the prize fails to consider literature written,
as he said, in "the many languages that sustain the cultural and literary
lives of these countries" ("Ghosh Letter"). He also objected to the use of
the term "Commonwealth" in the title of the award, suggesting one
might as well rename English literature as literature of the Norman
Conquest. He explains that

> this phrase anchors an area of contemporary writing not within the
> realities of the present day, nor within the possibilities of the future, but
> rather within a disputed aspect of the past. . . . That the past engenders

the present is of course undeniable; it is equally undeniable that the reasons why I write in English are ultimately rooted in my country's history. Yet, the ways in which we remember the past are not determined solely by the brute facts of time: they are also open to choice, reflection and judgment. ("Ghosh Letter")

Similarly, in a 1997 essay for a *New Yorker* issue dedicated to celebrating the jubilee of India's independence, Ghosh complicated the popular infatuation with Gandhi's nonviolent efforts by writing about the Indian National Army's contribution, a militant effort not typically included in stories of India's independence.

In *The Calcutta Chromosome*, Ghosh is less concerned with unsettling national myths than with undermining the very premise of Western individualism and Western knowledge. As Bishnupriya Ghosh observes, under colonialism, "folk and popular religious and medical knowledge becomes invisible, silent, ephemeral," but Ghosh's novel calls back the ghosts and imagines a very different world (199). In *The Calcutta Chromosome*, characters in the outer frame story are reincarnations of characters from embedded stories, others reappear holographically, and both the history of tropical medicine and Indian folks tales are repurposed and woven together. Mrs. Aratounian, from whom Murugan rents a room in Calcutta in August 1995, seems to be the reincarnation of Mangala, the fictional assistant Ghosh adds to the account of Ross's 1895 laboratory work in Calcutta. Phulboni, a Calcutta poet, seems to have had an experience in the 1930s at a train station that links him to Laakhan, a lab assistant of D. D. Cunningham, the colonial medical researcher whose lab Ross inherits, picked up at a train station in 1895. These transmigrations are never clarified nor are they the point of the novel. Rather, they force us to become aware of how we make sense of the bits and dust, the evidence, all around us. We are all like Antar, Ross, Urmila (the Calcutta journalist who helps Murugan), and especially Murugan, who is named after the Hindu god who holds power over chaos and is always present but also beyond space and time, feverishly rushing about trying to make sense out of the detritus of information, fragments of history, and stories that cross our paths.

Ghosh is committed to expanding the range of evidence we value, and thus collect, and the types of causal relations we accept as meaningful. In writing about a friend who died of brain cancer, Ghosh reflects on the fact that his friend's mother also died of brain cancer. Ghosh wonders if perhaps the friend's intense identification with his mother had led, even though brain cancer is not hereditary, to the son having the same disease as the mother. Ghosh writes,

> Even the thought appears preposterous in the bleak light of the Aristotelian distinction between mind and body, and the notions of cause and effect that flow from it. Yet there are traditions in which poetry is a world of causality entire unto itself, where metaphor extends beyond the mere linking of words, into the conjugation of a distinctive reality. ("'The Ghat'")

In *The Calucutta Chromosome*, Ghosh considers what we might learn by spending some time in that preposterous world beyond the bleak light of Western science.

As part of this project, Ghosh challenges the ideal of the scientific laboratory as a perfectly managed place sealed off from external influences. As Diane M. Nelson suggests, for Ghosh the laboratory is, in fact, a "network of unruly actants." Nelson describes *In an Antique Land: History in the Guise of a Traveler's Tale*, Ghosh's account of his archeological project to recover details about the life of a twelfth-century Indian slave who worked for a Jewish master in Egypt, as a "resolute search for unpredictable multiconductors via the global north and south" (255). Scientific knowledge, she suggests, is, like archeological knowledge, also the result of a "vast network of knowledge and practice." Offering as examples work done on malaria in Guatemala and Honduras and by scientists who are also active in indigenous politics on such problems as screening blood donations for malaria, Nelson observes, "science may pass through the obligatory passage points of big-S science and acknowledge the immense power of troops and Big Pharma . . ., but it's also weedy and promiscuous" (256). Ross's laboratory, in Ghosh's novel, is a site of accidents, manipulation, misunderstandings, and competing projects and paradigms. Similarly, the sequence of events that put Ross in a malaria laboratory with the right set of assumptions and questions to solve the problem of malaria transmission is the result of the confluence of unrelated, small decisions by assorted individuals in pursuit of various personal goals.

In fact, Ghosh challenges not only the paradigm of the scientific laboratory and scientific progress, but core Western assumptions about the transmission of knowledge, practices, and even genetic material. Mangala, at least according to Murugan, is not "hampered by the sort of stuff that might slow down someone who was conventionally trained. . . . She didn't care about formal classifications" (246). In Hindu astrology, Mangala is the name for Mars; he represents war, physical energy, drive, impulsiveness, and he is a teacher of the occult sciences. In Ghosh's novel, Mangala, though female, is true to her namesake, and her occult science is just a small step beyond established science. Murugan hypothesizes that Mangala was, in part, interested in malaria as a treatment for syphilis, a treatment that was used in the early twentieth century and led to Julius Wagner-Jauregg winning the 1927 Nobel Prize for Medicine for his work in this area. Mangala is also interested in the "weird neural effects" that accompany malaria fever, and, as Murugan explains, she seemed to think that the "strange personality disorders . . . weren't really disorders but transpositions . . . a crossover of randomly assorted personality traits" (249). She hypothesizes that because of its recombinatory powers and the constant transmission via mosquito from human host to human host, the malaria parasite might also transmit information that makes "some tiny little rewiring in the host's wetware" (252).

Significantly, Murugan names this carrier of information the Calcutta chromosome, explaining that it "is an item that is to the standard Mendelian pantheon of twenty-three chromosomes what Ganesh is to the gods; that is, different, non-standard, unique—which is exactly why it eludes standard techniques of research. And which is why I call it the Calcutta chromosome" (250). Murugan also calls Urmila, the journalist who joins him on his mad dash around the city to uncover the story of Ross and Mangala, "Calcutta." Throughout the novel, networks play a key role. Phulboni's life-changing experience at the train station in Renupur occurs because he is sent there by his firm, "a well known British firm . . . famous for its extensive distribution network, which reached into the smallest towns and villages" (256). The city, for Ghosh, is a network that makes possible transmissions that exceed the rules of scientists and planners. In 2001, Ghosh visited Sir Arthur C. Clarke in Sri Lanka. In an essay about this meeting, Ghosh writes about his love of science fiction. As a child, he reports, "my appetite for the genre was sustained I think, largely by the ethos of my birthplace, Kolkata, which has a passionate, if curiously ambiguous, relationship with the sciences" (Ghosh, "On Arthur C. Clarke").

Ultimately, Ghosh weaves together two cities and two tales of discovery to tell a tale of "counter-science." One is based on Murugan's mad dash around Calcutta and the movement of others across India's landscape and history, as Murugan seeks not only to tell the story of Ross and Mangala, but also to become a part of the latter's experiment, as he, too, suffers from the residual fevers of both syphilis and malaria. The second is based on Antar's archeological dig via technological networks as he sits in his New York City apartment. This outer frame story has the feel of a sci-fi dystopian world with *Blade Runner*-like watchful screens, empty buildings, and massive bureaucracies. The setting leads us to expect a novel about surveillance, environmental degradation, and obsessive pursuits of power. Formerly, Antar worked for "a small but respected non-profit organization that served as a public health consultancy." Now, he works for the International Water Council, a global conglomeration that has absorbed such independent agencies into its "mammoth public health wing" as it seeks to manage the world's water supplies (9). But what is noteworthy about Ghosh's novel is the suggestion that the vibrant nexus of people, histories, knowledge, and cultures that we associate with urban settings and global communications is not merely oppressive. Compared to the manic energy of Murugan's 1995 Calcutta, New York City of the near future is a melancholy, decaying city as the families of Kurds, Afghans, and Tajiks move out, and empty apartments become warehouses. But in this bleak setting, Antar finds relief in the "brilliantly lit passageways" of Penn Station and its "surging crowds around the ticket counters, the rumble of trains under one's feet, the deep, bass hum of a busker's didgeridoo throbbing in the concrete like an amplified heartbeat" (14), and an Egyptian tea shop that offers syrupy sweet tea.

Undoubtedly, as an image of the future, New York City, Antar's fully networked apartment, and the efforts of the Investigation Officers of the International Water Council to "run everything they could find" through a computer because they "saw themselves making History with their vast water-control experiments" serve as warnings about power and networks (7). But Antar's archeological inclinations and the availability of technological detritus, from audiocassettes to answering machine messages, as well as his memories and relationships, build networks beyond the reach of technocratic control. Similarly, Mangala's "counter-science" challenges the claims of traditional science for its explanatory powers. Mangala's Calcutta chromosome, much like Calcutta and Antar's NYC apartment, offers a means of transmission that cannot be controlled. Networks exceed all efforts to plan and constrain what is transmitted, by whom and when; and all knowledge, much like the protein information encoded in DNA, is constantly recombining and mutating.

Ghosh's effort to complement tales of global science by creating a richly imagined account of local science and "counter-science" is akin to Horton's call for "horizontal programs" and recent emphases on making sure public health is embedded in local data and practices because execution is typically more successful with this approach and because local knowledge is integral and essential to the scientific project and not merely contextual.

In 1999, during the humanitarian disaster that followed East Timor's vote for independence, Xanana Gusmão, the de facto president of East Timor, declared:

> Let us not be tempted to build and develop modern hospitals that are costly and in which only half a dozen people benefit from good treatment. Let us concentrate above all on planning intensive campaigns of sanitation, prevention, and the treatment of epidemics and endemics for the whole population.

As one health official noted, the previously centralized system "was based on a standard that was not relevant to local population needs, situation, or their capacity to maintain it." With the help of the World Health Organization/Roll Back Malaria and the British NGO Merlin, East Timor built local systems for collecting data and then used the data to develop protocols for malaria treatment and control (cf. Morris).

A recent letter in *PLoS Medicine*, an online, open-access peer-reviewed medical journal that focuses on global health issues, made the same point in a rebuttal to claims by scientists that there are ready-to-hand nanotechnologies that can address at least five of the eight UN Millennium Development Goals, including nanosensors that can fine-tune the dosage of water and fertilization to plants. The letter notes that "the efficiency and implications of the application of technology depend on the social context" and that the technologies that are adopted and supported with significant investment of dollars are not necessarily the ones that best meet the needs of the poor (Foladori and Invernizzi). Thus, while it may be true that nanotechnology can help manage malaria, through such technologies as social mobilization, fumigation, mosquito nets, and traditional medicines based on artemisinin, China reduced malaria in one province by 99 percent between 1965 and 1990 and Vietnam reduced malaria-related deaths by 97 percent between 1992 and 1997 (cf. Foladori and Invernizzi).

Ghosh's novel also underscores the unruly transmission and mutability of knowledge, or, as Nelson puts it, that "[h]umans make science but not as we choose" (260). The story of the origin of the HIV pandemic underscores this. Jacques Pepin's epidemiological analysis makes a convincing case for the role of large-scale IV treatment of tropical diseases in the 1930s for the initial amplification of occasional cases of infection caused by a hunter's contact with chimpanzee blood. Pepin notes that transmission of HIV is ten times more effective through needles and syringes than sexual intercourse, and that sexual trans-mission was an unlikely contributor to the amplification of HIV infection until the 1950s, when colonial work camp policies that were unwelcoming to wives led to high-risk prostitution (i.e., the provision of sexual services to several men every day). Even then, Pepin suggests that it was the syphilis treatment by injectable drugs of prostitutes—many of whom tested positive because they had yaws as a child, which leaves behind the same syphilis antibody—that led to widespread infection. In just one hospital in 1953, he explains, more than 150,000 injections were administered by syringes and needles that were only rinsed between treatments. As Pepin concludes, it was the 50-year lag between the development of IV treatments and the realization that accidental IV transmission of viruses might occur at the same time that created a pandemic that has killed more than 25 million people.

In the open-access pages of *PLoS Medicine*, Paul Farmer joins colleagues in Rwanda in making an urgent plea for "biosocial understandings of medical phenomena." He writes, "the holy grail of modern medicine remains the search for the molecular basis of disease." The results of this work have been enormous, but the "exclusive focus on molecular-level phenomena has contributed to the increasing 'desocialization' of scientific inquiry: a tendency to ask only biological questions about what are in fact *biosocial* phenomena" (Farmer et al.,

"Structural Violence"). Literature has a contribution to make to the resocialization of medicine and to understanding in particularly powerful and rich ways both the particular material realities of structural violence and what James Gilligan describes as the "ubiquitous social structures, normalized by stable institutions and regular experience" that make structural violence all too often invisible (306). Farmer and others agree there are solutions and that what is required is social and political will. Adiga's and Ghosh's novels contribute to this effort, as may our field of literature and medicine if we are willing to take up these issues.

Works Cited and Consulted

Adiga, Aravind. *The White Tiger: A Novel*. New York: Simon, 2008. Print.

Ashcroft, Bill, Gareth Griffiths, and Helen Tiffin. *The Empire Writes Back: Theory and Practice in Post-Colonial Literatures*. 2nd ed. New York: Routledge, 2002. Print.

Brown, Tim, and Morag Bell. "Imperial or Postcolonial Governance? Dissecting the Genealogy of a Global Public Health Strategy." *Social Science and Medicine* 67.10 (2008): 1571-79. Print.

Chambers, Claire. "Postcolonial Science Fiction: Amitav Ghosh's *The Calcutta Chromosome*." *Journal of Commonwealth Literature* 38.1 (2003): 57-72. Print.

Driver, Felix, and Luciana Martins. *Tropical Visions in an Age of Empire*. Chicago: U of Chicago P, 2005. Print.

Farmer, Paul. *Pathologies of Power: Health, Human Rights, and the New War on the Poor*. Berkeley: U of California P, 2005. Print.

Farmer, Paul E., Bruce Nizeye, Sara Stulac, and Salmaan Keshavjee. "Structural Violence and Clinical Medicine." *PLoS Medicine* 3.10 (24 Oct. 2006): e449. Web. 26 Nov. 2012.

Fernandes, Jorge Luis Andrade. *Challenging Euro-America's Politics of Identity: The Return of the Native*. New York: Routledge, 2008. Print.

Foladori, Guillermo, and Noela Invernizzi. "Nanotechnology for the Poor?" *PLoS Medicine* 2.8 (2005): e280. Web. 26 Nov. 2012.

Ghosh, Amitav. Personal web site. *Amitav Ghosh*. Web. 26 Nov. 2012.

---. *The Calcutta Chromosome: A Novel of Fevers, Delirium and Discovery*. New York: Harper, 1995. Print.

---. "'The Ghat of the Only World': Aga Shahid Ali in Brooklyn." *Amitav Ghosh*. Essays Section. Web. 26 Nov. 2012.

---. "India's Untold War of Independence." *New Yorker* 23 June 1997: 104-21. Print.

---. "Ghosh Letter to Administrators of Commonwealth Writers Prize." *eZipangu*. 18 Mar. 2001. Forwarded as open email posting by Yuko Ohnaka on 28 May 2001. Web. 26 Nov. 2012.

---. "On Arthur C. Clarke." *Amitav Ghosh*. Essays Section. 1 Nov. 2001. Web. 26 Nov. 2012.

Ghosh, Bishnupriya. "On Grafting the Vernacular: The Consequences of Postcolonial Spectrology." *boundary 2* 31.2 (2004): 197-218. Print.

Gilligan, James. *Violence: Reflections on a National Epidemic*. New York: Vintage, 1997. Print.

Haynes, Douglas Melvin. *Imperial Medicine: Patrick Manson and the Conquest of Tropical Medicine*. Philadelphia: U of Pennsylvania P, 2001. Print.

Horton, Richard. "Mr. Thornton's Experiments: Transformations in Culture and Health." *Literature and Medicine* 25.2 (2006): 194-215. Print.

---. "Stopping Malaria: The Wrong Road." *New York Review of Books* 24 February 2011. Web. 15 Mar. 2011.

Jones, Gavin. *American Hungers: The Problem of Poverty in U.S. Literature, 1840–1945*. Princeton: Princeton UP, 2007. Print.

---. "The Truths of Poverty in Fiction." *The Human Experience: Inside the Humanities at Stanford University*. Stanford University. Web. 26 Nov. 2012.

Kich, Martin. "Mosquito Bites and Computer Bytes: Amitav Ghosh's *The Calcutta Chromosome*." *Notes in Contemporary Literature* 30.4 (2000): 9-12. Print.

King, Nicholas B. "Security, Disease, Commerce: Ideologies of Postcolonial Public Health." *Social Studies of Science* 32.5-6 (2002): 763-89. Print.

Leer, Martin. "Odologia Indica: The Significance of Railways in Anglo-Indian and Indian Fiction in English." *Angles on the English-Speaking World: Unhinging Hinglish: The Language and Politics of Fiction in English from the Indian Subcontinent*. Ed. Nanette Hale and Tabish Khair. Vol. 1. Copenhagen: U of Copenhagen and Museum Tusculanum P, 2001. 41-61. Print.

McCoy, David, Gayatri Kembhavi, Jinesh Patel, and Akish Luintel. "The Bill and Melinda Gates Foundation's Grant-Making Programme for Global Health." *Lancet* 373.9675 (2009): 1645-53. Print.

Morris, Kelly. "Growing Pains of East Timor: Health of an Infant Nation." *Lancet* 357.9259 (2001): 873-77. Mar. 2001. Web. 26 Nov. 2012.

Nelson, Diane M. "A Social Science Fiction of Fevers, Delirium and Discovery: *The Calcutta Chromosome*, the Colonial Laboratory, and the Postcolonial New Human." *Science Fiction Studies* 30.2 (2003): 246-66. Print.

Pepin, Jacques. *The Origins of Aids*. Cambridge: Cambridge UP, 2011. Print.

Ramraj, Ruby S. "*The Calcutta Chromosome*: A Novel of Fevers, Delirium and Discovery—A Tour de Force Transcending Genres." Sankaran, ed. *History* 191-204. Print.

Sankaran, Chitra, "Sharing Landscapes and Mindscapes: Ethics and Aesthetics in Amitav Ghosh's *The Calcutta Chromosome*." Sankaran, ed. *History* 109-20. Print.

---, ed. *History, Narrative, and Testimony in Amitav Ghosh's Fiction*. Albany: State U of New York P, 2012. Print.

Sen, Amartya. Foreword. *Pathologies of Power: Health, Human Rights, and the New War on the Poor*. By Paul Farmer. Berkeley: U of California P, 2005. xi-xvii. Print.

Smith, Sidonie. "Narrating the Right to Sexual Well-being and the Global Management of Misery: Maria Rosa Henson's *Comfort Woman* and Charlene Smith's *Proud of Me*." *Literature and Medicine* 24.2 (2005): 153-80. Print.

Thompson, Hilary. "The Colonial City as Inverted Laboratory in *Baumgartner's Bombay* and *The Calcutta Chromosome*." *JNT: Journal of Narrative Theory* 39.3 (Fall 2009): 347-68. Print.

United Nations. *Universal Declaration of Human Rights*. (1948). United Nations. Web. 26 Nov. 2012.

World Health Organization. *Closing the Gap in a Generation: Health Equity through Action on the Social Determinants of Health*. Final Report of the Commission on Social Determinants of Health. Geneva: World Health Organization, 2008. Print.

PART II:

SUBVERTING

THE

MEDICAL PROFESSION

CARLA BITTEL

A Literary Physician?
The Paris Writings of Mary Putnam Jacobi

In September of 1867, Mary Putnam, a young American medical student in Paris, wrote a letter to her father, the well-known publisher George Palmer Putnam.[*] Back in New York, her father was re-launching his publication, *Putnam's Monthly*, and invited her to make contributions. Mary Putnam was torn. She needed to publish to finance her stay in Paris, and yet, she worried about writing fiction, for she had a "real dread of becoming a 'literary physician,'" just as she was trying to establish herself as a scientific practitioner. Referring to other famous physician-writers, such as Oliver Wendell Holmes, Sr., who was a medical practitioner, poet, and novelist, she commented, "Such men are never worth anything for medicine or science" (Putnam Jacobi, *Life and Letters* 147).

But Putnam continued to write. In fact, in Paris alone, she published three works of fiction, several essays of social commentary, 170 pages of medical journalism, and numerous anonymous reports for the *New York Evening Post*. She also detailed her experiences in private letters home to her family. This body of written work encompassed the public and the personal, the political and the scientific. Taken together, they form a travel narrative, not just of her experience in a foreign land, but of both personal and intellectual transitions. In Paris, Putnam tried to reconcile her literary upbringing with her medical education. As she

---

[*] This article is adapted from *Mary Putnam Jacobi and the Politics of Medicine in Nineteenth-Century America* by Carla Bittel. Copyright ©2009 by the University of North Carolina Press. Used by permission of the publisher: www.uncpress.unc.edu.

perceived it, fiction-writing and positivist science had become divergent, if not contradictory endeavors. Telling stories now seemed at odds with the real work of medicine and the serious nature of revolutionary politics. But while Putnam tried to draw a line between fact and fiction, the line blurred, over and over. This article explores the continuity of science and politics with fiction writing in Putnam's Paris years. It will show how Putnam wrote about the human body as both anatomical specimen and political metaphor to mediate her scientific studies and fictional compositions. As a result, her writing in France expressed the inextricable bond between science and politics.

Between 1866 and 1871, Mary Putnam lived in Paris with the goal of expanding her medical education; she eventually became the first woman to gain admission to the École de Médecine and would be the second woman to graduate. While Putnam's education was clinical and scientific, it was equally political; she was a witness to the Franco-Prussian War and the Paris Commune of 1871.[1] Thereafter, her career combined science and politics, as she served as both a physician, researcher, and activist in New York City for more than three decades, and became one of America's leading women practitioners of scientific medicine.[2]

Histories of Women Physicians

Historians have described the "struggles and strategies" of women like Putnam as they made their way into the scientific and medical professions, coded masculine in nineteenth-century America (cf. Rossiter). Although women had long served as midwives and healers in

---

[1]   For other treatments of Putnam in Paris, cf. Bonner, *To the Ends of the Earth*; Harvey, "'Faithful to Its Old Traditions'?"; Harvey, "La Visite"; Harvey, "Medicine and Politics"; Warner, *Against the Spirit of System*; Wells, *Out of the Dead House*.

[2]   Additional treatments of Mary Putnam Jacobi include Gartner, "Fussell's Folly"; Harvey, "Clanging Eagles"; Horowitz, "The Body in the Library"; Morantz-Sanchez, *Sympathy and Science*; Morantz, "Feminism, Professional-ism, and Germs"; Sicherman, "Paradox of Prudence"; Truax, *The Doctors Jacobi*.

the family, they found themselves on the margins of medicine as it professionalized. After Elizabeth Blackwell became the first woman in the United States to attain a medical degree in 1849, other women followed her lead, but faced many barriers (cf. Sahli; Wilson). Inside and outside of medicine, there was great opposition to women becoming physicians, as critics cited impropriety, female intellectual inferiority, and the violation of "separate spheres" of influence. The graphic and indelicate nature of medical training and practice seemed incompatible with Victorian conceptions of femininity. American critics also feared that medicine might masculinize women, inhibit reproduction, and threaten the future of the "race" (cf. Abram; Morantz-Sanchez; M. Walsh).

Rejected from "regular" or orthodox schools, some women attended sectarian institutions for training in homeopathy, hydropathy, or botanic medicine. Others enrolled at emerging women's medical colleges, such as the Female (later Woman's) Medical College of Pennsylvania in Philadelphia and after 1868, the Woman's Medical College of the New York Infirmary in Manhattan, founded by Elizabeth Blackwell. Women made gains by the late nineteenth century and began to access co-educational institutions, winning admission to, for instance, the Johns Hopkins School of Medicine in Baltimore, which opened in 1893. By 1900, women physicians had also grown in numbers; there were approximately 7,000 women physicians in the United States, representing about 5 percent of the physician population (cf. Morantz-Sanchez, *Sympathy* 232).

Scholars have analyzed the contradictions of being a woman physician in the late nineteenth century, and how notions of Victorian "true womanhood" both combined and clashed with emerging scientific medicine. In her groundbreaking work, *Sympathy and Science: Women Physicians in American Medicine*, Regina Morantz-Sanchez describes a variety of women's approaches to medical practice, from the "sympathetic," maternalist, spiritual approach of Elizabeth Blackwell, to the rational, positivist, laboratory-based inclinations of Mary Putnam Jacobi.[3] Morantz-Sanchez shows how the tensions between "sympathy

---

[3] Cf. Morantz, "Feminism, Professionalism, and Germs" and "Perils of Feminist History"; Morantz-Sanchez, "Feminist Theory." Besides Mary Put-

and science" encapsulated debates about the nature of medicine and definitions of womanhood itself (Morantz-Sanchez, *Sympathy*). In her book, *Restoring the Balance: Women Physicians and the Profession of Medicine, 1850-1995,* Ellen S. More argues that many women physicians actually combined "professional and feminine cultures" (8), and balanced sympathy and science. Finally, in *Out of the Dead House: Nineteenth-Century Women Physicians and the Writing of Medicine*, Susan Wells examines how these women "intervened in medical discourse" and used it to insist on or elide their gender (12). She argues that women physicians "performed" gender, either rhetorically "masquerading" as men or emphasizing their womanhood to incorporate feminine characteristics into medicine (Wells 59-60).[4] As all of these scholars show, through both actions and discourse, women physicians negotiated their gender identities to make a place for themselves in late nineteenth-century medicine.

Mary Putnam as Pioneer Woman Doctor

As one of these "pioneer" women doctors, Mary Putnam Jacobi was one of the most significant medical voices of the late nineteenth century. Born Mary Corinna Putnam in 1842, she was the first child of George Palmer Putnam, the famous American publisher who helped develop New York into a literary capital (cf. Greenspan). Of Protestant New England stock, they were descendants of other famous Putnams, including some accusers in the Salem witch crisis. Growing up in the world of literature, Mary Putnam was expected by her family to become a writer. She began composing short pieces in her youth and published

---

nam Jacobi, other women physicians chose scientific identities and rejected the notion of feminized medicine. For example, on Mary Dixon Jones, cf. Morantz-Sanchez, *Conduct Unbecoming a Woman* and "Female Patient Agency." On Marie Zakrzewska, cf. Tuchman, "'Only in a Republic,'" *Science Has No Sex,* "Situating Gender."

[4] Wells analyzes Mary Putnam's writings as gender performance and "rhetorical cross-dressing," as Putnam shifted between masculine and feminine voices and personas. Cf. Wells 5-6. Also on discourses, cf. Theriot, "Women's Voices."

her first story in 1860 ("Found and Lost"), at the age of seventeen. Surrounded by other women novelists, encouraged by her father, and intellectually precocious, Mary Putnam seemed destined to live by the work of the pen (cf. Putnam Jacobi, *Life and Letters*). Writing domestic and didactic literature fit within the realm of middle-class feminine respectability. But for Putnam, writing became a vehicle of resistance. At an early age, she used short stories to express dissatisfaction with Victorian notions of femininity as well as religious principles. And though pushed by her grandmother to embrace evangelicalism, she instead "converted" to science, and made it her faith. Her own conversion narrative, documented at age twenty, used cell theory and the concept of "reparative growth" to challenge notions of original sin and human damnation (cf. Bittel, *Politics of Medicine* 32).

Ultimately, Putnam acquired an education that equaled or surpassed that of many medical men, earning three degrees. She began her training at the New York College of Pharmacy in 1861 and was the institution's only woman student at the time. She disliked the idea of female separatism, but when faced with few options for continuing her medical education, she turned to the Female Medical College of Pennsylvania in Philadelphia, where she received her second degree and graduated in 1864 with a thesis, written in Latin, on the function of the spleen (cf. Putnam, "Theorae").

Like many American male and female students of medicine in the mid-nineteenth century, she traveled to Paris, then considered the center of the medical universe, as historian John Harley Warner has shown (cf. *Against the Spirit of System*). Putnam used the Paris clinics to access patients and cadavers. But she also worked in the laboratories, and was most influenced by her time with Louis-Antoine Ranvier, an assistant to Claude Bernard (cf. Bernard; Holmes), and André-Victor Cornil (cf. Cornil and Ranvier). Her tissue studies with Ranvier inspired her thesis at the École de Médecine de Paris, which described how fat (in cells) led to cellular degeneration (Putnam, "De la graisse"). The culture of experimentalism in France would have tremendous influence on her later work.[5]

---

[5] On experimentalism in France, cf. Lesch, *Science and Medicine*.

Paris also provided her with a political education. During this volatile time, she became interested in both republicanism and socialism. She was particularly influenced by her friendship with Elisée Reclus, the socialist geographer.[6] For Putnam, Reclus articulated and illustrated the inseparability of science and political thought; his maps of the world reflected his belief in natural boundaries and the sovereignty of the people in particular regions, rejecting monarchical or church power (cf. Dunbar; Fleming; Ishill). Reclus modeled for Putnam how to merge scientific practice and political philosophy.

Returning to New York in 1871, Putnam worked at the New York Infirmary for Women and Children, founded by Elizabeth Blackwell, and taught at its affiliated Woman's Medical College. This would be her home base for much of her career. While she worked in a women's institution, she also accessed several medical societies and worked in hospital clinics dominated by men. Through one of those societies, she met Abraham Jacobi, a German-Jewish exile from the 1848 revolutions in Prussia, who is now considered the "father of pediatrics" (cf. Viner). The couple shared a commitment to combining science and politics and improving the health of children. They married in 1873, and thereafter she became known as Mary Putnam Jacobi.

At a time when the meaning of science in medicine was under debate, Mary Putnam Jacobi became active in the effort to "scientize" medicine, pushing the medical community to use the laboratory to advance clinical care. Her advocacy of science is seen in her numerous medical publications from her career in New York. She was most famous for her prize-winning essay, *The Question of Rest for Women during Menstruation*, published in 1877. In this essay, she sought to disprove notions of female fragility during menstruation. Instead, she argued for women's vitality and used experiments and testing to prove her point. In 1888, Mary Putnam Jacobi also famously wrote on hysteria, the malady that seemed to plague so many women. She showed that hysteria resulted from a lack of physical and mental exercise, not

---

[6] For another view of Reclus's influence on Putnam, cf. Harvey, "Medicine and Politics." Harvey describes some ways in which Putnam's exposure to revolutionary politics in France inspired her later battles on behalf of women in medicine and suffrage.

excessive activity, and rejected principles of the "rest cure" (cf. Putnam Jacobi, *Essays on Hysteria*). In these and other writings, she argued against oppositional sex differences and maintained that men and women were more alike than different (cf. Putnam Jacobi, "Case of Absent Uterus"). Strategically, she performed expertise in her medical writings, with overt demonstrations of her knowledge and scientific skill, in an effort to demonstrate the bias of her opponents and prove women's ability to do science (cf. Bittel, "Women's Health Research"). Positivist readings of nature became her main priority, as she moved away from writing fiction once she returned to New York.

Paris Writing

Putnam's Paris years mark an important point of transition, as she stood with one foot in her father's world of literature and with one foot in her new world of medical science. Literary work was financially necessary, but intellectually distracting, taking precious time away from her medical studies. It also threatened her carefully constructed persona as a dedicated American woman of science. Determined to be taken seriously as a physician, in France and back in the United States, Putnam closely protected her reputation. She asked her mother not to disclose her literary activities "*to anybody*," for association with such "frivolities," she said, "injures the reputation of a medical student . . ." (Putnam Jacobi, *Life and Letters* 190).[7] As a solution, Putnam discreetly published essays and fiction based on scientific themes, and used popular writing as a way to mediate between medicine and literature. As she navigated between genres, she negotiated gender identities as well.

Putnam fashioned herself into an acceptable feminine participant in French medicine by balancing a strong professional air with the demeanor of a respectable lady. She rejected norms of femininity in France and constructed her identity as foreign and American. Emphasizing character over appearance, modesty over coquetry, Putnam reported that French observers saw her as more "*gentille*" than beautiful,

---

[7]   Mary Putnam to Victorine Haven Putnam, 22 September 1868, in Putnam Jacobi, *Life and Letters* 190.

which was to her advantage, since, she said, prettiness got in the way of attending at the hospitals. With a "greater coldness of temperament and reliability of character," American women seemed less feminine and lacking passion, and therefore, less of a temptation to men (Putnam Jacobi, *Life and Letters* 121).[8] Ironically, an American woman became acceptable in France for the same reason female professionals seemed unacceptable in the United States: She appeared less womanly.[9]

Putnam recognized the importance of her gender identity, and for that reason, she was very careful about the words she put in print. For most of 1867, she sent correspondence to the *New York Evening Post*, summarizing French news, including scientific developments.[10] But the paper wanted Putnam to lighten the content and focus more on "'gossip'" and "scandalous stories," which she found a "dreadful bore" (Putnam Jacobi, *Life and Letters* 112-13).[11] Again, Putnam dismissed expectations that, as a woman, she would write society page columns. She wanted to avoid writing anything too light, fanciful, or overtly feminine. Rather, she preferred to put her new medical experience to use, with no indication of her gender.

In the spring of 1867, though Putnam had not yet gained admission to the École de Médecine, she could attend and observe clinical rounds and had found work in the histology lab of Ranvier. Putnam used her access to clinics and laboratories to report medical news from Paris to American physicians, becoming the "special correspondent" for the *Medical Record*.[12] In her column "Medical Matters in Paris," she described the latest clinical reports, medical theories, and debates being published in French medical journals and gazettes. Using the

---

[8] Mary Putnam to Victorine Haven Putnam, 16 April 1867, in Putnam Jacobi, *Life and Letters* 121.

[9] Cf. Margadant; McMillan.

[10] Putnam's letters in the *New York Evening Post* were unsigned. Although difficult to verify, several entries cover topics of interest to her. Cf., for example, *New York Evening Post* 7 Jan., 8 Jan., 21 Jan., 4 Feb. 1867. On the challenges of writing for the *Post*, cf. Putnam Jacobi, *Life and Letters* 151, 153, 157.

[11] Mary C. Putnam to Edith Putnam, 21 February 1867, Putnam Jacobi, *Life and Letters* 112-13.

[12] Cf. P.C.M., "Letters to the Medical Record."

pseudonym P.C.M. (a reversal of her initials), Putnam disguised herself, and her gender, to her reading audience. George Frederick Shrady, founder and editor of the *Medical Record*, accepted her first report in June of 1867 and published her columns regularly for the next two years. A respected surgeon and leading medical journalist in Manhattan, Shrady served as medical editor for the *New York Herald* for many years and probably had professional ties to Putnam's father.[13]

Addressing American men of medicine, many of whom had studied in Paris, Putnam's articles in the *Medical Record* described the technical and theoretical developments emerging from the Paris clinics.[14] She conveyed her first-hand observations of working on clinical rounds and relayed the methods, procedures, and approaches of her instructors.[15] Putnam's letters to the *Medical Record* focused on clinical reports, but they also addressed matters of pathology as well as developments in the laboratory. For example, in her reporting on the debate over Bright's disease (a disease of the kidney), Putnam described microscopical investigations to illustrate debates over whether certain physical conditions represented distinct diseases or steps in the evolution of a chronic disease.[16] Her coverage of this debate over disease specificity spoke to her growing interest in the laboratory as a locale for diagnosis. Her writing for the *Medical Record* made her a leading voice of intellectual exchange across the Atlantic, as she translated French medicine for American audiences. And while these columns sustained her financially, she did not earn enough to cover books and other expenses in Paris, and thus needed other sources of income (cf. Putnam Jacobi, *Life and Letters* 147).

Despite her reservations, Putnam agreed to compose work for her father's revived *Putnam's Monthly*. A compendium of art, science, and literature, the magazine encapsulated the *belles lettres* style of the age. Mary Putnam felt honored by George Putnam's eager invitation and saw

---

[13] Cf. "George Frederick Shrady" 680-81; J. Walsh 350.

[14] For another discussion of Putnam's letters to the *Medical Record*, cf. Harvey, "'Faithful to Its Old Traditions'?" and "La Visite."

[15] For example, cf. P.C.M. [Mary C. Putnam], "Letters to the Medical Record," *Pathfinder* 4, 12, 17, 51.

[16] Bright's disease was characterized by a renal lesion, albuminuria, and dropsy.

a financial opportunity. Yet, she still maintained reservations about publishing non-medical work. She described the literary world as one of "folly and vanity and uncertainty." And while she often boasted about her medical skills, she said of writing, "[I] have no confidence in my own powers." But, finally, she conceded, writing seemed to be her "destiny" (Putnam Jacobi, *Life and Letters* 144, 145, 147). In 1868, she published her first contribution to *Putnam's Monthly*. Ultimately, her father's magazine published five works; two additional articles appeared in *Scribner's Monthly*, which took over the Putnam title in 1871 due to the magazine's financial difficulties.[17]

1868 was a pivotal year for Mary Putnam. After two years of persistent campaigning and finally appealing to the reform-minded minister of public instruction, Victor Duruy, she officially gained admission to the École de Médecine de Paris (cf. Bittel, *Politics of Medicine*; Duruy; Harvey; Horvath-Peterson). She also fostered strong friendships with the Reclus family and their circle of socialists and feminists. As she pursued her studies and engaged with political activists, science and socialism came together for Putnam, just as she began to write for her father's magazine.

Medical Fictions

Mary Putnam intended to write pieces for *Putnam's Monthly* that walked the line between "science and popularity," as she put it. At first, she proposed several non-fiction essays, many on scientific subjects accessible to a lay audience, such as the nature of scientific proof, nervous diseases, and epidemics. As she claimed, "I cannot write stories"; rather, she needed inspiration from "real life" (Putnam Jacobi, *Life and Letters* 145). But these "real" science-based topics did,

---

[17] Several articles from Paris were later published under the name Mary Putnam Jacobi in *Stories and Sketches*. In *Putnam's Monthly*, cf. "Imagination and Language" (March 1868), "A Study of Still-Life, (Paris)" (December 1868), "A Sermon at Notre-Dame" (February 1869), "A Martyr to Science" (August 1869), and "Concerning Charlotte" (January-March 1870). Putnam also contributed "Some of the French Leaders" (August 1871) and "The Clubs of Paris" (1871) to *Scribner's Monthly*.

eventually, become the basis of her fiction. Two stories, "A Sermon at Notre-Dame" and "A Martyr to Science," are set in France and capture tensions between science and faith in the "age of positivism" at the end of the Second Empire (cf. Charlton; Simon). Both stories use bodies—the corporeal human body and the socio-political body—to convey the virtues of positivist science and socialism, and to criticize clericalism, monarchism, and individualism. They also served Putnam as a writer, mediating between medical and fictional writing, and at the same time, illustrating the interrelationship of science and politics.

Putnam combined criticism of the Catholic Church with enthusiasm for socialism in a short story, "A Sermon at Notre-Dame," published in February of 1869 in *Putnam's Monthly*. This fable takes place in Paris during the onslaught of a cholera epidemic and depicts the failures of organized religion and the triumph of public health measures. The story opens at Notre Dame Cathedral, where one of the city's most famous preachers delivers a sermon on the immortality of the soul. The preacher calls upon the people to ignore "materialists and men of science" (179). The service ends, and as the congregation leaves the cathedral, they witness a scuffle between a policeman and a young man posting placards that read: "Cholera!!! Citizens, the plague has again broken out in our midst" (187). The posters call on citizens to stop the epidemic. As the crowd erupts in a panic and the preacher tries to suppress their fears, the government ministers and the citizens "recognised at that moment that no one of them believed in the Immortality of the Soul!" (195). Then a leader emerges from the crowd and calls upon the people to defend themselves from the plague just as they would defend themselves from a foreign invader. For seven days and seven nights, the people work to depopulate the city, remove its "pestilence" (206), and transport people to the countryside. Committees are enthusiastically born and organized, "with as much effective precision as organs shape themselves out of the fluid mass of an embryonic body," wrote Putnam, using biological metaphors (210). In the story, the people save themselves and the city, for, as the narrator remarks, "life alone, intense, mobile, overflowing, could resist the threatened stagnation and paralysis of death" (209). The people then gather before the cathedral to rejoice in the power of humanity.

Putnam's "A Sermon at Notre-Dame" promoted faith in socialism and science over faith in religion. It is "the people" and not a preacher, public health measures, not passive prayer, that ultimately resolve an impending health crisis. Despite the preacher's attack on "materialists," it is material knowledge and science that triumph in the story. Putnam clearly wanted Americans to know that "it [was] the hour for socialism" in France (Putnam Jacobi, *Life and Letters* 201). Her story portrayed France as a country burdened by its religious institutions; it also served as a warning to those Americans who privileged religious interpretations over scientific and positivist readings of nature.

"A Martyr to Science," published in *Putnam's Monthly* in August of 1869, tells the story of a man who takes experimentation too far. This physician, who also has a crisis of religious faith, rejects Catholicism in favor of science. He becomes obsessed with learning about the "movements of the human heart" (222) and reads a book that describes experiments on live human subjects, conducted by sixteenth-century anatomist Andreas Vesalius. The doctor, now so absorbed by the prospect of making history, decides to conduct a human vivisection, on himself. In the name of "supreme heroism," the physician wants "undying fame," to sacrifice himself to science, and to be remembered with a "reverent homage" (233). But before he can become a martyr to science, his students place him in an asylum.

In this dark, yet amusing, mad-scientist story, Putnam scoffed at her character's egotism, but showed some understanding for the all-consuming desire for discovery. The character embodies her own faith in science, and yet, his fate in the asylum is the result of his own self-absorption. "A Martyr to Science" mocks individualism and the physician's privileging of the single body over the social body. His desire to cut up his own body for personal recognition violates the collective body and the premise that science serves the people. His obsession with his own body stands in opposition to seeing science for the good of the whole.

"A Martyr to Science" also foreshadows Putnam's own support of vivisection, but on animal subjects, instead of human. She, too, became engrossed with the internal movements of the heart and found the view inside the living body awe-inspiring. Her vivisection on a live frog prompted her to write about "the streaming movement" inside of him as "indescribably powerful" (Putnam Jacobi, *Pathfinder* 462). Later, Putnam argued that surgical experiments on live animals were necessary for teaching physiology, and even testified before a congressional committee in defense of vivisection (cf. *Vivisection*). She believed the rational physician should support animal experimentation to educate and save physicians from serious mistakes on patients. Animals should be martyrs to science, not humans, she insisted.[18]

The Social Organism

Putnam's medical fictions reflected the intersection of science and politics in her medical studies and intellectual life. Her ongoing research in the laboratories of Paris amalgamated with her growing feminist, socialist, and republican views, so that her understanding of cells shaped, and was shaped by, her outlook on the social order. Ultimately, her fictional stories of ineffectual sermons and scientific martyrdom were parables of the "social organism." Based on the congruence between the socio-political body and the human body, the social organism concept was central to positivist and socialist thinking in the mid- and late-nineteenth century. Thus, Putnam's short stories built on a combination of influences, including her education in scientific medicine, her philosophical readings, and her relationship with the Reclus family.

Putnam's study of cell theory and cellular pathology, even before she arrived in Paris, provided a scientific premise for her belief in the social organism. Cell theory argued that the cell was the basic form of human life and that cells generated from preexisting cells. The latter idea is associated with Rudolf Virchow, German physician and pathologist, who famously promoted the aphorism "*omnis cellula e cellula*," or "each cell stems from another cell" (Ackerknecht 57-58; Virchow). Virchow also became famous for his studies of cellular pathology, which attributed certain diseases to cellular abnormalities. Finally, Virchow theorized the social organism by equating cell organization with human relations. "Cellular pathology showed the body to be a free state of equal individuals, a federation of cells, a democratic cell state"

---

[18] On Mary Putnam Jacobi and vivisection, cf. Bittel, "Science, Suffrage, and Experimentation." On the history of vivisection, cf. Lederer, *Subjected to Science* and Rupke, *Vivisection in Historical Perspective*.

or "a social unit composed of equals" (Ackerknecht 45). While Putnam referenced Virchow in her Philadelphia thesis on the spleen, it was in Paris that his principles of cellular pathology influenced both her medical studies and political thought. Citing Virchow, her French thesis addressed the physiological impact of cellular degeneration and how failed cellular nutrition affected a body's general health and "vital powers" (cf. Putnam, "Theorae"; Putnam, "De la graisse"). Thus, like the human body, the social body depended on the health and nutrition of each cell, or each person.

The Reclus family also influenced Putnam's understanding of the social organism. Socialist, feminist, and anti-clerical, they shaped her opinions about state politics, religion, and the bourgeoisie (cf. Dunbar; Fleming; Harvey; Ishill). Putnam met the Reclus family's two eldest brothers, Elie and Elisée, in the spring of 1868, on the heels of her admission to the École de Médecine. Elisée Reclus, as a geographer and scientist himself, had the most profound impact on her. He drew parallels between the natural world and the political, influencing Putnam, who overlapped her own views about the physiological body and an egalitarian body politic.

Elisée Reclus was one of the chief architects of radical thought in France during the resurgence of socialist activity in late nineteenth-century Europe. In the late 1860s, he participated in a number of related movements and associations, including the cooperative movement, Freemasonry, the Free Thinkers, and the International Working Men's Association (cf. Fleming, *Anarchist Way* 67-70). Reclus worked within the existing political and social structures to promote an evolution in social thinking that would lead to revolution, the overthrow of the emperor, and the establishment of a government led by the people's associations. Although Elisée Reclus became an anarchist after 1871, he was a revolutionary socialist in the years leading up to the Franco-Prussian War; he hoped for the establishment of a "social republic" in France and abroad that would end the tyranny of centralized government and allow people to directly govern themselves through communal associations (Fleming, *Anarchist Way* 71-72).

The study of geography was an integral component of Elisée Reclus's political activism. Reclus, once called "the father of modern geography in France," made his field central to the study of the relationship between humans and the physical world (cf. Dunbar).

Putnam's time with Reclus had a profound effect in shaping her own integration of politics and science because he cultivated and reinforced her interest in rationalism and, more importantly, positivism. During her stay in Paris, Putnam energetically read French philosophy, especially the writings of Enlightenment thinkers, such as Rousseau and Voltaire. She also studied Auguste Comte and his positivist writings. She had started reading Comte before arriving in France and discussed his work at length with her brother, Haven (cf. Putnam Jacobi, *Life and Letters* 105).[19] But it was in Paris that positivism became the philosophical underpinning of her daily studies of medical science. Putnam, like many physicians and scientists of her generation, selectively adopted Comtean principles, embracing his ideals of observation and investigation and neglecting his criticisms of experimentation and statistics. Moved by Comte's unification of science and faith, she interpreted his thought to create an epistemological foundation for her work in Paris, and later in New York (cf. Putnam Jacobi, *Value of Life*).[20]

As Reclus mapped the earth to reflect socialist principles, Putnam learned to construct the human body as an ideal representation of human relations. Inspired by Comte, she began to see that the socio-political body, or social organism, grew, functioned, and sustained itself much like living organisms, through the contributions of all its interdependent parts. Nature, in other words, required the inclusion and work of all people, including those who had been on the margins, especially women. It also meant that all parts of the social organism had a stake and a role in shaping society. Putnam grew to understand nature as a model for collectivism and republicanism, a metaphor for Reclus's social republic.

Feminism and socialism also came together for Putnam during her time in Paris and with the Reclus family. Their support for women's

---

[19]   In a letter to her mother, Mary Putnam refers to discussions of Comte with her brother. Mary C. Putnam to Victorine Haven Putnam, 9 December 1866, in Putnam Jacobi, *Life and Letters* 105.

[20]   On Comte's use and criticism of certain sciences and their methods, cf. Pickering, *Auguste Comte,* vol. 1: 561-624. On positivism and American responses to Comte, see Harp, *Positivist Republic* and Leach, *True Love and Perfect Union.*

rights and education affirmed her both personally and intellectually, as they strongly encouraged her academic and scientific pursuits. In their company, she also studied the work of utopian socialist Charles Fourier, a vocal critic of industrialism, Catholicism, patriarchy, marriage, and the traditional family structure, and an advocate of female emancipation. He believed humanity was evolving toward "Harmony," a state of being characterized by equality between the sexes in which men and women would be similarly educated, productive, and free to express their "passions." Harmony could be achieved through "associationist communities," in which all members contributed equal labor, and through the liberation of women, who would lead the task of social reform (cf. Guarneri; Moses; Taylor). Putnam was very intrigued with Fourier's idea that men and women were born equal, but made unequal by society, a concept that influenced her later work (cf. Putnam Jacobi, *Life and Letters* 191).[21]

Socialist, positivist, and feminist concepts of the social organism shaped Putnam's fictional writing in Paris, but also informed her non-fiction writing. As she carried on with her medical studies, Putnam became more attuned to the growing political unrest and more hopeful about radical change in France. When the Franco-Prussian War subsided, and the Commune did arise, Putnam hoped for its success; she was disappointed at its failure and the return to conservative rule in France.[22] She expressed her frustrations in letters home to her family and in a critical essay, "Some of the French Leaders," published in *Scribner's Monthly* after the fall of the Commune. Though disappointed with political progress in France, she did leave Paris satisfied with her own education; she completed her degree with honors and compliments from her male professors.

---

[21] Mary C. Putnam to Victorine Haven Putnam, 22 September 1868, in Putnam Jacobi, *Life and Letters* 191. On the intersection of socialism and science in America and influences on her later work, cf. Pittenger.

[22] On the Paris Commune, cf. Eichner; Gullickson; Katz; Shafer; Tombs.

Conclusion

In some ways, Mary Putnam's writing dilemmas in Paris were unique to her; she was the daughter of a publisher destined for writing and, simultaneously, one of the first women to access the masculine bastion of Paris medicine, a specific combination of identities. She engaged in very particular negotiations of gender and was selective about her modes of writing and outlets for publication. But while her experience was not typical, many pioneering women physicians in Britain and America also had to negotiate their gender identities carefully; they too used writing as a way to publicly pronounce their abilities and promote their acceptability in the field. Clearly, both men and women physicians wrote medicine and engaged with other literary genres, but women did so conscious of their subordinate professional position. They wrote, aware that their words had consequences not only for themselves, but for how readers perceived women in medicine and beyond. Putnam knew this too and made every effort to reach a popular audience without compromising her professional identity.

Putnam returned to New York in the fall of 1871 and would thereafter treat medicine and politics as inseparable. As the physician, Mary Putnam Jacobi, she focused her writing on scientific papers, calls for women's rights and education, and, many times, a combination thereof. From then on, she abandoned fiction writing for public consumption. As a working physician, she no longer needed the financial compensation. But more importantly, fiction writing did not fit her identity as a practitioner of scientific medicine. Working to fight prejudices against women in medicine, she had to perform expertise and objectivity; publishing fiction had no place in this performance.

But although she saw herself as divorced from fiction, medical writing did have several familiar literary elements. Medicine consisted of case reports and research summaries, essentially narratives of illness. Her writing contained metaphor, for the anatomical body and the social body stood constantly in dialogue. Combining science and politics, many of her writings contained positivist parables, told through physiological studies. Whether she liked it or not, Mary Putnam Jacobi remained a literary physician.

Works Cited

Abram, Ruth J. *"Send Us a Lady Physician": Women Doctors in America, 1835-1920*. New York: Norton 1985. Print.

Ackerknecht, Erwin H. *Rudolf Virchow: Doctor, Statesman, Anthropologist*. Madison: U of Wisconsin P, 1953. Print.

Bernard, Claude. *An Introduction to the Study of Experimental Medicine*. 1865. Trans. Henry Copley Greene. New York: Dover, 1957. Print.

Bittel, Carla. *Mary Putnam Jacobi and the Politics of Medicine in Nineteenth-Century America*. Chapel Hill: U of North Carolina P, 2009. Print.

---. "Mary Putnam Jacobi and the Nineteenth-Century Politics of Women's Health Research." *Women Physicians and the Cultures of Medicine*. Ed. Ellen S. More, Elizabeth Fee, and Manon Parry. Baltimore: Johns Hopkins UP, 2009. 23-51. Print.

---. "Science, Suffrage, and Experimentation: Mary Putnam Jacobi and the Controversy over Vivisection in Late Nineteenth-Century America." *Bulletin of the History of Medicine* 79.4 (2005): 664-94. Print.

Bonner, Thomas Neville. *To the Ends of the Earth: Women's Search for Education in Medicine*. Cambridge: Harvard UP, 1992. Print.

Charlton, Donald G. *Positivist Thought in France during the Second Empire, 1852-1870*. Oxford: Clarendon, 1959. Print.

Cornil, André-Victor, and Louis-Antoine Ranvier. *A Manual of Pathological Histology*. Trans. E. O. Shakespeare and J. Henry C. Simes. Philadelphia: Henry C. Lea, 1880. Print.

Dunbar, Gary S. *Élisée Reclus: Historian of Nature*. Hamden: Archon, 1978. Print.

Duruy, Victor. *Notes et souvenirs, 1811-1894*. Vol. 2. Paris: Hachette, 1902. Print.

---. "Une Conquête du féminisme sous le Second Empire: Fondation d'une école pour l'instruction medical des femmes." 1870. Bulletin enseignement public au Maroc 41 (1954): 51-61. Print.

Eichner, Carolyn J. *Surmounting the Barricades: Women in the Paris Commune*. Bloomington: Indiana UP, 2004. Print.

Fleming, Marie. *The Anarchist Way to Socialism: Elisée Reclus and Nineteenth-Century European Anarchism*. London: Croom Helm, 1979. Print.

---. *The Geography of Freedom: The Odyssey of Elisée Reclus*. Montreal: Black Rose, 1988. Print.

Gartner, Carol B. "Fussell's Folly: Academic Standards and the Case of Mary Putnam Jacobi." *Academic Medicine* 71.5 (1996): 470-77. Print.

Greenspan, Ezra. *George Palmer Putnam: Representative American Publisher*. University Park: Pennsylvania State UP, 2000. Print.

Guarneri, Carl J. The Utopian Alternative: Fourierism in Nineteenth-Century America. Ithaca: Cornell UP, 1991. Print.

Gullickson, Gay L. *Unruly Women of Paris: Images of the Commune*. Ithaca: Cornell UP, 1996. Print.

Harp, Gillis J. *Positivist Republic: Auguste Comte and the Reconstruction of American Liberalism, 1865-1920*. University Park: Pennsylvania State UP, 1995. Print.

Harvey, Joy. "Clanging Eagles: The Marriage and Collaboration between Two Nineteenth-Century Physicians, Mary Putman Jacobi and Abraham Jacobi." *Creative Couples in the Sciences*. Ed. Helena M. Pycior, Nancy G. Slack, and Pnina G. Abir-Am. New Brunswick: Rutgers UP, 1996. 185-95. Print.

---. "'Faithful to Its Old Traditions'? Paris Clinical Medicine from the Second Empire to the Third Republic (1848-1872)." *Constructing Paris Medicine*. Spec. issue of *Clio Medica* 50 (1998): 313-35. Print.

---. "La Visite: Mary Putnam Jacobi and the Paris Medical Clinics." *French Medical Culture in the Nineteenth Century*. Spec. issue of *Clio Medica* 25 (1994): 350-71. Print.

---. "Medicine and Politics: Dr. Mary Putnam Jacobi and the Paris Commune." *Dialectical Anthropology* 15.2-3 (1990): 107-17. Print.

Holmes, Frederic Lawrence. *Claude Bernard and Animal Chemistry: The Emergence of a Scientist*. Cambridge: Harvard UP, 1974. Print.

---. "Claude Bernard, the Milieu Intérieur, and Regulatory Physiology." *History and Philosophy of Life Sciences* 8 (1986): 3-25. Print.

Horowitz, Helen Lefkowitz. "The Body in the Library." *The "Woman Question" and Higher Education: Perspectives on Gender and Knowledge Production in America*. Ed. Ann Mari May. Cheltenham: Elgar, 2008. 11-31. Print.

Horvath-Peterson, Sandra. *Victor Duruy and French Education: Liberal Reform in the Second Empire*. Baton Rouge: Louisiana State UP, 1984. Print.

Ishill, Joseph, comp. and ed. *Elisée and Elie Reclus: In Memoriam*. Berkeley Heights: Oriole, 1927. Print.

Katz, Philip M. *From Appomattox to Montmartre: Americans and the Paris Commune*. Cambridge: Harvard UP, 1998. Print.

Leach, William. *True Love and Perfect Union: The Feminist Reform of Sex and Society*. Middletown: Wesleyan UP, 1989. Print.

Lederer, Susan E. *Subjected to Science: Human Experimentation in America Before the Second World War*. Baltimore: Johns Hopkins UP, 1995. Print.

Lesch, John E. *Science and Medicine in France: The Emergence of Experimental Physiology, 1790-1855*. Cambridge: Harvard UP, 1984. Print.

Margadant, Jo Burr, ed. *The New Biography: Performing Femininity in Nineteenth-Century France*. Berkeley: U of California P, 2000. Print.

McMillan, James F. *France and Women, 1789-1914: Gender, Society, and Politics*. New York: Routledge, 2000. Print.

Morantz, Regina Markell. "Feminism, Professionalism, and Germs: The Thought of Mary Putnam Jacobi and Elizabeth Blackwell." *American Quarterly* 34.5 (1982): 459-78. Print.

---. "The Perils of Feminist History." *Journal of Interdisciplinary History* 4.4 (1974): 649-60. Print.

Morantz-Sanchez, Regina. *Conduct Unbecoming a Woman: Medicine on Trial in Turn-of-the-Century Brooklyn*. New York: Oxford UP, 1999. Print.

---. "Female Patient Agency and the 1892 Trial of Dr. Mary Dixon Jones in Late Nineteenth-Century Brooklyn." *Women Physicians and the Cultures of Medicine*. Ed. Ellen S. More, Elizabeth Fee, and Manon Parry. Baltimore: Johns Hopkins UP, 2009. 69-88. Print.

---. "Feminist Theory and Historical Practice: Rereading Elizabeth Blackwell." *History and Theory* 31.4 (1992): 51-69. Print.

---. *Sympathy and Science: Women Physicians in American Medicine*. New York: Oxford UP, 1985. Print.

More, Ellen S. *Restoring the Balance: Women Physicians and the Profession of Medicine, 1850-1995*. Cambridge: Harvard UP, 1999. Print.

Moses, Claire Goldberg. *French Feminism in the Nineteenth Century*. Albany: State U of New York P, 1984. Print.

P.C.M. [Mary C. Putnam]. "Letters to the Medical Record, 1867-1870." Rpt. in Putnam Jacobi, *Pathfinder* 1-170. Print.

Pickering, Mary. *Auguste Comte: An Intellectual Biography*. Vol. 1. Cambridge: Cambridge UP, 1993. Print.

Pittenger, Mark. *American Socialists and Evolutionary Thought, 1870-1920.* Madison: U of Wisconsin P, 1993. Print.

Putnam, Mary C. "The Clubs of Paris." *Scribner's Monthly* Nov. 1871: 105-09. Print.

---. "Concerning Charlotte." *Putnam's Monthly* Jan.-March 1870: 38+ (serial publ.). Rpt. in Putnam Jacobi, *Stories and Sketches* 262-389. Print.

---. "De la graisse neutre et des acides gras." Diss. Faculté de Médecine de Paris. Paris: A. Parent, 1871. Trans. for the author by Andrew J. Cain. Print.

---. "Found and Lost." *Atlantic Monthly* April 1860. Rpt. in Putnam Jacobi, *Stories and Sketches* 1-49. Print.

---. "Imagination and Language." *Putnam's Monthly* Mar. 1868: 301-10. Rpt. in Putnam Jacobi, *Stories and Sketches* 97-125. Print.

---. "A Martyr to Science." *Putnam's Monthly* Aug. 1869: 137-53. Rpt. in Putnam Jacobi, *Stories and Sketches* 212-61. Print.

---. "A Sermon at Notre-Dame." *Putnam's Monthly* Feb. 1869: 185-200. Rpt. in Putnam Jacobi, *Stories and Sketches* 166-211. Print.

---. "Some of the French Leaders." *Scribner's Monthly* Aug. 1871: 366-83. Rpt. in Putnam Jacobi, *Stories and Sketches* 390-443. Print.

---. "A Study of Still-Life (Paris)." *Putnam's Monthly* Dec. 1868: 688-701. Rpt. in Putnam Jacobi, *Stories and Sketches* 126-65. Print.

---. "Theorae ad lienis officium." Diss. Female Medical College of Pennsylvania, 1864. MS. Archives and Special Collections on Women in Medicine and Homeopathy, Drexel University College of Medicine. Trans. for the author by Andrew J. Cain. Archival Manuscript.

Putnam Jacobi, Mary. "Case of Absent Uterus: With Considerations on the Significance of Hermaphroditism." *American Journal of Obstetrics and Diseases of Women and Children* 32 (1895): 510-44. Print.

---. *Essays on Hysteria, Brain-Tumor, and Some Other Cases of Nervous Disease.* New York: Putnam's, 1888. Print.

---. *Life and Letters of Mary Putnam Jacobi.* Ed. Ruth Putnam. New York: Putnam's, 1925. Print.

---. *Mary Putnam Jacobi, M.D.: A Pathfinder in Medicine, with Selections from Her Writings and a Complete Bibliography.* Ed. Women's Medical Association of New York City. New York: Putnam's, 1925. Print.

---. "The Practical Study of Biology." *Boston Medical and Surgical Journal* 120 (1889): 631-36. Rpt. Putnam Jacobi, *Pathfinder* 458-62. Print.

---. *The Question of Rest for Women during Menstruation*. New York: Putnam's, 1877. Print.

---. *Stories and Sketches*. New York: Putnam's, 1907. Print.

---. *The Value of Life: A Reply to Mr. Mallock's Essay, "Is Life Worth Living?"* New York: Putnam's, 1879. Print.

Rossiter, Margaret W. *Women Scientists in America: Struggles and Strategies to 1940*. Baltimore: Johns Hopkins UP, 1982. Print.

Rupke, Nicolaas A. *Vivisection in Historical Perspective*. London: Croom Helm, 1987. Print.

Sahli, Nancy Ann. *Elizabeth Blackwell, M.D., 1821-1910: A Biography*. New York: Arno, 1982. Print.

Shafer, David A. *The Paris Commune: French Politics, Culture, and Society at the Crossroads of the Revolutionary Tradition and Revolutionary Socialism*. New York: Palgrave, 2005. Print.

"George Frederick Shrady." *Dictionary of American Medical Biography*. Vol. 2. Ed. Martin Kaufman, Stuart Galishoff, and Todd L. Savitt. Westport: Greenwood, 1984. 680-81. Print.

Sicherman, Barbara. "The Paradox of Prudence: Mental Health in the Gilded Age." *Journal of American History* 62.4 (1976): 890-912. Print.

Simon, Walter Michael. *European Positivism in the Nineteenth Century: An Essay in Intellectual History*. Ithaca: Cornell UP, 1963. Print.

Taylor, Keith. *The Political Ideas of the Utopian Socialists*. London: Cass, 1982. Print.

Theriot, Nancy M. "Women's Voices in Nineteenth-Century Medical Discourse: A Step toward Deconstructing Science." *Signs* 19 (1993): 1-31. Print.

Tombs, Robert. *The Paris Commune, 1871*. New York: Longman, 1999. Print.

Truax, Rhoda. *The Doctors Jacobi*. Boston: Little, 1952. Print.

Tuchman, Arleen Marcia. "'Only in a Republic Can it be Proved that Science Has No Sex': Marie Elizabeth Zakrzewska (1829-1902) and the Multiple Meanings of Science in the Nineteenth-Century United States." *Journal of Women's History* 11.1 (1999): 121-42. Print.

---. *Science Has No Sex: The Life of Marie Zakrzewska, M.D.* Chapel Hill: U of North Carolina P, 2006. Print.

---. "Situating Gender: Marie E. Zakrzewska and the Place of Science in Women's Medical Education." *Isis* 95.1 (2004): 34-57. Print.

Viner, Russell. "Abraham Jacobi and German Medical Radicalism in Antebellum New York." *Bulletin of the History of Medicine* 72.3 (1998): 434-63. Print.

---. "Abraham Jacobi and the Origins of Scientific Pediatrics in America." *Formative Years: Children's Health in the United States, 1880-2000.* Ed. Alexandra Minna Stern and Howard Markel. Ann Arbor: U of Michigan P, 2002. 23-46. Print.

---. "Healthy Children for a New World: Abraham Jacobi and the Making of American Pediatrics." Diss. University of Cambridge, 1997. Print.

Virchow, Rudolf. *Cellular Pathology as Based Upon Physiological and Pathological Histology.* Trans. Frank Chance. 1858. New York: Dover, 1971. Print.

Vivisection: Hearing Before the Senate Committee on the District of Columbia, February 21, 1900, on the Bill S. 34, For the Further Prevention of Cruelty to Animals in the District of Columbia. Washington, D.C.: GPO, 1900. Print.

Walsh, James J. *History of Medicine in New York: Three Centuries of Medical Progress.* Vol. 2. New York: National Americana Society, 1919. Print.

Walsh, Mary Roth. *"Doctors Wanted; No Women Need Apply": Sexual Barriers in the Medical Profession, 1835-1975.* New Haven: Yale UP, 1977. Print.

Warner, John Harley. *Against the Spirit of System: The French Impulse in Nineteenth-Century American Medicine.* Princeton: Princeton UP, 1998. Print.

Wells, Susan. *Out of the Dead House: Nineteenth-Century Women Physicians and the Writing of Medicine.* Madison: U of Wisconsin P, 2001. Print.

Wilson, Dorothy Clarke. *Lone Woman: The Story of Elizabeth Blackwell, the First Woman Doctor.* Boston: Little, 1970. Print.

ANTJE DALLMANN

"Doctors Are Never Mistaken": Doctor Romances and Re-Negotiations of the *Nature* of Marriage in Late Nineteenth-Century America

The "doctor romance," as it emerged in postbellum America, can be understood as a genre in which a re-negotiation of the private sphere, and particularly of marriage, was promoted. Within this genre, novels featuring female doctors occupy a special place. These female protagonists may leave the private sphere or reconcile private and public without jeopardizing their status as ladies. At the same time, the reference to biomedicine allows for an increase in narrative authority.[1]

I intend to show that this appropriation of medical authority in "doctor romances" does not necessarily entail that these texts subscribe fully to the patriarchal logic of Foucauldian biopolitics. In "doctor romances," a straightforward naturalization of the social on the basis of biomedical tenets is often subverted and questioned through the very authority of medicine—the authoritative "medical gaze"—which the texts appropriate and gender. Thus, arguably, one of the central

---

[1] By "biomedicine," I refer to medicine in a modern sense that, beginning with the eighteenth century, was increasingly transformed into a discipline that relied on laboratory research and that introduced the clinic as most important site of health care and professional medical training. It is the interrelation between society and emerging biomedicine which is central to Michel Foucault's analyses of biopolitics and biopower, since, as Roy Porter puts it, "[b]iomedicine claimed an explanatory monopoly over the body, its exploration, and its treatment" (95).

symbolic concerns of this emerging genre is to find a "cure" for the pressing question of how to re-imagine the social space by re-negotiating women's role in it.

Marriage Plots and Women Doctors

Nan "went closer to the river, and looked far across it and beyond it to the hills. . . . suddenly she reached her hands upward in an ecstasy of life and strength and gladness. 'O God,' she said, 'I thank thee for my future'" (Jewett 274). In these closing lines of Sarah Orne Jewett's *A Country Doctor* (1884), the book's heroine contemplates a future from which every shadow of inconclusiveness is removed. For Nan, her life to come emerges as preordained; a natural, foreseeable, and therefore secure space, tangible already in the distance.

The proper space for a female within Victorian ideology was, of course, the private sphere of the home; and the means by which to reach this supposedly safe haven was marriage. In narrative fiction from the eighteenth century onward, the marriage plot is a correspondingly central device, according to Nancy Armstrong, gendering and individuating social and political structures, which it both naturalizes and obscures.[2]

Yet Kathy Alexis Psomiades importantly points out that, due to the advent of Victorian theories of anthropology, "[n]ovels written from 1865 to the end of the century drew upon theories about the relationship between marriage and larger social structures that ultimately inflected their metaphorical and structural uses of marriage" (54). At the same time, around the middle of the nineteenth century, the state of individual marriage increasingly became a subject of criticism (cf. Bourke 422). Elizabeth Cady Stanton, for instance, stated that "there is one kind of marriage that has not been tried, and that is a contract made by equal

---

[2]   The marriage plot also lends itself to symbolizations which go beyond the creation and simultaneous depoliticization of the private sphere—a tendency which is obvious in its use as a trope for an American national reunion (cf. Keely), which underlines the importance of marriage as social institution that gives order not only to the individual, but also to the body politic.

parties to lead an equal life with equal restraints and privileges on either side" (qtd. in Pateman 422).

It is in this discursive context that the marriage plot is used in contemporary American fiction, which arguably cannot escape from reflecting the repercussions these political and theoretical discussions had on the understanding of the relation between gender, sex, and the opposition of public versus private sphere. To negotiate this relation, the motif of female professional activity gains importance, since it allows pertinent questions to be raised concerning the contractual nature of marriage and the domestication of sexuality, while also highlighting both the problematizations and also the possibilities of women entering the public sphere, as well as providing a general critique of the division between private and public.

Jewett's *A Country Doctor* belongs to a group of texts which pursue this negotiation. The book's main plot revolves around the protagonist's search for her "natural" place in life and in society. Medical science provides the authority that allows a critical inspection of this state of "nature." While Nan briefly contemplates marriage, it is not family life but the career of a doctor which she anticipates in the epiphanic vision quoted above. Thus, Jewett inverts the marriage plot by not leading the protagonist into the formulaic ultimate embrace of family life. The narrative's individualizing gesture allows questions of sexuality to be implicitly raised in a mode that mixes realist and non-realist narrative conventions. Of foremost importance, however, is Nan's choice of profession: Through Nan's becoming a doctor, the negative implications of social descent often invoked by the motif of female employment are reduced, at the same time allowing a maximum of authority to be seized in a society that was in the process of undergoing a wave of medicalization. Furthermore, to be a doctor allows Nan to make use of qualities that were understood to be "naturally" female: compassion, a talent for healing, and a privileged understanding of the health problems of women and children.

In the course of the second half of the nineteenth century, the figure of the doctor gained more and more importance in American culture, not least due to a broader public's increasing interest in medical topics and to medicine's growing authority. Significantly, this fictional doctor is not so much the protagonist of the "humanitarian narrative" which, according to Thomas W. Laqueur, from the eighteenth century on "describes particular suffering and offers a model for precise social action" (178). Rather, this physician is located at the center of romantic entanglements culminating in marriage plots. Thus, the marriage plot, Tabitha Sparks argues, effectively "harness[es] the empirical mindset, as represented by the doctor, into a conventionally romantic story" (2).

By drawing authority from biomedicine, the doctor romance also dramatizes, at the levels of narration and character constellation, one of the elements of modern medicine that Michel Foucault, in *The Birth of the Clinic,* deems especially important in modern medicine: the seemingly disinterested medical gaze. Thereby, the doctor romance also invests in the cultural project of "romantic materialism," which Janis McLarren Caldwell describes as "negotiating between two distinctly different ways of knowing: between, that is, personal experience and scientific knowledge of the natural world" (1). By using the character of the doctor, female authors could implicitly revoke the parallelization of the medical gaze as male gaze (cf. Schmieder in this volume).

By referring to the genre as "doctor romance," I emphasize that these texts, even while they establish a reference to modern science, are also close to the narrative conventions of romance. While marriage is a formulaic cornerstone of realist fiction, it is equally important within so-called non-representational literature. Thomas H. Fick pertinently argues that the attempt to categorize works of nineteenth-century fiction in the mode of either romance *or* realism overlooks that this literature often makes reference to both traditions. The often merely programmatic relation to realism establishes, even at an architextual level,[3] a claim to the veracity of the narrated world, which it in turn naturalizes.

In the 1880s and early 1890s, a number of books were published that all made use of the marriage plot as narrative formula, that all had female doctors at their center, and that all drew authority from the reference to biomedicine through a voice that parallels the Foucauldian disinterested, coldly analyzing instance of the clinical physician. By putting female doctors at the center of these narratives, the equation of

---

[3] Gérard Genette introduced the term architext or architextuality to encompass "the entire set of general or transcendent categories . . . from which emerges each singular text" (1). "Novel" as generic reference serves as an architextual signal.

medical and male, which was becoming more and more pronounced under the influence of professionalizing medicine, is undermined. William Dean Howells's *Dr. Breen's Practice* (1881), Elizabeth Stuart Phelps's *Doctor Zay* (1882), Jewett's *A Country Doctor* (1884), and Annie Nathan Meyer's *Helen Brent, M.D.: A Social Study* (1892) make use of these structures.[4] In the following I will argue that, by referring to medicine as authoritative discourse, these narratives, while employing conventional formulaic structures, discuss and re-negotiate a range of questions related to the on-going broader problematization of marriage as a legal, social, and political institution and as a symbolic order which creates gender-specific spaces.

"Under the Shelter of Her Husband's Name": Howells's *Dr. Breen's Practice*

The first broadly received "doctor novel" with a female protagonist was William Dean Howells's *Dr. Breen's Practice*. This title turns out to be ironic, since the eponymous Dr. Grace Breen has no practice to speak of: From the beginning, she is depicted as unfit for the profession of a physician that she has chosen not as a "vocation" but as the result of an unhappy engagement. "What was certain was that she was rich enough to have no need of her profession as a means of support, and that its study had cost her more than the usual suffering that it brings to persons of sensitive nerves" (7).

After graduation, Breen visits Jocelyn's, a hotel in a small New England seaside resort. At Jocelyn's, Breen is joined by Louise Maynard, an old friend who suffers from some little specified disease and who has run away from her allegedly abusive husband. In the course of the narrative, Maynard contracts pneumonia. Breen tries to cure her, but the other woman's state deteriorates, and she finally exclaims: "'I can't be trifled with any longer. I want a man doctor!'" (28). After some

---

[4]   Other texts, such as Henry James's *The Bostonians* (1885), Rebecca Harding Davis's "A Day with Doctor Sarah" (1878), and Phelps's "Hannah Colby's Chance" (1873) and "Zerviah Hope" (1880), use female doctors as minor characters and/or in shorter narratives.

hesitation, Breen seeks the counsel of the local Dr. Rufus Mulbridge, who, however, declines to consult with her, not because she is a woman but because she is a homeopath and his medical code forbids consultation with so-called non-regular practitioners. Eventually, Breen decides to fully give up her friend's case to the care of the male doctor and reverts to nursing her. In the end, Maynard is saved and also reconciled with her husband, thanks to Mulbridge's superior medical knowledge and to Breen's natural, "womanly" capacities to nurse her friend and to reconcile the spouses.

> Mulbridge is depicted as being a successful and thoroughly professional medical doctor exactly because he is a "tyrant" (107) used to ordering his patients around, mostly women from the city whom he covertly despises. Yet while Mulbridge's violent character, the text argues, is helpful and necessary in practicing medicine, he is unsuited as a husband and thus Breen declines his marriage proposal, which had been presented with overawing directness and not a little emphasis on financial considerations.

The narrative suggests that Breen lacks professionalism as a physician exactly because she is a natural woman, averse to lying, conscientious, and compassionate: female qualities that are depicted as detrimental to professional success. Physically, Breen becomes weak when pressed for a decision: She feels "as if she were giddy" (44), and Mulbridge quickly comes to her rescue, putting his "finger . . . instantly on her wrist" (44). Finally, Breen reverts to the role best suited for her as a woman: She marries her second suitor, the wealthy Mr. Libby, and gives up her job, although she eventually dedicates her efforts to the care of the children of the workers in her husband's factory, now protected "[u]nder the shelter of her husband's name" (114).

By emphasizing that Breen has not become a doctor out of economic necessity, the novel affirms a clear-cut class ideology. In using the profession of a woman doctor, fictional texts of the second half of the nineteenth century refer to the life choices of upper-middle-class women.[5] This symbolic appropriation of the female doctor as epitome of

---

[5]   In her influential book *Sympathy and Science*, Regina Morantz-Sanchez has argued that the small group of women doctors of the second half of the nineteenth century was by no means homogenous, and not all of them "called

upper-middle-class sensibilities does not allow engagement in a discussion of the economic possibilities involved in pursuing the career of a doctor. Rather, the "woman doctor" is a symbol of an upper-middle-class, financially secure American woman, a lady. Thereby, the character of the woman doctor itself confirms Victorian gender roles that posit the male as breadwinner. In Howells's narrative, the "Cult of True Womanhood" (Welter) reigns supreme, and the "lady" is the ideal woman: "[T]here is nothing better for a girl, even a girl who is a doctor of medicine, than a ladylike manner" (41), Breen contemplates. Mulbridge, who declares his intention to take up practice together with a prospective wife, accordingly disqualifies himself as not being a "gentleman," an idea which even his mother suggests (87). Libby, on the other hand, is well-off and thus suitable for Breen. Initially, however, Libby is introduced as a lazy young man who is brought to his senses by a woman's, i.e., Breen's, healing powers: She is able to convert him to a life of industrious labor, not by virtue of being a doctor, but as a future wife (36).

Contemporary narrative conventions did not allow for a discussion of "indelicate" bodily details (cf. Skinner). There is hardly more corporeal evidence of Louise Maynard's disease than a few drops of blood on her handkerchief that, according to Breen, "mean . . . nothing worth speaking of" (28). The book in fact suggests that Maynard's problem is mental rather than physical, and lies in her refusal to accept the controlling hand of her husband in particular and social control in general. (The cause of her acute pneumonia is suggested as lying in an unchaperoned boat ride with Libby.) When Breen exclaims: "You forget that you are married, and ill, too" (10), it is implicit that the two conditions are in some way related. Accordingly, curing Maynard's

---

themselves feminists" (4). At the same time, class did play a role in the choice of this profession, and not only for women, since, especially with the increasing professionalization and institutionalization of medical education, it also became more expensive to pursue this subject of study. This is one explanation for the divided interest of women who chose medical careers from the 1880s onward, who, according to Karen E. Campbell and Holly J. McCammon's empirical analysis, went for both the careers of doctor and nurse: The choice was preconditioned by the respective women's economic situation.

body introduces her eventual reconciliation with her husband, which entails Maynard's acceptance of her role as wife and mother and the appropriate behavior this status demands.

Far more central to *Dr. Breen's Practice* than realist "actualities" (Howells, "Editor's Study" 641) are romantic plot twists, which position the text's heroines within entanglements of love, family, and (prospective) marriage, and also render them minor characters within a story of patriarchal / biopolitical order disturbed and re-established. It is for this very re-establishment that the authority of medicine is claimed: Through an authoritative medical perspective, which the heterodiegetic narrator adopts, the social emerges as a realm of biomedical fact, and not only are female and male characters subject to a potential biomedical analysis, but the institution of marriage, too, falls into the realm of the natural, which biomedicine explains and cures. Thus, the intricate link between romance and realism here serves the function of naturalizing the social within conventional structures of a division between public and private as "natural" division between family and profession.

Typical of the emerging genre of the doctor romance, *Dr. Breen's Practice* is set in a remote rural place. Female physicians at the time, in the majority of cases, took up practice in big cities, where they treated women and children (cf. Campbell and McCammon). Nevertheless, the doctor in "doctor romances" is often a country doctor. The rural setting makes the physician appear less related to objective, distanced science and more attached to his (or her) individual patients. The plight of a country doctor is shown to be extremely strenuous, and it is not surprising that the metaphor of the night-time visit could be used to epitomize the unsuitability of a doctor's career for a woman.

Furthermore, placing the aspiring female doctor within a rural wilderness, within nature, forcibly advances the question of the "naturalness" of a woman pursuing a career. In Howells's narrative, women do not command nature, as male physicians do, since they are themselves part of nature—from which they depart when they live in the city, and thereby become afflicted by a range of illnesses that a doctor like Mulbridge cures. Thus, *Dr. Breen's Practice* invests in a nostalgic, anti-urban, anti-modern agenda while, at plot level, addressing the modern topic of professionalizing medicine.

Yet published barely twenty years after the end of the Civil War, in a country which was still deeply divided, the setting also posits New

England as peaceful, quintessential paradigm of American reality. The social Other, especially the African American Other, exists only in its blatant absence.[6] The narrative thus offers a phantasmagoric model for female middle-class propriety, not least in leaving out Otherness. Libby, when contemplating joining his father's business, proclaims: "[T]here's nothing so irreproachable as cotton for a business" (63), just as if slavery had never existed in the United States.[7] Thus, *Dr. Breen's Practice* makes use of the marriage plot at different levels, and thereby further emphasizes the symbolic appropriation of this constellation to negotiate and (en)gender a national space.

The romanticizing marriage plot in domestic fiction traditionally affirms the status quo of a gender-specific division between private and public, and tellingly ends with a marriage, closing off the private from the publicly visible, the text, even at the level of plot formula. Introducing a woman doctor as protagonist draws attention to contemporary discussions of marriage—as individual practice and as social institution with a character which shapes the fabric of the whole body politic. As discussed above, the state of marriage was central on the agenda of contemporary feminists, and famous women doctors from Elizabeth Blackwell to Mary Edwards Walker addressed the topic, discussing it with an authority clearly enforced by their own medical expertise.[8] The medical authority that the narrator of *Dr. Breen's*

---

[6] Implicitly, the marriage plot would, for the contemporary reader, evoke a reference to Civil War romances with their typical symbolic marriage plots that reunited, and thus healed, the republic, for "[b]y the 1880s, 'the South was the most popular setting in American fiction'" (Hubbell qtd. in Keely 623).

[7] Next to this, the only reference to the Civil War in the book is the discussion of Mulbridge's early return from his post as army surgeon, suggesting that the war experience is indicative of a man's character, and Mulbridge was deficient in some element of honor or bravery (cf. 77).

[8] As Bourke shows, advice literature in the second half of the nineteenth century discussed sex as an element of married life and often censured male (sexual) violence, which was legal within marriage. Blackwell, the first woman to receive a medical degree from an American medical college, wrote an advice book for married life, *The Human Element in Sex* (1894), which openly addresses female needs and sensibilities, taking recourse to her

Practice adopts equally allows for a discussion of marriage, as much as of female and male character, as "natural."

Dr. Breen's Practice takes a complex, and thoroughly traditional, position in its "biomedical" negotiation of marriage. If Howells's better-known narratives, which are understood to belong to his brand of "smiling realism," have often been criticized for their exclusive focus on the better-off parts of American society, *Dr. Breen's Practice* can be understood as a study in class-consciousness in the sense that patriarchal upper-middle-class sensibilities are a norm so deeply naturalized in this book that every Other to this norm is either obliterated (both African Americans and poor locals, especially females) or pathologized, as Mulbridge's rich female patients. Zooming in on Maynard's "case," it is obvious that the ill the narrative seeks to heal is not so much that of an individual body but rather of a body politic out of its "natural" order: its division of private and public jeopardized by female emancipation. The narrative censures visible violence, as exemplified by Mulbridge, which it characterizes as necessary in the treatment of disease, yet inadequate as the basis for marriage. Thus, the notion of equality between the sexes in marriage gets paid only lip service. Yet this equality is a matter of the husband's discretion within the closed realm of the private sphere. Thus, the newly converted Breen propagates, under the influence of her own impending engagement to Libby: "'Marriage must change people. . . . It ought to be so much easier to forgive any wrong your husband does you than to punish it; for that perpetuates the wrong, and forgiveness ends it, and it's the only thing that can end a wrong'" (75).

The narrative's recourse to biomedicine, and the adoption of biomedical authority by the narrative voice, thus attempt to negotiate the social as naturally given, as subject to the doctor's analysis. Yet the nostalgic tinge which dominates the text tells the story of a social realm that is already in an irreversible process of change and that cannot be understood from the isolated perspective of patriarchal upper-middle-

---

medical authority to legitimize the treatment of questions otherwise considered highly "indelicate." Mary Edwards Walker, believed to be the only woman who served as an Army surgeon during the Civil War, wrote at length about the moral implications of marriage and the right of divorce in her autobiographic *Hit* (1871), which also draws heavily on her authority as respected physician.

class implicitness any more, if this was ever possible. In the following, it will become clear how diverse the spectrum of disagreement with these norms had become.

"[D]reaming a Dream": Phelps's *Doctor Zay*

Elizabeth Stuart Phelps's *Doctor Zay* takes up a constellation very similar to Howells's novel. Yet while the two narratives turn out to be much alike in their character constellations, they are also very different in their respective use of subject matter.

As a women's rights activist, Phelps was outspoken in her protest against what she perceived as antiquated gender restrictions. The "True Woman" of reigning ideology, she argued, "is the gauntest scarecrow ever posted on the rich fields of Truth to frighten timid birds away" ("True Woman" 269). Phelps was a proponent of both modern and alternative medicine and of the woman doctor's place in it. There were, she argued, "few things more womanly or more noble" than to be a physician ("What Shall They Do?" 523).

Thus, Phelps takes up a rhetorical stance in her defense of women entering the field of medicine that Carolyn Skinner describes as typical of nineteenth-century self-help books by female physicians, who "used specific strategies to capitalize on . . . femininity in order to reassure readers of their normalcy, despite the risqué topics they addressed: human sexuality, pregnancy, abortion, . . . among others" (106). Phelps draws authority from women's morally superior position in nineteenth-century gender ideology and is legitimized by her reference to medicine.

In *Doctor Zay*, Waldo Yorke, a young, idle, yet good-natured lawyer, embarks on a journey to Sherman, Maine, to claim an inheritance. Sherman is depicted as a remote place which Yorke experiences as idyllic (4). Yet Yorke, just arrived from the city, is unable to understand this natural "Maine wilderness" (7), gets hopelessly lost, and finds Sherman only after a young woman, "unmistakably, a lady" (8), has shown him the way.

Soon after, Yorke has an accident, in the course of which he is badly injured (26).[9] He experiences a visit from a doctor in a feverish state of half-consciousness. Only when looking at the globules the doctor has left behind, Yorke realizes that he is in the care of a homeopath. Falling in and out of consciousness, Yorke gathers that "this unseen, unknown, being" (22), his doctor, is called Zay. He feels a woman's touch only to realize that it "does not caress; it tears" (18), introducing his realization that he is virtually in "*[a] woman's hand*" (23; my emphasis). While disturbed at first, Yorke realizes that he is in fact in the "firm hands" (41) of a very competent female physician, and he slowly but steadily recovers.

Early on, the reader realizes that Yorke is in awe of his doctor's competence and hard work, yet had already fallen in love with her when he had first met her on his way to Sherman. In *Doctor Zay*, in contrast to *Dr. Breen's Practice*, it is the woman who loves nature and is in command of it as a physician.[10] Yorke is introduced as well-off and idle. He admits bitterly: "'I have never been busy in my life. . . . Instead of being successful, I have been rich'" (45). He goes back to Boston after his dislocated ankle is healed, yet returns to Sherman later on. In the novel's final scene, roles are reversed, as Jean Carwile Masteller argues: Yorke is healthy and confident while Zay is weak after a winter of illness and a tough night attending to a patient. Yet this reversal of roles is not irrevocable: When Zay takes the reins of the buggy from Yorke, he responds: "'I don't care who has the reins . . . as long as I have the driver'" (256).

---

[9] Like *Dr. Breen's Practice*, *Doctor Zay* refrains from going into detail concerning Yorke's injuries, with one exception: Soon after he has regained consciousness and Zay is first introduced to him as his physician, he starts to bleed from a severed artery. While he "grew giddy and faint," Zay is in full control, "ligat[ing] the artery . . . with a firm and fearless touch" (27). This scene obviously intends to demonstrate Zay's full capacity as a doctor, even when confronted with critical realities.

[10] For Zay to be acceptable, she is introduced in a contradictory way: While she gives Yorke instructions which amount to commands, with Yorke "rebelling at her authority" (35), she is also a "beautiful and obedient machine" (37) whom Yorke "orders" to come to his bedside (25).

This ending implies an impending marriage, and thus advances the argument that a woman can have both a career and a family.[11] Timothy Morris argues that to Phelps's contemporary readers, this plot twist "must have seemed like a secular Utopia" (141). Yet the book's ending, surprising as it is when considered outside of the conventions of romance, has a very important rhetorical function, Morris shows. While Zay is presented as a competent, self-sufficient professional throughout the novel, the final plot twist allows for her to be also considered "womanly" and "natural."

At a symbolic level, the novel proposes a concept of the private and public realms altogether other than Howells's: Arguing that family and career for a woman can be reconciled, the novel advances a perception of the public as modeled after the private, under the moral authority of women. This is especially important since with Yorke a character is introduced who, once again, symbolizes a crisis of male agency that, the narrative argues, can be overcome by female influence. For this, biomedicine as a discourse is instrumental, since it naturalizes the social, and, through the character of a woman doctor, gives scientific, moral, and emotional authority to women.

Thereby, the text also appropriates and genders the medical gaze, rendering it less universal and at the same time more comprehensive. Furthermore, by reversing the gendered roles of patient and doctor, the female body is no longer the symbol of illness and becomes a sign of power, symbolized as well by Zay's hands, which treat Yorke. Even Zay's final weakness can be read as accentuating the claim that she is the better doctor precisely because she is herself a physical being, in contrast to the figure of the cold and distanced male physician. This ambivalent appropriation and re-signification of the doctor figure as personification of the medical gaze is evident from Zay's first appearance as doctor. Here, she remains invisible, yet not because she stands for the distanced physician, but because she is a woman and has to enact this role. Nevertheless, the narrative describes the doctor's

---

[11] This, in fact, was in accordance with Phelps's belief and her research on the marital status of women doctors. "[O]ut of twenty-nine women in one medical school class [seventeen] were married," if most of them to other medical doctors, Wegener quotes Phelps (4).

distance to her patient as a necessary, if male, stance: She looks at Yorke, searching for "symptoms," categorizing Yorke's love for her as consequence of a concussion. "'*Symptoms!*'" Yorke moans, "'There are new symptoms every day'" (63). Love as a link between individuals thereby becomes the subject of the diagnosis made by Zay, as doctor. On the other hand, however, Zay's relation to Yorke as doctor to patient is, from the beginning, referred to through the metaphor of "hands," not "eyes," emphasizing her care as "tactile" and therefore less distanced.

Still, *Doctor Zay* remains ambiguous in its emancipatory agenda. While arguing for women in professional careers, it is, once again, not about careers chosen out of economic necessity. *Doctor Zay* uses the figure of the lady doctor to promote the claim of female participation in the public sphere, and marriage as an institution is clearly considered its central pillar, linking the individual to the body politic. Importantly, this claim not only rests on moral, but also on scientific—biomedical— authority, personified by the narrative's heroine.

"'Most of my patients are women and children. That is as I prefer it,'" Zay states (47). According to the narrative, it is the woman doctor's foremost task to prevent women from what physician Emma Frances Angell Drake, author of *What a Young Wife Ought to Know* (1901), was to call "the terrible wrong" (Drake 125), namely abortion, which Blackwell called the "gross perversion and destruction of motherhood" and which she felt dishonored the term "female physician" (*Pioneer Work* 30).[12] The "terrible wrong" is in *Doctor Zay* imagined to take place outside of the protagonist's social sphere. The narrative thereby engages in a discussion which had become highly politicized by the 1880s, and which carried with it clear overtones of class sensibility. Blackwell's honorable female physician, as much as the fictional Zay, take a pronounced stance against abortion as an immoral practice, as did most contemporary women's rights activists who were anti-abortionists,

---

[12] When Blackwell and Marie Zakrezewska finalized their plans for an all-women's hospital, they argued that the practice of medicine should be kept out of "ignorant or unworthy hands," by which they targeted both irregular practitioners (as homeopaths) and female abortionists (cf. Tuchman 81). Phelps, an ardent believer in homeopathy, obviously intended to discard the notion that homeopathy and "Restellism" had anything in common.

since they "argued that such practices allowed men to avoid responsibility for their sexual behavior" (Tuchman 81).[13]

Doctor Zay establishes a close link between female health and marital security, and argues for the woman doctor's authority in both fields. This argument becomes especially pronounced when Molly is introduced, a young, pregnant, unmarried woman. Molly seems to hope for an abortion, and Zay sighs: "'Why, she clings to me as if she thought I could undo it all,—could make her what she used to be again!'" (79). While abortion is out of the question for Zay, she still finds a way to help her young patient: Just after Zay has left Molly's house, the doctor is summoned to resuscitate a lumberman who was dragged out of a mill-pond and is considered dead. The man turns out to be Molly's lover. Zay perseveres and the man finally comes back to life. Then, she forces him to immediately marry Molly, arguing with the reluctant minister that "'[s]omething might go wrong with the case yet'" (86). Yorke, who witnesses the scene, is shocked: "Nothing could have revealed to him [better] the gravity and sacredness of her work" (79).

Here, the narrative favorably compares the work of a doctor to that of a minister, and Zay in fact ardently believes in the sacredness of marriage. "'Next to the love between man and his Creator,'" she preaches, "'the love of one man and one woman is the loftiest . . . ideal that has been set before the world. A perfect marriage is like a pure heart: those who have it are fit to see God'" (144). On these grounds, she rejects Yorke's marriage proposal, arguing that she has experienced too many unhappy marriages. She concludes, "'[y]ou and I are dreaming a dream. It has a wakening, and that is marriage'" (144).

---

[13] Abortion was at the time euphemistically known as "Restellism," named after Madame Restell, a former poor immigrant who had become a health practitioner who provided abortions. In 1873, influenced by the death of a young woman who allegedly had been killed by an abortion provided by Madame Restell, abortion was officially outlawed in the U.S. (cf. Reagan). The discourse against abortion thus found the issue to belong to the lower social classes with greedy immigrant practitioners, personified by Restell, and innocent poor victims. Yet Restell's house also bespeaks the fact that her clients were by no means only poor and uneducated: It was, according to Nicola Beisel, "the sins of the upper class [which] were rendered invisible in one of the most visible and notorious houses of the city" (36).

Thus, using the concepts of "family," "marriage," and "naturalness" as the symbolic cornerstones of an emancipatory discourse, *Doctor Zay* advances an argument in favor of female agency outside the private realm. It thus opposes Howells's reductive contrast between family and profession. It is the mode of romance which makes this conciliation possible since it not only allows for the implausible to happen, but also offers formulaic closure through the plot twist of marriage, which, in this case, prescribes an enduring happy ending, irrespective of the probabilities. Yet the new public sphere envisioned by the narrative is thoroughly reigned in by bourgeois sensibilities, which are enforced and naturalized by both the medical discourse and the narrative mode of romance. Furthermore, by advocating the institution of marriage as a means for female security, as in the case of Molly, the narrative refrains from acknowledging the reality of violence in marriage, at which *Dr. Breen's Practice* at least hints. Both narratives thus also use their remote settings to place their stories within a fairy-tale reality of upper-middle-class sensibilities in which the social Other is barely more than a foil against which the "lady's" claim of doing charitable work is projected. In the following, however, I will argue that the "doctor romance" also allows for a critical discussion of the link between marriage and enforced sexuality.

"[T]o Work with Nature": Jewett's *A Country Doctor*

Sarah Orne Jewett's *A Country Doctor*, which offers a very pronounced alternative to women's restriction to the private sphere, is arguably the most hybrid of the texts discussed so far. On the one hand, the narrative depends heavily on formulas of sentimental and gothic fiction[14] and of the fairy tale.[15] On the other hand, its depiction of a

---

[14] The gothic element is especially obvious in the first chapter, where Adeline, Nan's mother, returns home to die, already contemplating suicide on her way. She advances in the twilight like a threatening ghost (which underlines the narrative's opposition between the city's corrupting influences and the idyllic and innocent countryside), "stumbl[ing] among the graves" (3), to finally attract her mother's attention by uttering "a strange little cry" (14).

country doctor's practice is comparatively realistic.[16] I argue that it is this convergence of romance and realism which allows for the text's positive treatment of alternative female biographies.

As the title indicates, *A Country Doctor* is set in a rural location, Oldfields. At the book's beginning, the reader makes the acquaintance of three nice, elderly countrywomen—Mrs. Thacher and her two friends—who are spending a chilly evening together when a young woman, her small baby girl in her arms, suddenly appears and turns out to be Adeline, Mrs. Thacher's long-lost daughter. Adeline dies that very night, due to consumption, to her addiction to alcohol, and to a "touch of insanity" (78); the little girl, Nan Prince, grows up with her grandmother. When the latter dies, too, the local Dr. Leslie takes Nan into his care. She turns out to be a compassionate and intelligent young woman who shows a talent for healing. Even though the locals ridicule women doctors (69), Nan announces: "'I should like best to be a doctor'" (69). She accompanies Leslie on his rounds, and the doctor starts to contemplate the career of a doctor for her, Nan becoming "the patient in charge whose welfare seemed to the doctor so dependent upon his own decisions" (70). Thus, the naturalness of Nan's emerging choice to become a doctor is substantiated by Dr. Leslie's medical authority.

Nan goes to medical school when she decides to finally contact her paternal aunt Nancy Prince, whom she has not yet met. Nan soon receives an invitation to her aunt's mansion in Dunport. While the latter had dreaded the encounter, fearing that her niece could have taken after her mother, Nan turns out to be "a lady," and Miss Prince starts to hope that the young woman will not return to Oldfields. When a romance between Nan and George Gerry, Aunt Prince's protégé, develops, it is thoroughly encouraged. Nan, however, ends her visit and the young man's advances, claiming that she cannot give up her vocation.

A Country Doctor takes a complex position concerning the issue of work and female ambition. Clearly, as documented by the positive interpretation of the countrywomen's life at the narrative's beginning,

---

[15] Nan is the Prince(ss), Dr. Leslie the kind surrogate father, and Nancy Prince a fairy aunt (cf. Gale 54).

[16] This is often attributed to the fact that Jewett's father was a doctor whom she frequently accompanied on his rounds.

the book invests in a nostalgic, anti-urban view on social change. The narrative does not find the ideal American (woman) in the city, and it does not propagate women's relegation to the house as "natural." Rather, by focusing on countrywomen, the broader responsibility of the woman for the complex household of the farm is evoked. In a Crèvecœurian sense, it finds the true American (woman) on a farm, and as far as it is depicted to be desirable to be a lady, this term refers to a moral education and a standard of manners that is irrespective of wealth.

Through the character of Adeline, the book critically inspects the concept of ambition and dismisses marriage, as a road open to women, for bettering one's social status. "'[H]er ambitions,'" one of the elderly women notes, "'ain't what they should be'" (6). To leave one's home town, and thereby to leave one's social position, in order to marry is not an option the countrywomen find feasible, and, from their stance, they describe Adeline's attempt to leave Oldfields behind as ill-starred. "'If she'd got a gift for anything special'" (6), they continue, arguing that a special talent might justify taking such a risk. Thus, from the beginning, the narrative questions the unconditional "naturalness" of marriage a lady-friend of Nan's aunt is to propagate: "'[I]t [becoming a doctor] is quite unnatural,'" she claims. "'A woman's place is at home. . . . The best service to the public can be done by keeping one's own house in order and one's husband comfortable . . .'" (221). By juxtaposing the perspective of the countrywomen to that of the Dunport ladies, the text also critically inspects the ideological precepts of the concept of True Womanhood, whose class-conscious perspective is naturalized by the narratives I have discussed earlier.

In the light of this problematization of prevailing conceptions of marriage as implicitly informed by class sensibilities, Nan's choice to embark on the career of a doctor, in contrast to seeking security through marriage, emerges as the more "natural." This is especially true when the narrative's investment in fairy-tale formulas is taken into consideration. As a young girl, Nan dreams of a life at her aunt's house, heralded by "a carriage drawn by a pair of prancing black horses [which] might be seen turning up the lane, and that lovely lady might alight and claim her as her only niece" (53). It is such a vision which implicitly informs the question: "'[Y]ou surely don't mean to let her risk her happiness in following that career?'" (81). But when Nan chooses her profession, it is explicitly not—as in the case of Howells's Dr.

Breen—out of irresolution, but is rather the well-conceived plan of a mature woman. While for Nan marriage is the golden dream which can never be redeemed, as the case of her mother shows, a career is the promising, and realistic, option for future happiness. Furthermore, *Dr. Breen's Practice* and *Doctor Zay* adopt a narrative mode which allows for the heroines to escape the perils of violence, broken marriage, and unwanted pregnancy they discuss and aim to heal, since these perils are imagined as not belonging to a lady's social sphere. Nan Prince, on the other hand, is herself the subject of the narrative instance's pseudo-medical examination: "It seemed, too, as if she could do whatever she undertook, and as if she had a power which made her able to use and unite the best traits of her ancestors, the strong capabilities which had been unbalanced or allowed to run to waste in others" (54).[17]

By no means does *A Country Doctor* dismiss marriage as an institution. Yet in its argument that usefulness should equal happiness, marriage and professional career are equally means to an end. Nan often implies that, for various reasons, she is not in a position to marry. "'I do not wish to be married, and do not think it right that I should be,'" she says (221). One of these reasons is explained as the "touch of insanity" which runs in her family: "'I know the wretched inheritance I might have had from my poor mother's people'" (248).

Yet the text implicitly hints at more than this, not least when Dr. Leslie, one of Nan's potential suitors, according to the formula of romance, "sadly" argues: "'Nan is not the kind of girl who will be likely to marry. . . . I believe that it is a mistake for such a woman to marry. Nan's feeling toward her boy-playmates is exactly the same as toward the girls she knows'" (108). Arguably, *A Country Doctor* here implies a lack of erotic interest in males on Nan's part, and for this reason recommends abstaining from marriage and from socially enforced heteronormative marital sexuality.

Morris argues that "*Doctor Zay* is radical with respect to gender roles, conservative with respect to sexuality" (142). *A Country Doctor*

---

[17] While the influence of her mother's family is emphasized, the importance of her father's inheritance is pointed out later as explanation for her lady-like demeanor and her talent for healing: Her father had also been a doctor (cf. 77).

implicitly takes up where *Doctor Zay* falls short. As Valerie Fulton shows, Jewett makes it possible to think beyond the narrative plot patterns of a "necessary marriage" as social and often financial imperative to female security (252). If the ending of Jewett's narrative seems unrealistic, Fulton posits, this has to do with the canonization of the marriage plot in contemporary novels of manners, particularly by Henry James. In his *The Bostonians*, the end of what he called a Boston marriage[18] between two women's rights activists is brought about by the emergence of an unsympathetic and utterly conservative young man who nevertheless convinces one of the women, the beautiful but strangely "empty" Verena, to give up her cause in order to marry him. This implausible ending is often read as symbolizing the impossibility of women avoiding marriage. Yet it also complies with reigning notions that conceive of female sexuality exclusively within patterns of heterosexual marriage or depict the Other as "asexual," as with the female physician Dr. Prance in James's novel. While *The Bostonians*, Aaron Shaheen argues, allows for homosexual desire to exist between two women, it "succumb[s] to heteronormative whiteness" (Shaheen 293) at the narrative's end. *A Country Doctor*, on the other hand, allows for no such final closure: The narrative grants the female protagonist privacy through the introduction of ambiguity, while the conventional plot pattern, by marrying off the heroine, paradoxically destroys her privacy by her entry into the private sphere, since, from that point on, she has to succumb to a fixed model of gender roles. Nan Prince's medical expertise as much as her distanced position as physician allow her to claim the freedom to dismiss marriage as adequate life choice for herself, and thus "to work with nature" (84): both by healing others and by remaining true to herself.

---

[18] Jewett's long relationship to Annie Adams Fields is often referred to as real-life model for the concept of the Boston marriage (cf. Gardner). Yet Phelps's relation to Dr. Mary Briggs Harris is also sometimes mentioned in this context (cf. Castle 499).

"Almost Fairyland": Meyer's *Helen Brent, M.D.* and the Re-Negotiation of Marriage

Of the narratives discussed so far, Annie Nathan Meyer's is arguably the one which adheres most closely to conventions of realist writing. Set in New York City, *Helen Brent, M.D.* leaves behind the stock character of the country doctor and turns to a woman, Helen Brent, who, as in the case of James's Dr. Prance, practices medicine in a big city. It is, however, indicative of the very strong convergence of doctor narratives and romance patterns that, here, again, romantic plots and the problematization of marriage are central.

Helen Brent is introduced *in medias res* of her professional duties as president of the new and prestigious Root Memorial Hospital, an institution dedicated to the professional medical training of women, giving an address in front of an "enthusiastic audience" (14). She is a "very handsome . . . woman, surely not past thirty . . ." (16). Yet she has also "performed . . . difficult gynecological operations . . .—operations that required nerve, coolness, daring, skill, a steady hand and a delicate one . . ." (15). Despite her professional detachment, however, Brent has tears in her eyes at the end of her address and turns "pale, so pale that someone offered her a chair" (22): She has seen her former fiancé in the audience.

While touching on the topic of women's freedom of education, which Meyer actively propagated (cf. Meyer, "The Higher Education"), the narrative's central plot element is the romantic relationship between Brent and Harold Skidmore. The two got engaged as young adults, but Skidmore broke the engagement, claiming that, as a doctor, Brent would not be able to "'attend to household duties,'" and asking: "'how much of yourself could you give up to home life, without giving up your practice?'" (28).

The narrative's main argument focuses on dismantling the dishonesty of Victorian gender conceptions, which require women to give up "their earnestness in taking up a profession," while, for a man, marriage "mean[s] renewed effort, a greater stimulus for [professional] success" (36). While the text still invests in the notion that "men and women [are] born to marry" (37), and Brent contemplates that "life was not complete to her" without a family (53), it argues that the nature of marriage has to change to allow for women's self-fulfillment not only as mothers and wives, but also in their own right pursuing a career outside the home.

Yet, as does *Doctor Zay*, *Helen Brent, M.D.* nevertheless posits a need for female doctors who dedicate their care to women in more conscientious ways than their male colleagues, thereby also restoring the health of the body politic.[19] Dr. Brent takes up the care of a pregnant unmarried woman who has lost her child due to an infection with syphilis, at which the text hints. The father of the child is considered the "handsomest" (68) and best-off bachelor in New York. His infection goes undiscovered, and he proposes marriage to the society girl Rose, a daughter of one of Brent's patients. The latter tries to persuade Rose's mother to break off the engagement, arguing, "'you [will] kill your daughter . . . by [not] breaking off this match'" (79). But the mother is not convinced, muttering, "'[d]octors [are] sometimes mistaken—think they know everything'" (79). Yet Brent is not mistaken, of course, and consequently the young wife gives birth to a stillborn child and, soon after, dies herself.

Nevertheless, the narrative argues in favor of marriage. The moral authority over marriage as institution fundamental to society should, however, be with well-trained and progressive women. In due course, at the narrative's end, Skidmore, humbled by a severe illness, sends Brent a letter in which he implicitly begs her to take him back into her healing care. The narrative thereby allows for a happy ending, an ending that "'scents of fairyland'" (30). For *Helen Brent, M.D.*, even if it carries the subtitle *A Social Study*, also belongs in the genre of doctor romances.

"'[I]s it not the man that is the *natural* breadwinner?'" (32; my emphasis), Skidmore asks in the course of an argument with Brent, and thereby sheds further light on the deeper symbolic meaning of doctor romances. The male doctor as stock character attains increasing importance in nineteenth-century literature because he negotiates between nature and civilization and between religious belief and scientific certainty. It is his command over the scientific and the natural alike which makes him so attractive as potential spouse, since he is the link between very different belief systems, which he, through his person, reconciles. Marrying a doctor in popular fiction thus means to bring

---

[19] In *The Crux* (1911), Charlotte Perkins Gilman advances a similar argument.

order to modern society, to virtually heal the confusing realities of a changing social world.

For the same reason, the woman doctor is introduced in nineteenth-century fiction. She, like no other character, can be used to illustrate the vicissitudes of social change, especially concerning the division between private and public sphere. As a character, she commands over "nature," and whether or not it is "natural" for a woman to pursue a career is accordingly the most pressing question posed by all the narratives discussed here. These texts wrest authority from the increasingly important discourse of biomedicine, dissecting the social realm of the private, of family, and of marriage as natural sphere over which they claim control, and thereby go beyond the necessary depiction of women pursuing important professional careers as role models for female ambition outside the home. The narratives' use of conventions of both realism and romance plays an important role in making it possible to advance this argument, since the hybridity of narration allows for a broad spectrum of different positions. While Howells dismisses professional careers for women, Phelps, Jewett, and Meyer all argue in favor of it. Yet the crucial common element of these texts is their treatment of marriage as an issue of public, not only private, interest. It is the discourse of biomedicine which is used to justify female intrusion in and authority over this public realm, and what is perceived as "natural" is subject to the doctor's discretion. And, as with Helen Brent, the doctor is never mistaken.

Works Cited

Armstrong, Nancy. *Desire and Domestic Fiction: A Political History of the Novel.* Oxford: Oxford UP, 1987. Print.

Beisel, Nicola. *Imperiled Innocents: Anthony Comstock and Family Reproduction in Victorian America.* Princeton: Princeton UP, 1997. Print.

Blackwell, Elizabeth. *The Human Element in Sex: Being a Medical Inquiry into the Relation of Sexual Physiology to Christian Morality.* London: J. and A. Churchill, 1894. Print.

---. *Pioneer Work in Opening the Medical Profession to Women: Autobiographical Sketches.* New York: Longmans, Green, 1895. Print.

Bourke, Joanna. "Sexual Violence, Marital Guidance, and Victorian Bodies: An Aesthesiology." *Victorian Studies* 50.3 (2008): 419-36. Print.

Caldwell, Janis McLarren. *Literature and Medicine in Nineteenth-Century Britain: From Mary Shelley to George Eliot.* Cambridge: Cambridge UP, 2004. Print.

Campbell, Karen E., and Holly J. McCammon. "Elizabeth Blackwell's Heirs: Women as Physicians in the United States, 1880-1920." *Work and Occupations* 32.3 (2005): 290-318. Print.

Castle, Terry. "Elizabeth Stuart Phelps." *The Literature of Lesbianism: A Historical Anthology from Ariosto to Stonewall.* Ed. Castle. New York: Columbia UP, 2003. 499-504. Print.

Cott, Nancy F. "Giving Character to Our Whole Civil Polity: Marriage and the Public Order in the Late Nineteenth Century." *U.S. History as Women's History: New Feminist Essays.* Ed. Linda K. Kerber, Alice Kessler-Harris, and Kathryn Kish Sklar. Chapel Hill: U of North Carolina P, 1995. 107-21. Print.

Davis, Rebecca Harding. "A Day with Doctor Sarah." *Harper's Magazine* Sept. 1878. Web. 20 July 2011.

Drake, Emma Frances Angell. *What a Young Wife Ought to Know.* Philadelphia: Vir, 1901. Print.

Fick, Thomas H. "Genre Wars and the Rhetoric of Manhood in *Miss Ravenel's Conversion from Secession to Loyalty.*" *Nineteenth Century Literature* 46.4 (1992): 473-94. Print.

Foucault, Michel. *The Birth of the Clinic: An Archaeology of Medical Perception.* 1963. New York: Vintage, 1994. Print.

Fulton, Valerie. "Rewriting the Necessary Woman: Marriage and Professionalism in James, Jewett, and Phelps." *Henry James Review* 15.3 (1994): 242-56. Print.

Gale, Robert L. *A Sarah Orne Jewett Companion.* Westport: Greenwood, 1999. Print.

Gardner, Carol Brooks. "Boston Marriages." *Encyclopedia of Gender and Society.* Vol. 2. London: Sage, 2009. 87-88. Print.

Genette, Gérard. *Palimpsests: Literature in the Second Degree.* 1982. Trans. Channa Newman and Claude Doubinsky. Lincoln: U of Nebraska P, 1997. Print.

Gilman, Charlotte Perkins. *The Crux.* 1911. Introd. Dana Seitler. Durham: Duke UP, 2003. Print.

Howells, William Dean. *Dr. Breen's Practice*. 1881. Middlesex, UK: Echo Library, 2009. Print.

---. "Editor's Study." *Harper's New Monthly Magazine* 73.463 (1886): 639-44. Library of Congress: American Memory. Web. 9 Dec. 2012. <http://memory.loc.gov/ammem/ndlpcoop/moahtml/title/lists/harp_V73I43 6.html>.

James, Henry. *The Bostonians*. 1885. London: Penguin, 1986. Print.

Jewett, Sarah Orne. *A Country Doctor*. 1884. New York: Random, 2008. Print.

Keely, Karen A. "Marriage Plots and National Reunion: The Trope of Romantic Reconciliation in Postbellum Literature." *Mississippi Quarterly* 51.4 (1998): 621-48. Print.

Laqueur, Thomas W. "Bodies, Details and the Humanitarian Narrative." *The New Cultural History*. Ed. Lynn Hunt. Berkeley: U of California P, 1989. 176-204. Print.

Masteller, Jean Carwile. "The Women Doctors of Howells, Phelps, and Jewett: The Conflict of Marriage and Career." *Critical Essays on Sarah Orne Jewett*. Ed. Gwen L. Nagel. Boston: Hall, 1984. 135-47. Print.

Meyer, Annie Nathan. *Helen Brent, M.D.: A Social Study*. 1892. Charleston: BiblioBazaar, 2008. Print.

---. "The Higher Education for Women in New York City." *The Nation* 26 January 1888: 68. Web. 7 June 2011.

Morantz-Sanchez, Regina. *Sympathy and Science: Women Physicians in American Medicine*. New York: Oxford UP, 1985. Print.

Morris, Timothy. "Professional Ethics and Professional Erotics in Elizabeth Stuart Phelps' *Doctor Zay*." *Studies in American Fiction* 21.2 (1993): 141-52. Print.

Pateman, Carole. *The Sexual Contract*. Stanford: Stanford UP, 1988. Print.

Phelps, Elizabeth Stuart. *Doctor Zay*. 1882. Bel Air: Dodo, 2008. Print.

---. "Hannah Colby's Chance." *Our Young Folks* Oct.-Dec. 1873: 595+. Print.

---. "The True Woman." 1871. *The Story of Avis*. Ed. Carol Farley Kessler. New Brunswick: Rutgers UP, 2001. 269-72. Print.

---. "What Shall They Do?" *Harper's New Monthly Magazine* Sept. 1867: 519-23. Print.

---. "Zerviah Hope." *Scribner's Monthly* Nov. 1880: 78-88. Print.

Porter, Roy. "What Is Disease?" *The Cambridge Illustrated History of Medicine*. Ed. Porter. Cambridge: Cambridge UP, 2006. 82-117. Print.

Psomiades, Kathy Alexis. "The Marriage Plot in Theory." *Novel* 43.1 (2010): 53-59. Print.

Reagan, Leslie J. *When Abortion Was a Crime: Women, Medicine, and Law in the United States, 1867-1973*. Berkeley: U of California P, 1997. Print.

Shaheen, Aaron. "'The Social Dusk of that Mysterious Democracy': Race, Sexology, and the New Woman in Henry James's *The Bostonians*." *ATQ* 19.4 (2005): 281-300. Print.

Skinner, Carolyn. "'The Purity of Truth': Nineteenth-Century American Women Physicians Write about Delicate Topics." *Rhetoric Review* 26.2 (2007): 103-19. Print.

Sparks, Tabitha. *The Doctor in the Victorian Novel: Family Practices*. Burlington: Ashgate, 2009. Print.

Tuchman, Arleen Marcia. *Science Has No Sex: The Life of Marie Zakrzewska, M.D.* Chapel Hill: U of North Carolina P, 2006. Print.

Walker, Mary Edwards. *Hit*. 1871. Breinigsville: General, 2011. Print.

Wegener, Frederick. "'Few Things More Womanly or More Noble': Elizabeth Stuart Phelps and the Advent of the Woman Doctor in America." *Legacy* 22.1 (2005): 1-17. Print.

Welter, Barbara. "The Cult of True Womanhood: 1820-1860." *American Quarterly* 18.2 (1966): 151-74. Print.

Kirsten Twelbeck

How Far Could They Go?
Imprisoned Nurses, Unsexed Angels, and the Transformation of True Womanhood in Civil War America

Introduction

The first half of the 1860s was not only the most fundamental rupture in American history since the Revolution but also a watershed moment for the country's gender relations. The Civil War enabled a majority of Americans to experience a different organization of family relationships: With their husbands at the front for several years, more and more women became responsible for managing family farms, plantations, and businesses. By and by, Americans came to understand that such activities did not necessarily corrupt a woman's character. Brought about by necessity rather than as a result of feminist struggles, these new experiences contributed crucially to the gradual transformation of True Womanhood and, thus, eventually to the formation of a new, modern figure, the New Woman.

Women's experiences during the American Civil War have been discussed by various scholars of nineteenth-century gender relations,[1] yet few have paid attention to the debates among the women themselves. This article argues that legal, political, and social transformations that took place during the first half of the 1860s encouraged feminists to engage in a surprisingly nuanced public debate about "how far"

---

[1]   A selection includes titles by Catherine Clinton, Drew Gilpin Faust, Sarah E. Gardner, Mary Elizabeth Massey, Nina Silber, and LeeAnn Whites.

American women could—and should—go at this point. The discussion was most articulate in the North, where, under the influence of feminist victories in the field of law as well as the Emancipation Proclamation, the feminists and abolitionists Louisa May Alcott and Sarah Emma Edmonds engaged in a textual conversation whose overarching topic was the organization of difference within the social fabric of the nation. American readers followed their conversation in large numbers: Alcott's *Hospital Sketches* (1863) and Edmonds's *Nurse and Spy in the Union Army* (1864)[2] had gone through several reprints by the end of the century. An intertextual analysis of the two works sheds light not only on a particularly female tradition of political debate but also on its emotional dimension.

When *Hospital Sketches* and *Nurse and Spy* first appeared, American women were still reeling from the 1860 Earnings Act and its partly revised 1862 version known as the Married Women's Property Act. These legal reforms had given women control over their own possessions and thereby changed "the terms defining a True Woman dramatically" (Kraus 208). For a younger generation of women, including Alcott and Edmonds, these changes were the beginning of a new era. Faced with the horrors of the Civil War, Victorian women like Alcott and Edmonds no longer accepted that their influence should be limited to the domestic realm, and many of them transgressed the institutionalized border that separated them from the men at the front: Between 1862 and 1865, thousands of white, middle-class women volunteered as nurses in what came to be termed the "army in white."[3]

As Jane E. Schultz explains in her historical analysis of female Civil War hospital workers, women's exposure to "male nudity, profanity, and lechery" was originally seen as compromising their natural "delicacy" (*Women at the Front* 123). Female nurses met such prejudices by fashioning themselves as "born nurturers," arguing that "nursing was," after all, "domestic work" (*Women at the Front* 123). After an initial phase of resistance from surgeons and doctors, female

---

[2]   For the remainder of this essay I will designate these two texts as "*HS*" and "*NaS*" in my parenthetical citations.

[3]   For an account of the introduction of female nurses into Civil War hospitals, cf. Freemon 54. Regarding the use of military jargon in female accounts of the war, cf. Leonard, *Yankee Women* xvii.

hospital workers were eventually welcomed, not least because their sheer presence "acted symbolically to remind soldiers of the civilizing influence of home and hearth" (*Women at the Front* 91). In the context of the Civil War, in other words, domesticity became a predominantly moral category that was—at least potentially—without spatial limitations. Interestingly, however, women themselves debated the flexibility of the concept of domesticity and the extent to which it should remain linked to the trope of Civil War nursing.

This was at least partially due to the transformation of American race relations that became visible as more and more so-called "contrabands"[4] poured into Union camps and hospitals seeking shelter and work. The hospital quickly became an interracial "contact zone"[5] complete with the social tensions that the concept entails. When on January 1, 1863, these black men and women celebrated the Emancipation Proclamation, many white female nurses sympathized wholeheartedly. Yet, while many nurses were abolitionists, they did not necessarily support the notion of full racial equality. Like their sons, husbands, and fathers, white Northern women tended to oppose the formation of black regiments because allowing African Americans to serve would make it impossible to deny them full political representation once the war was over.[6] In this situation, white feminists in particular faced an ideological dilemma: Wary of demanding full political rights for African Americans, they nevertheless jumped on the bandwagon of emancipation to remind their fellow citizens that white women were still waiting to be "freed" from an ideology that limited their social mobility and political options. In light of these often unconscious ambivalences and social fears, it is hardly surprising that the feminist debate on how

---

[4] The term was originally applied to runaway slaves from Confederate territory who were not returned to their owners because the Union army considered them "[g]oods deemed to benefit an opponent and therefore subject to seizure" (Garrison 55). The object status expressed in this definition was, of course, problematic: "contraband" labor was used to the point of exploitation in Union camps and hospitals. In the course of the war and Reconstruction, the term became synonymous with all former slaves (cf. Gerteis).

[5] I have borrowed this term from Mary Louise Pratt.

[6] The formation of black regiments had been a core motivation for Abraham Lincoln's Emancipation Proclamation. Cf. Foner 48-49.

far women could—and should—go was linked, somewhat uncomfortably, to negotiations regarding the place of African Americans in American society.

The textual site for this debate was the nursing narrative, a literary fad whose popularity went back to Florence Nightingale's 1859 *Notes on Nursing*. During the American Civil War this essentially autobiographical mode appeared in a variety of genres, including letters, essays, and full-fledged narratives, some of which merged non-fictional and fictional elements. According to an estimate by Schultz, "66 women wrote monographs about military relief work and 42 of them sought publication" ("Performing Genres" 78, note).[7] If all of these women aimed at a fuller acknowledgement of female hospital workers, some also employed the nursing narrative to discuss more general questions: What should be the political consequences of the fact that both white women *and* African Americans had sacrificed their health and (sometimes) lives for their love of the nation? And what was their future place within the social configuration?

Louisa May Alcott and the Silent Scream of the Isolated Nurse

That Louisa May Alcott should struggle at all with the notion of a truly egalitarian, multiracial democracy is somewhat surprising. The daughter of the famous reformer and anti-slavery activist Bronson Alcott and his politically active wife, Abigail May, Louisa May Alcott not only opposed slavery but also flirted with the notion of her own "African" traits. As Elizabeth Young has argued, the author described herself "in mixed-race terms" in her private correspondence, thereby making "an attempt to escape the constraints of white femininity" in her self-representation (80). *Hospital Sketches*, too, relies on this logic when its narrator, Tribulation Periwinkle, construes African Americans as "other" in order to "project her own unruly desires while safely displacing them elsewhere" (Young 82).

---

[7]   Schultz adds that among the 42, "11 were former Confederate, 31 former Union citizens" ("Performing Genres" 78).

Interestingly, Alcott was quite aware that emancipation posed a challenge to this mechanism and concept: The abolition of slavery was a specifically African American experience that could not easily be appropriated to a white woman's psychological needs. *Hospital Sketches* solves this problem by pursuing a two-fold strategy: In a much-quoted scene, it acknowledges the newly won agency and individual independence of a group of freedmen who celebrate the Emancipation Proclamation, while at the same time it represents them as a "site of psychic release" (Young 82). Significantly, the group of African Americans is not at the center of this description; the focus of the scene is the author's alter ego, Nurse Periwinkle, who watches from a window above: "As the bells rung midnight, I electrified my room-mate by dancing out of bed, throwing up the window, and flapping my handkerchief, with a feeble cheer, in answer to the shout of a group of colored men in the street below" (*HS* 82).

On the one hand, the historical event causes the abolitionist to temporarily shake off the credo of white self-discipline: Periwinkle throws open the (literal and metaphorical) window that cuts her off from the "real world" of historical change and—with a "feeble cheer"—grants herself a brief moment of activity in which she is, significantly, "acting black." As Young has argued, this was "a would-be proclamation of emancipation for Alcott herself' (82). At the same time, however, the story insists almost painfully on the spatial distance and social hierarchy between the two groups, thereby preserving the white woman's female respectability. Flapping her handkerchief like an onlooker on the mezzanine, the nurse is staged as a privileged member of an enthusiastic white audience that has made the performance below possible in the first place. The image represents a deeply ambiguous idea of racial inclusion; while, on the one hand, it acknowledges and embraces the "shout" as a unique expression of African American culture,[8] on the other hand, it emphasizes the white woman's superior self-control: After all, she manages to muffle her cheer and stay where she is. In what is essentially

---

[8]   Also known as a "ring-shout," this ritual was very often described during the war years as Northern whites for the first time came into contact with slaves from the South. During a shout, participants worship God by moving in a circle, stomping their feet, and clapping their hands.

an exercise in female self-restraint, the nurse validates the racial and
gendered norms of antebellum society. What this means with regard to
an egalitarian society, however, is ultimately left open: It was up to
American readers to draw their own conclusions from the intercultural
encounter.

What must have attracted the reader's attention as much then as it
does now is the white woman's "feeble cheer." In some ways more
pronounced than the freedmen's "shout,"[9] it is also, I argue, a cry for
help. Periwinkle is a sort of prisoner in the room above the street after
the "youngest surgeon in the hospital," a "paternal" yet "kind-hearted
little gentleman who seemed to consider [her] a frail young blossom"
(*HS* 66) sends the coughing and feverish Periwinkle off duty, thereby
returning her to the state of "uselessness" that had made her join the
army in white in the first place. And yet she is not locked in, in the
actual sense of the term: The true metaphorical illness that keeps
Periwinkle from joining the men below is her internalization of
Victorian norms of female behavior. Framed by the window, the
memorable image of the nurse who flaps a handkerchief as she emits her
muted cheer highlights white women's involuntary uselessness in an era
of otherwise massive political change.

Hospital Sketches therefore depicts not only a woman's triumphant
victory over her "unruly" impulses but also the pain of recognition:
Distinguishing sharply between the before and after of her trip into the
"real world" of the Civil War hospital, the protagonist learns that her
expectations were mere illusions. The idealized hospital that Periwinkle
initially imagined as a space where she "would be in charge, not only
caring for male soldiers but also governing race relations" (Young 93)
turns out to welcome women as an unpaid workforce only: Periwinkle
learns that she is ultimately excluded from what David Quigley has
termed the "democratic game" of the 1860s and 1870s (ix). When the
nurse's father eventually shows up at the hospital to re-integrate his
metaphorically invalid daughter into the paternal household, a defiant
yet obedient "Miss Periwinkle" takes refuge in the nineteenth-century
realm of female self-realization, her imagination: "The next hospital I

---

[9]   This is particularly true if one considers that the ring-shout did not
necessarily include shouting. It is possible that Alcott was not aware of this.

enter will, I hope, be one for the colored regiments, as they seem to be proving their right to the admiration and kind offices of their white relations, who owe them so large a debt, a little part of which I shall be proud to pay" (*HS* 96).

That Periwinkle imagines herself as the freedmen's most devoted servant is a concession to Victorian gender norms, albeit one that, due to its racial component, aims at raising objections among its white readership. By declaring a white woman a servant of black men, *Hospital Sketches* provocatively highlights the extent to which Victorian ideology had turned white women into "prisoners" of ideals of self-sacrifice and servitude.

In her further Civil War oeuvre, Alcott continued to develop the trope of the hospital as the natural home for America's self-sacrificing white women in the contact zone.[10] The best-known of these texts is a story, originally published as "The Brothers" in 1863 and then re-titled "My Contraband" in 1869,[11] about a white nurse and her "contraband" helpmate that is essentially a continuation of *Hospital Sketches*.[12] Here the reader learns what "Nurse Periwinkle" would have done if her father had not prevented her from following her impulse to cross the racial divide: Cast as the similarly self-regulated "Nurse Dane," Alcott's protagonist manages to suppress her obvious erotic attraction to a freedman as she convinces him to join the Union Army.

In both *Hospital Sketches* and "The Brothers / My Contraband," Alcott, in other words, relied on the nursing narrative to refute the idea that a True Woman put her purity at risk once she left the safe bounds of the domestic sphere. If in *Hospital Sketches* the hospital was still

---

[10] Among the titles are "The Brothers" (1863, re-titled "My Contraband" in 1869) and "Nelly's Hospital" (1865).

[11] My analysis relies on a copy of the 1869 edition, information about which can be found in the bibliography. Both versions are identical. For details on the publishing history of "The Brothers / My Contraband," cf. Alcott, *The Journals* 124, note.

[12] As Young has argued, Alcott's stories are "related versions of a revitalized body politic" that seeks to overcome the cultural hierarchy between male doctor and female nurse (*Disarming* 93). Yet, instead of interpreting them merely as *variations* on a theme I understand their creation as a *systematic* problem-solving strategy.

predominantly white, "The Brothers / My Contraband" depicts it as the racially and politically heterogeneous place that it actually was. By placing a young white woman in the social laboratory of the wartime hospital, where she was confronted with a broad array of men from different classes, races, and ethnicities, Alcott indirectly claimed a woman's right to influence society through national healing. She did not, however, severely challenge the notion of True Womanhood.

Sarah Emma Edmonds and a Cross-Dresser's Response

Some of Alcott's contemporary readers may have heard the muted cry for help that is always an aspect of Alcott's narratives about what Young has termed the "civil wars within women" (70). Sarah Emma Edmonds, I argue, responded to Alcott's desperation by challenging the spatial prerequisites of nursing without questioning the paradigm of compassionate care. In *Nurse and Spy*, in other words, the female prisoner is set free.

The historical Edmonds was an extremely mobile figure. Born in Nova Scotia, Canada, she was raised as the son her father never had (Lee 56).[13] By the time Edmonds ran away from home to work as a milliner she was not only well-equipped with the performative means to embody the role of a man but had also learned that female self-realization and survival depended on the strategic transgression of nineteenth-century gender norms. When her tyrannical father tracked her down to marry her off to a man far older than herself, she fled again, this time across the border to the United States. There she made a living selling Bibles door-to-door, conducting her business while posing as a man, "Franklin Thompson"—a role that allowed her a degree of security and personal freedom.[14] In 1861, Edmonds (alias "Private Frank

---

[13] Elizabeth D. Leonard offers a slightly different explanation for Edmonds's "male" behavior, claiming that "as was typical for nineteenth-century farm girls, she and her sisters participated in all the same activities and performed all the same chores as her brother: tending to the animals, chopping wood and milking cows, planting, harvesting, and so forth" (*All the Daring* 170).

[14] Laura Leedy Gansler, who has written a biography of Edmonds, suggests that "Emma discovered that not only could she pass herself off as a young man,

Thompson") was accepted into the Union Army as a male nurse,[15] later becoming a regimental mail carrier and, as she claims in her novel, a spy for the Union army.[16] After several years during which she supposedly adopted no less than eleven different personae, including the roles of nurse, male soldier, African American "contraband" (male and female), Irish peddler woman, Canadian boy, Union spy, and four others (including the role of dead soldier), in 1864 she crossed the line once again to take up the occupation of writer. This, however, was not a voluntary act: Edmonds deserted from the military for fear of being detected as a woman. She was as successful an author as she had been a salesman: First published in 1864 under the title *Unsexed; or, the Female Soldier* and subtitled *The Thrilling Adventures, Experiences, and Escapes of a Woman, as Nurse, Spy and Scout, in Hospitals, Camps, and Battle-Fields*,[17] her novel became an immediate marketing success. The

---

but that she was happy doing it. Life as the 'enemy' was not too bad. She relished the freedom it gave her to go where she wanted, do what she wanted, earn what she could, without the nagging constraints society placed on an unattached woman" (12). More scholarly sources on Edmonds include Hall; Lee; and Fladeland. Cf. also Leonard, *All the Daring* 170-81.

[15] She was one of several hundred women who passed as men in both armies. Cf. Sizer 114-25 as well as Bullough and Bullough 157-64.

[16] As Gansler has pointed out, there is historical evidence that Edmonds did spend considerable time working as a spy. Yet it remains unclear whether she really went behind enemy lines in the various guises that she describes in her novel. A number of her tales have been "contradicted by known facts," at least in part, and "some of her claims are simply too audacious to be believed" (Afterword 221). It is neither within the scope nor is it the aim of this paper to provide closure regarding this issue.

[17] Subsequent editions appeared under different titles such as *Soldier, Nurse, and Spy in the Union Army* (1864 and 1865). This article relies on the 1865 reprint of the 1864 W. S. Williams Hartford edition that (in an aberration of the actual title) was brought out under the title *Soldier, Nurse and Spy in the Union Army* (2006). The 1865 Hartford "original" can also be found online at http://www.archive.org/details/nurseandspyinun03edmogoog. In terms of content, the editions are all identical.

Regarding the editorial history of the novel, cf. the scholarly edition of the memoir, edited by Elizabeth D. Leonard, as well as Schultz, "Performing Genres" 78.

1865 edition of *Nurse and Spy* sold a reported 175,000 copies, making it a bestseller for its time.[18] Although poorly edited, the number of copies sold of Edmonds's presumably autobiographical account was "three times greater than any nursing narrative" (Schultz, "Performing Genres" 78). Just like Alcott, in other words, the Canadian immigrant seems to have successfully fulfilled the cultural needs of at least one generation. Yet if in Alcott's far more cautious narrative the nurse resists her unruly impulses by holding on to the norms of True Womanhood, Edmonds's heroine confides that she is not only a true American patriot but "naturally fond of adventure, a little ambitious and a good deal romantic" (*NaS* 51).[19] Ten years younger than Alcott and far more independent of the cultural norms and debates that the New Englander had imbibed,[20] the immigrant author took the credo that "all men and women are created equal," first formulated in the 1848 Seneca Falls *Declaration of Sentiments,* to surprisingly radical ends.

Providing a backdrop of chaos and social disintegration "owing to a combination of circumstances entirely beyond the control" of those officially in charge (*NaS* 6-7), the Civil War hospital figures as an ideal starting point for Edmonds's radical endeavor. Looking back on her experiences, the narrating "I" remembers the hospital as a machine that deprived her of the basic categories upon which her identity was built. Described as the "most important and most interesting" labor in her "life's history" (*NaS* 165), work in the hospital reduces the white, Canadian, and Anglican woman to the fundamentals of human existence: "There is no cessation, and yet it is strange that the sight of all this suffering and death does not affect me more. I am simply eyes, ears, hands and feet" (*NaS* 23). In a somewhat subversive reversal of the

---

[18] Fladeland 562. The first edition of *Uncle Tom's Cabin* sold a reported 300,000 copies.

[19] The notion of pleasure is glossed over by the apologetic "Publisher's Notice" that links Edmonds's masquerades to the "purest motives and most praiseworthy patriotism." The "Publisher's Notice" acknowledges "cultural anxiety regarding a woman disguised as a man" by reminding readers of the reasons that made her temporarily switch identities (cf. Laffrado 164-65).

[20] As Young puts it, Alcott had grown up under a "self-regulating pedagogy" that "re-wrote the implicitly male credo of Emersonian self-reliance as female self-denial" (77).

language of amputations and loss that marks most nursing narratives, the heroine is symbolically freed from the deficits associated with the female gender, such as frailty and mental inferiority. Symbolically renewed, she is able to proceed wherever she wants to go.

Interestingly, the function of the hospital as a locus of symbolic renewal also extends to the racial other. Unlike Alcott, who could not imagine black women in the South possessing individual agency,[21] Edmonds explicitly acknowledges an African American freedwoman as an active agent of history. This woman, who still identifies as a slave, is celebrated by white Union soldiers, whom she offers "packages of tea, cans of fruit, pears and peaches, lint, linen for bandages, and pocket handkerchiefs," as one of their own race: They "looked with wonder and admiration on the old colored woman, and soon a hundred voices cried out 'God bless you, aunty! You are the only white woman we have seen since we came to Winchester'" (*NaS* 173-74). While the equation of whiteness with patriotism, humanitarian values, and Christianity is of course problematic from today's point of view, the scene was exceptionally radical even among the abolitionist literature of the Civil War era.

Yet although Edmonds attaches a particular moral dimension to the hospital, this is not the only place where a woman can nurse a sickly nation. Once her heroine has shed her nursing uniform she nevertheless remains the "selfless" person the hospital made her: The multifaceted, patriotic spy approaches her changing environments with the motivation to help and care for the weak. Thus, when in one of her later roles she "procure[s] the dress and outfit of an Irish female peddler, following the army, selling cakes, pies, etc., together with a considerable amount of brogue, and a set of Irish phrases, which did much toward characterizing me as one of the 'rale ould stock of bog-trotters'" (*NaS* 64), the nurse-turned-Union spy simply expands the former nurse's sphere of influence beyond the hospital ward. Upon entering a deserted farmhouse, she

---

[21] This even holds true with regard to "An Hour" (1864), the only one of Alcott's Civil War stories that centers on a female African American protagonist. The rebellious slave woman Milly eventually acts under the soothing influence of her white benefactor. The reader never learns what becomes of her in the end.

encounters a "rebel" soldier "who [lies] upon a straw-tick on the floor in a helpless condition" (*NaS* 66). The encounter immediately eliminates the many differences between the two, making room for a declaration of humanitarian commitment:

> It is strange how sickness and disease disarm our antipathy and remove our prejudice. There lay before me an enemy to the Government for which I was daily and willingly exposing my life and suffering unspeakable privation; he may have been the very man who took deadly aim at my friend and sent the cruel bullet through his temple . . . but [I] looked upon him only as an unfortunate, suffering man . . . and I longed to restore him to health and Strength [sic]; not considering that the very health and strength which I wished to secure for him would be employed against the cause which I had espoused. (*NaS* 67)

The scene is one of the most memorable in the narrative, reminiscent of the famous fourth chapter in *Hospital Sketches,* where Periwinkle watches at the deathbed of her favorite patient, the "brave Virginia blacksmith" John (*HS* 65),[22] yet far more ideologically explicit. Interestingly, the focus is neither on the nurse's identification with the concept of True Womanhood nor on patriotism as the driving force behind her actions: Throughout the narrative, Edmonds follows the higher calling of a Christian God who preaches the love of neighbor.[23]

For all the differences in focus, allusions to *Hospital Sketches* are a constant presence in *Nurse and Spy.* Telling her story in a straightforward and lively manner, and staging herself as the type of nurse who "was not in the habit of going among the patients with a long, doleful face," instead making "cheerfulness" her "motto" (*NaS* 24), Edmonds's alter ego must have reminded nineteenth-century readers of the equally cheerful Tribulation Periwinkle, whose self-descriptions relied on similar word choice. Yet, in addition to such indirect connections, there are also direct references to *Hospital Sketches:*

> As I sat in my tent, roasting or shivering as the case might be, I took a strange pleasure in watching the long trains of six mule teams which

---

[22]   For an in-depth analysis of this scene in Alcott's work, cf. Young 90-91.

[23]   As I have elaborated elsewhere, Edmonds was a patriot in a very American, Christian sense: her aim was to establish the kingdom of God on earth.

were constantly passing and repassing within a few rods of my tent. As "Miss Periwinkle" remarks, there are several classes of mules. (*NaS* 30)

Such references to Alcott may have added "a measure of respectability" to Edmonds's "otherwise lurid tale" (Schultz, "Performing" 78),[24] and they may also have helped market the book: Edmonds was a very talented businesswoman who knew how to cater to the tastes of her audience (Gansler 12). More importantly, however, there is an intellectual dimension that marks all of Edmonds's references to Alcott. As Laura Leedy Gansler reminds us, Sarah Emma came from a rural working-class background but was nevertheless "highly educated" (28).[25] Edmonds's allusions to and quotes from *Hospital Sketches* may therefore be read as a Canadian's conscious intervention into the worldview of her American "sister." *Nurse and Spy,* I argue, initiated a system of internal and external references that paid homage to Alcott but at the same time challenged some problematic aspects of her ideology. The first example of such an intervention is the scene quoted above, where the "roasting or shivering" narrator of *Nurse and Spy* is reminded of a scene from *Hospital Sketches*, which she then quotes at length. While the story itself is identical in both books, its meaning is considerably changed by its recontextualization in Edmonds's presumably autobiographical text.

In *Hospital Sketches* the episode is described from the perspective of a nurse who feels like a prisoner in her own institution, the hospital. Commanded by a well-meaning doctor to stay in her bedroom, a sickly Periwinkle feels socially alienated as she views a street scene unfolding

---

[24] According to at least one critic, the 1863 edition of *Hospital Sketches* "allowed more Northerners than Southerners to serve without fear of reprisals" (Schultz, *Women at the Front* 53). On the other hand, *Hospital Sketches* was not without its critics: as Alcott remarks in her apologetic "Preface" to the postwar edition of *Hospital Sketches,* she had been heavily criticized for the light-hearted, tomboyish, ironic tone of her narrative and its perceived lack of Christian piety and rhetorical modesty (*HS* i).

[25] Edmonds's mother had insisted that she receive an education and had sent Emma and her siblings to a small parish school. Later on, Edmonds became an avid reader and bookseller, an occupation that gave her the opportunity to remain abreast of the literary developments of the era (Gansler 28).

beneath her window. She is particularly taken aback by the visible "uselessness" of the women, who "were so extinguished in three story bonnets, with overhanging balconies of flowers, that their charms were obscured." The men who participate in this "mammoth masquerade" "[do] the picturesque" with their

> Spanish hats, scarlet lined riding cloaks, swords and sashes, high boots and bright spurs, beards and mustaches, which made plain faces comely, and comely faces heroic; these vanities of the flesh transformed our butchers, bakers, and candlestick makers into gallant riders of gaily caparisoned horses, much handsomer than themselves; and dozens of such figures were constantly prancing by, with private prickings of spurs, for the benefit of the perambulating flower-bed. (*HS* 78)

The nurse feels doubly excluded here: As a True Woman at heart, she cannot identify with the immodest "vanities of the flesh" below her window, yet at the same time she is denied her favorite, morally superior occupation of compassionate care: "Being forbidden to meddle with fleshly arms and legs, I solaced myself by mending cotton ones, and, as I sat sewing at my window, watched the moving panorama that passed below . . . ." It is in this mood that she finds "especial delight" in a group of mules that passes below her window: While the situation of the "odd little beasts" that draw the army wagons is akin to her own, their "hopping like frogs through the stream of mud that gently rolled along the street" (*HS* 79) restores the nurse's sense of self as a member of a superior civilization.[26]

While the former passage is slightly different in *Nurse and Spy,* the following was virtually stolen by Edmonds; she did not alter it in any way:

> The coquettish mule had small feet, a nicely trimmed tassel of a tail, perked up ears, and seemed much given to little tosses of the head, affected skips and prances; and, if he wore the bells, or were bedizzened with a bit of finery, put on as many airs as any belle. The moral mule was a stout, hard-working creature, always tugging with all his might; often pulling away after the rest had stopped, laboring under the

---

[26] The racial implications that echo through this scene will be analyzed in more detail later in this essay.

conscientious delusion that food for the entire army depended upon his private exertions. I respected this style of mule; and, had I possessed a juicy cabbage, would have pressed it upon him, with thanks for his excellent example. The historical mule was a melodramatic quadruped, prone to startling humanity by erratic leaps, and wild plunges, much shaking of his stubborn head, and lashing out of his vicious heels; now and then falling flat, and apparently dying *a la* Forrest[27]: a gasp—a squirm—a flop, and so on, till the street was well blocked up, the drivers all swearing like demons in bad hats, and the chief actor's circulation decidedly quickened by every variety of kick, cuff, jerk and haul. When the last breath seemed to have left his body, and "Doctors were in vain," a sudden resurrection took place; and if ever a mule laughed with scornful triumph, that was the beast, as he leisurely rose, gave a comfortable shake; and, calmly regarding the excited crowd seemed to say—"A hit! a decided hit! for the stupidest of animals has bamboozled a dozen men. Now, then! what are you stopping the way for?" The pathetic mule was, perhaps, the most interesting of all; for, though he always seemed to be the smallest, thinnest, weakest of the six, the postillion, with big boots, long-tailed coat, and heavy whip, was sure to bestride this one, who struggled feebly along, head down, coat muddy and rough, eye spiritless and sad, his very tail a mortified stump, and the whole beast a picture of meek misery, fit to touch a heart of stone. The jovial mule was a roly poly, happy-go-lucky little piece of horse-flesh, taking everything easily, from cudgeling to caressing; strolling along with a roguish twinkle of the eye, and, if the thing were possible, would have had his hands in his pockets, and whistled as he went. If there ever chanced to be an apple core, a stray turnip, or wisp of hay, in the gutter, this Mark Tapley[28] was sure to find it, and none of his mates seemed to begrudge him his bite. I suspected this fellow was the peacemaker, confidant and friend of all the others, for he had a sort of "Cheer-up,-old-boy,-I'll-pull-you-through" look, which was exceedingly engaging. (*NaS* 31 and *HS* 79)

If Alcott inserted this passage to celebrate the nurse's imperturbable sense of rebellion, she could not hide from her readers the fact that such

---

[27] This is an allusion to Edwin Forest, the famous New York actor, who was most successful during the 1840s.

[28] A figure in Charles Dickens's *The Life and Adventures of Martin Chuzzlewit* (1843).

musings did not free her alter ego from her state of imposed passivity. Since, as a rule, mules are not able to reproduce, they were a perfect choice to represent the powerlessness of those whose wish for individual self-realization was continuously limited from without.[29]

As I hinted earlier, *Hospital Sketches* also racialized the idea of a disciplinary regime that linked the nurse/prisoner with mules: Reeling up bandages ("cotton ones"), the nurse-turned-patient attends to the raw material associated with slavery and also partakes in the daily routine of African American hospital workers. The link between nurse, mules, and slavery becomes more explicit when, in the book's next passage, Periwinkle describes what she calls "the genuine article" as "the sort of creatures generations of slavery have made them" (*HS* 80). And yet the connection between a Victorian woman's lack of agency and the slave system is made through a playful allusion rather than an immediate analogy: Through the metaphorical abstraction of the mule episode, Alcott adapted the antebellum formula of a white woman's "slave-like" existence to the new sensibilities of the post-emancipation era.

And yet American readers could easily recognize the racial component of the mule episode. As Robert E. Hemenway has pointed out, African Americans in the South used the term "mule" allegorically: Not only were these animals "bought and sold by massa" and "forced to work long hours just as slaves were," but they were also individualized, stubborn, strong, and unpredictable (222).[30] Alcott significantly translated this African American allegory into the language of white abolitionist feminism: After indirectly aligning the cotton-mending white woman's limited options with chattel slavery, Periwinkle distances herself from the "colored brothers and sisters" below her window. While she finds them "more interesting" than the "officers, ladies, mules, or pigs" on parade, she describes them in condescending terms. Slavery, she argues (in keeping with the racist discourse of her era), has made them "obsequious, trickish, lazy and ignorant." At the

---

[29] Alcott herself was, on the one hand, secretly fascinated with Thoreau's "On the Duty of Civil Disobedience," but, on the other hand, promoted female self-sacrifice and a disciplining of "unruly" impulses. Cf. Elbert, especially 151-53.

[30] He bases this observation on Zora Neale Hurston's research on the term "mule" in American slave society.

same time she represents them as a childlike race—"kind-hearted, merry-tempered, quick to feel"—fit to be the objects of white benevolence (*HS* 80). In the course of this long and multifaceted passage, in other words, the disempowered nurse manages to build up her largely demolished sense of agency through a fantasy of racial uplift: By metaphorically "grasp[ing] the black [hand]," Periwinkle represents what she calls "this great struggle for the liberty of both the races" according to the established hierarchy of superior whiteness.

Edmonds chooses a significantly different setting for this scene. While she, too, is a nurse here and equally ill, she is not cut off from her surroundings; on the contrary, in her function as a field nurse she is subject to the "breeze from the adjacent swamps and marshes." Feeling "the effects of the miasma which came floating" toward her from a hostile environment, bringing with it "fever and ague," the white nurse emerges from the "Virginia mud" as an independent, masculinized, and rough-tongued tent-dweller who takes "a strange pleasure" in the unfolding scene (*NaS* 30). As we will see, the "pleasure" of Edmonds-the-observer-figure-and-narrator is also the "pleasure" of Edmonds-the-writer, who watches, and eventually appropriates, Alcott's metaphorical mules.

Before taking a closer look at how Edmonds renders the scene, it is important to understand that in *Nurse and Spy* race is figured as a performative category: In a particularly memorable scene, the cross-dressing narrator turns into an African American man simply by the application of some coal, nitrate of silver, and a wig:[31]

> I purchased a suit of contraband clothing, real plantation style, and then I went to a barber and had my hair sheared close to my head.
>
> Next came the coloring process—head, face, neck, hands, and arms were colored black as any African, and then, to complete my contraband costume, I required a wig of real negro wool. But how and where was it to be found? There was no such thing at the Fortress, and none short of Washington. Happily I found the mail-boat was about to start, and hastened on board, and finding a Postmaster with whom I was

---

[31] The scene alludes to minstrelsy yet at the same time reads the tradition against the grain: nineteenth-century minstrelsy was an overwhelmingly male tradition of travesty (cf. Garber 276).

acquainted, I stepped forward to speak to him, forgetting my contraband appearance, and was saluted with:

"Well, Massa Cuff – what will you have?"

Said I: "Massa send me to you wid dis yere money for you to fotch him a darkie wig from Washington."

"What does he want a darkie wig?" asked the Postmaster.

"No matter, dat's my orders; guess it's for some 'noiterin' business."

"Oh, for reconnoitering you mean; all right old fellow, I will bring it, tell him." (*NaS* 45)

By reducing the need for camouflage to a minimum of items, the scene brims with the irony of an immigrant observer: According to Edmonds, the nineteenth-century American mind is easily deceived by a set of stereotypes.[32] If, as postulated by the reception theorist Wolfgang Iser, reading is a process of meaning-making based on the effort to integrate new passages into the experiences one has already had in the course of reading a particular text (and vice versa), it is safe to say that the implied reader of *Nurse and Spy* was expected to look at the narrative's various characters with a heightened sense of suspicion: nineteenth-century readers, I argue, had not only learned to "interpret *Nurse and Spy* as a fiction" (Schultz, "Performing Genres" 75), but they also enjoyed its fundamentally performative qualities. What the cross-dressed spy says on one occasion about herself, in other words, was understood to be true about the text as a whole: "I was not what my appearance indicated" (*NaS* 67).

In 1864, *Hospital Sketches* was so popular that Edmonds's textual appropriations could hardly have escaped American readers, but the text's hidden "identity" can only be disclosed through a close look at its different framing. Edmonds appears very unlike the sickly Periwinkle: While the latter was "forbidden to meddle with [the] fleshly arms and legs" of white and black men, nobody could keep the former from "visiting the contrabands," who "occupied a long row of board buildings near the fort" (*NaS* 29). After listening to an "old colored man" who

---

[32] The diary of Hannah Ropes is a good example of the era's obsession with such categories: overwhelmed by the difficulties she had with her male stewards, she sought refuge in anti-Semitism, regional prejudice, and anti-immigrant rhetoric (cf. Ropes 72).

preaches among the freedmen, the nurse, in the manner of a true soldier, returns to the fragile structure of her tent and nonchalantly accepts her illness as a nurse's badge of courage.[33] Unlike Nurse Periwinkle (whose soldiering qualities are merely rhetorical) Edmonds truly qualifies as a soldier. (The cross-dresser will in fact take this military role in the narrative's subsequent chapter).

By emphasizing that the mules "were constantly passing and repassing within a few rods of my tent" (*NaS* 30), the textual image constructs a close proximity between observer and observed, both of whom manage to preserve their individuality in a disciplinary context. Given the fact that Alcott relies on windows to represent the separation between the secluded world of white Victorian women and the public sphere, this is a rather significant alteration. While watching the mules, Edmonds is gripped with a "strange pleasure" (*NaS* 30) that differs from the "especial delight" that Periwinkle experienced when recognizing the limits of her own agency in the controlled and ultimately inconsequential rebelliousness of the mules. While Alcott's novel had cast white nineteenth-century women as inherently masochistic, Edmonds's "pleasure" derives from the triumph of rebellion over the human effort to discipline it. Edmonds leaves no doubt about the allegorical function of the mule episode; there is no magical shifting here between rebellious animals, white women, and slaves. Instead, the paragraph aligns the mules with black agency and assures readers that eventually their rebelliousness will succeed. The passage, significantly, is preceded by a poem about interracial brotherhood and solidarity. Inspired by a Christian theme, it is devoid of the condescension that Periwinkle attaches to *her* "brothers and sisters":

> Resolved, although my brother be a slave,
> And poor and black, he is my brother still;
> Can I, o'er trampled "institutions," save
> That brother from the chain and lash, I will. (NaS 30)

Nurse and Spy, in other words, does not manipulate the slavery metaphor to criticize the patriarchal structures with which Alcott is primarily concerned. By framing the mule episode between, on the one

---

[33] Regarding this trope in *HS*, cf. Young 87.

hand, celebratory descriptions of a charismatic African American preacher and an antislavery poem and, on the other, a story about a "faithful colored boy" who supports the Union in "most approved military style" (*NaS* 31), Edmonds's version emphasizes black agency. It is through her own example that she encourages white women to move beyond a narrow definition of nursing and to reconsider their options in an environment where categories like race, gender, ethnicity, and religious denomination fade in the face of destruction, suffering, and death.[34]

Interestingly, however, Edmonds also attaches a warning to this depiction of female freedom. In the second episode that I want to introduce here, Edmonds draws on *Hospital Sketches* and also on Harriet Beecher Stowe's *Uncle Tom's Cabin*[35] to remind white readers that a true democracy depends, as stated in the *Declaration of Independence*, on the "consent of the governed."

As Elizabeth Young has pointed out, *Uncle Tom's Cabin* "makes an appearance, as passing experience, extended reference, or implicit intertext" in "the majority of women's writings about the war" (24). Pro-Confederate and pro-Union authors competed in referencing the Topsy figure and Stowe herself, using both (to different ends) as "templates for new forms of national allegory" (Young 59). *Hospital Sketches*, too, was inspired by Stowe's "fictional creation of a feminized world"; yet in Alcott's novella the tension between female morality and the heroine's "topsy-turvy self" (Young 70) grows to larger, more dramatic dimensions.

Critically speaking, Alcott's abolitionist message relies on the same "suffocating and racist sentimentalism" that pervades *Uncle Tom's Cabin* (Young 70).[36] In the New Englander's nightmarish vision of an

---

[34] That these representations of African Americans are stereotypical as well is beyond question, but in light of Edmonds's overall performative strategy it would be too easy to read this as a straightforward romanticization of the freedmen. In its function as intertextual commentary the passage at least destabilizes Alcott's representation of African Americans as fundamentally helpless and dependent.

[35] Regarding the connections between Alcott and Stowe, cf. Young 69-72.

[36] Young refers to the "less sympathetic readers" of Alcott here, such as James Baldwin, who criticized both Stowe and the author of *Little Women* for their

interracial democracy (where African American women are left ubiquitously absent),[37] "black" traits become synonymous with a lack of "civilization" among men in general. Thus, when Periwinkle takes a day off to visit the Senate chamber (after the politicians have left) she finds "the Speaker's chair occupied by a colored gentleman of ten; while two others were on their legs, having a hot debate over the cornball question, as they gathered the waste paper strewn about the floor into bags; and several white members played leap-frog over the desks" (76).

Edmonds, too, readily ridicules the male members of an imaginary Senate (after confirming her admiration for the generation of the founders) but carefully avoids racial specification. She eschews allusions to future African American senators as quarreling children and instead shifts the reader's attention to a less hypothetical field, focusing on the recently freed slaves who seek shelter before the gates of the Senate. Describing them as "saucy, lazy, degraded creature[s]," Edmonds seems to have borrowed her vocabulary from Alcott, whose heroine was "tormented" by the sight of the "degraded and forsaken" freedpeople, many of them "lazy boys and saucy girls" (*HS* 81). Edmonds then introduces a well-known white character in equally stereotypical terms:

> I found a young lady there, from the North, who had come to Washington with the intention of nursing the sick soldiers, but her sympathies being divided between sick America and down trodden Africa, she decides to teach the contrabands instead. She seemed delighted with her employment, and the little black faces were beaming with joy as they gathered around her to receive instruction. (*NaS* 106)

The vocabulary hews closely to that of *Hospital Sketches;* nineteenth-century readers could easily identify the "young lady" as Nurse Periwinkle turned teacher among the freedmen. They also understood the allusions to Aunt Ophelia (the iconographic abolitionist Yankee cousin in Stowe's famous novel) that mark the dialogue that follows. By

---

racist self-righteousness. As I argued earlier, there is good reason to extend this criticism to *Hospital Sketches,* too (Young 70).

[37] I discuss this issue in a chapter on *Hospital Sketches* in my forthcoming book-length study of the debate about democracy during Reconstruction.

projecting Alcott's potentially disempowered nurse outside of the confines of the hospital and by merging this figure with an older image of white women's moral imperialism, *Nurse and Spy* confronts Periwinkle's naïve abolitionist fantasies with the complexities of American race relations after the Emancipation Proclamation.[38] In Edmonds's ironic commentary on *Hospital Sketches,* the narrated "I" of *Nurse and Spy* stands next to the Northern reformer and eventually takes over the conversation with the freedmen. This is how Edmonds stages the encounter:

> One colored man stood listening to the questions which were being asked [by the nurse] and answered [by other freedmen], and looked as if he would like to give in his testimony. I [Edmonds] turned to him, and asked:
> "How is it with you? Do you think you can take care of yourself, now that you have no master to look after you?" "Gosh a-mighty, guess I can! Ben taking car' of self and massa too for dis fifteen year. Guess I can take car' of dis nig all alone now." (*NaS* 106)

In this version of the famous Aunt Ophelia-Topsy conversation, a white observer figure (who has lived among a group of "contrabands" long enough to be considered an insider to their experience) interrupts the teacher-pupil constellation by asking a significantly different question. She thereby triggers the expression of an "original," "authentic"[39] African American viewpoint that ridicules the female reformer's benevolent discourse. While *Nurse and Spy* does not reject Alcott's civilizing mission *tout court*, it cautions its white readership not to

---

[38] While in *Hospital Sketches* the heroine merely *dreams* of nursing black soldiers, she actually *becomes* a teacher among Southern "contrabands" in "The Brothers." This, however, is merely mentioned in a subordinate clause toward the end of the story. Whether Edmonds had read "The Brothers" (or "My Contraband") and was aware of the sentence remains open to speculation.

[39] I place "authentic" and "original" in quotation marks to acknowledge that Edmonds's use of an "authentic" African American vernacular is of course stereotypical. And yet, the scene does not suggest a different interpretation: The fact that Edmonds interrupts an established white discourse on racial uplift is a strong indication of the author's critical viewpoint.

deprive African Americans of their sense of agency. As *Nurse and Spy* argues elsewhere, "colored men" did not need to be "uplifted" since their admission to the army had permitted them "to assume the privileges of rational beings." The same applied to "the negro woman" who, "as manifested in the hospital, is a perfect sample of the devotion of the contrabands, male and female, to the Union cause" (*NaS* 174). By explicitly acknowledging the patriotic contribution of both freedmen and freedwomen, *Nurse and Spy* challenges the sentimental narrative about the "rescue of the race" that figured so prominently in *Uncle Tom's Cabin, Hospital Sketches,* and most of Alcott's subsequent stories about the "civil wars within [white] women" (Young 70).

By appropriating other texts and roles, *Nurse and Spy* addressed a generation of young white women who identified with the dreams and drives of the age's most adventurous nurse, Tribulation Periwinkle. Moving beyond the latter's struggles to regulate her "unruly" impulses, Edmonds's *Adventures* challenged the ideology of female self-regulation and encouraged Victorian women to move beyond the walls of home and hospital. At the same time, however, the real-life cross-dresser and border-crosser also reminded female readers of the fundamentally democratic and religious basis of nursing in the age of Florence Nightingale: As the allegorical episode about the Irish peddler teaches the reader, God's kingdom can only come if the collective "we" of America's self-appointed nurses "remove our prejudice" (*NaS* 67).

Edmonds's radical vision—which is essentially an early formulation of the perceived "other's" democratic right to fully represent him- or herself as different from the ruling norms and positions—is founded on the idea that otherness is fundamental to the human experience: Anybody can become a patient. As the epitome of self-limitation and passivity, the prototypical patient relies on the selfless care of the professional nurse. In *Hospital Sketches*, this professional selflessness fades when the patient is a woman: Suggesting the theme of Charlotte Perkins Gilman's "The Yellow Wallpaper" (1892), Alcott's female patient is a prisoner of her imagination and remains there until the end of the narrative.[40] It is here that Edmonds interferes. Like Periwinkle (and Alcott herself), the spy, too, experiences a fundamental physical and

---

[40] For a different interpretation, cf. Young 86.

mental crisis in which she "could do nothing but weep hour after hour
. . . . All the horrid scenes that I had witnessed during the past two years
seemed now to be fore me with vivid distinctness, and I could think of
nothing else" (*NaS* 163).

Sick and exhausted, Edmonds finds herself stripped of all her
"soldierly qualities," sheds her male attire, and becomes "again a poor,
cowardly, nervous, whining woman" (*NaS* 163). The crisis removes the
spy from any association with the military realm: In line with the
deserter's actual experience, Edmonds leaves the army[41] and starts
writing her book, *Nurse and Spy,* instead. Yet, unlike Alcott, she scorns
the role of writer and proclaims that she will eventually leave her desk
behind to continue her work as an active shaper of history:

> To prove to my friends that I am not ambitious of gaining the reputation
> of that venerable general (Halleck) whose "pen is mightier than his
> sword,"[42] I am about to return to the army to offer my services in any
> capacity which will best promote the interests of the Federal cause—no
> matter how perilous the position may be. (*NaS* 174)

Given the fact that the general-in-chief of the Union Army, Henry
Wager Halleck (who was in fact a writer), was historically ridiculed as
being unmasculine, the passage is a clear indication of a nineteenth-
century woman's identification with the male norms of her era,
including a condescending attitude toward what Nathaniel Hawthorne
famously called the "damned mob of scribbling women."[43] In *Nurse and
Spy*, writing is an occupation for those who accept the role of patient as
permanent. This was a none too subtle attack on Alcott, whose
soldiering qualities were merely a matter of fiction. For Edmonds, both

---

[41] According to Gansler, Frank Thompson was "officially listed as a deserter on
his regimental muster rolls." Edmonds herself explained that she was ill and
denied a medical furlough, so "she felt she had no choice but to leave before
being discovered" (Gansler 172).

[42] Halleck wrote a number of books, among them *Military Arts and Science*
(1856), his best-known work. As Sizer has pointed out, the passage obscures
the fact that the historical Edmonds returned in women's dress to nurse the
wounded (126).

[43] The original quote stems from Hawthorne's January 19, 1855 letter to his
publisher, William D. Ticknor. For a published version see Nelson 152.

writing and fits of "feminine" weakness are a part of the human repertoire but not essential for a self-identified "Foreign Missionary" (*NaS* 5) from Nova Scotia who wishes to remind American readers of the promise that lies in their foundational text, the *Declaration of Independence,* and its follow-up, the *Declaration of Sentiments*. If "all men and women are created equal," then everybody is always already somebody else.

Conclusion

Alcott and Edmonds were approximately twenty and thirty years old when, in the early 1860s, the Earnings Act and the Married Women's Property Act opened up new options for their generation. When in 1863 the Emancipation Proclamation signaled a further step toward a more democratic, egalitarian society, the two writers grasped the opportunity to analyze the status quo of the warring nation, suggest a set of rules for the "democratic game" that was about to begin, and project their respective visions of a "healthier," more perfect future. Cast in the rhetoric of illness, nursing, and healing, their visions were clearly gendered yet also tinged with their individual experiences and cultural education: While Alcott struggled with the deeply contradictory messages imparted by her New England upbringing, Edmonds based her ideas on the many years that she had spent moving between and across the borders of countries, gender roles, and professions.

By staging her alter ego in the role of adolescent girl, Alcott was able to represent a woman's "unruly" and self-reliant behavior without sanction. Periwinkle's coming-of-age in the hospital is, essentially, a balancing act between "carnival and discipline" (Young 70) that results in the heroine's return to her father's house and thereby to the female realm of dreaming of and writing about a world shaped by women. The book's emphasis on the almost unbearable tension between dreams and reality, female agency and paralysis, struck a cord among a wartime readership that could in many ways identify with these discrepancies. Edmonds, too, admired Alcott, but as an immigrant the former also saw the problematic aspects that laced the American's feminist agenda, particularly with regard to the implications it had for women and race relations. Edmonds's critical gloss on *Hospital Sketches* defies both female self-denial and racial subordination and replaces them with a concept of unprejudiced selflessness that transcends the notions of gender, race, ethnicity, and denomination.

The Civil War hospital figures largely in the making of this concept: The overpowering encounter with suffering humanity reminds Edmonds (and the reader) of the fundamental commonality of all people. Cast as a machine that turns both patients and nurses into "eyes, ears, hands, and feet," the hospital as multiracial contact zone also reminds Americans of the fact that moral goodness exists independently from a person's race. This is also the lesson taught by the "Irish" woman in disguise: Cast in the role of a Catholic immigrant, the spy conveys to her Virginian patient that compassion knows neither country nor religion nor political opinion. The scene significantly severs nursing from the spatial and temporal confines of the Civil War hospital and replaces it with a universal notion of altruism that exists independently of the gendered and ethnicized hierarchies that structured that institution. Having moved beyond the institutional and spatial confines of the hospital and been forced to survive in a hostile environment that threatens to turn her into a patient herself, Edmonds is symbolically authorized to see beyond the limitations of the disempowered. It is from this position that *Nurse and Spy* disrupts the narrative of white female benevolent action that marks interracial relations in Stowe's influential *Uncle Tom's Cabin* and Alcott's *Hospital Sketches*, and confronts it with the self-assured voice of an African American man who no longer wishes to be controlled. As Edmonds reminds her readers, freedom implies the right to disagree.

In this and other passages, *Nurse and Spy* shifts the focus from structural limitations to individual agency. Contrary to the "imprisoned" Periwinkle, who experiences a strange, almost sadomasochistic "delight" when she watches the group of struggling mules, Edmonds celebrates their strong-willed character and stubborn opposition. When Edmonds eventually falls ill and has to leave the army, the nurse-turned-spy is as stubborn as the proverbial mule: Much like Periwinkle, she seeks to maintain her agency by emphasizing the temporariness of her crisis, yet her insistence seems far more determined, as she devalues writing as an inadequate means to influence the course of history in a time of crisis. By aligning writing with femininity, and femininity with illness, *Nurse and Spy* problematically aligns itself with the misogynist devaluation of female authorship that pervaded the era.

If in *Hospital Sketches* women remain subject to the norms and structures that limit their agency, *Nurse and Spy* projects an individual identity that transcends the confines of normative identity categories. If, according to Alcott's novella, a woman's influence in society depends on a rigid regime of self-discipline, in Edmonds's novel, it is a matter of individual transformation. If Nurse Periwinkle remains a prisoner of Victorian ideology, Edmonds is a true "angel in white": Unsexed and transgressive, the nurse-turned-spy combines the roles of messenger and healer, mediator and prophet. And yet, she chooses to not travel alone. In an erotically charged scene that incorporates short passages from *Hospital Sketches* into the story of the spy's temporary return to the hospital, Edmonds pays tribute to a nurse who very much resembles her literary predecessor[44]: "She was a splendid woman, and had the best faculty of dispelling the blues, dumps and dismals of any person I ever met" (*NaS* 110).

Works Cited

Alcott, Louisa May. *Hospital Sketches*. Boston: James Redpath, 1863. Print.

---. "An Hour." 1864. *Louisa May Alcott on Race, Sex, and Slavery*. By Alcott. Ed. Sarah Elbert. Boston: Northeastern UP, 1997. 47-67. Print.

---. "My Contraband" ["The Brothers"]. 1869. *Civil War Memories: Nineteen Stories of Glory and Tragedy*. Ed. S.T. Joshi. New York: Gramercy, 2000. 75-92. Print.

---. *The Journals of Louisa May Alcott*. Ed. Joel Myerson and Daniel Shealy. Athens: U of Georgia P, 1997. Print.

Bullough, Vern L., and Bonnie Bullough. "Joining the Battle at Home and at War." *Cross-Dressing, Sex, and Gender*. By Bullough and Bullough. Philadelphia: U of Pennsylvania, 1993. 157-64. Print.

Clinton, Catherine, and Nina Silber, eds. *Battle Scars: Gender and Sexuality in the American Civil War*. New York: Oxford UP, 2006. Print.

---

[44] The scene clearly aligns the woman called "Nellie" with Nurse Periwinkle by quoting from *Hospital Sketches*.

Edmonds, Sarah Emma. *Memoirs of a Soldier, Nurse and Spy.* 1864. Ed. Elizabeth D. Leonard. DeKalb: Northern Illinois UP, 1999. Print.

---. *Soldier, Nurse and Spy in the Union Army.* Three Rivers, Cornwall: Diggory, 2006. Print.

Elbert, Sarah. *A Hunger for Home: Louisa May Alcott's Place in American Culture.* New Brunswick: Rutgers UP, 1987. Print.

Faust, Drew Gilpin. *Mothers of Invention: Women of the Slaveholding South in the American Civil War.* Chapel Hill: U of North Carolina P, 1996. Print.

Fladeland, Betty L. "Edmonds, Sarah Emma Evelyn." *Notable American Women, 1607-1950.* Ed. Edward T. James. Vol. 1. Cambridge: Belknap, 1980. 561-62. Print.

Foner, Eric. *Forever Free: The Story of Emancipation and Reconstruction.* New York: Random, 2005. Print.

Freemon, Frank R. *Gangrene and Glory: Medical Care During the American Civil War.* Urbana: U of Illinois P, 2001. Print.

Gansler, Laura Leedy. *The Mysterious Private Thompson.* Lincoln: U of Nebraska P, 2007. Print.

Garber, Marjorie. *Vested Interests: Cross-Dressing and Cultural Anxiety.* New York: Routledge, 1992. Print.

Gardner, Sarah E. *Blood and Irony: Southern White Women's Narratives of the Civil War, 1861-1937.* Chapel Hill: U of North Carolina P, 2004. Print.

Garrison, Webb, with Cheryl Garrison. "Contraband." *The Encyclopedia of Civil War Usage.* Nashville: Cumberland House, 2001. 55. Print.

Gerteis, Louis S. *From Contraband to Freedman: Federal Policy toward Southern Blacks, 1861–1865.* Westport: Greenwood, 1973. Print.

Hall, Richard. *Patriots in Disguise.* New York: Paragon, 1993. Print.

Hemenway, Robert E. *Zora Neale Hurston: A Literary Biography.* Chicago: U of Illinois P, 1980. Print.

Iser, Wolfgang. *Der Akt des Lesens.* Munich: Fink, 1976. Print.

Kraus, Natasha Kirsten. *A New Type of Womanhood.* Durham: Duke UP, 2008. Print.

Laffrado, Laura. "'I am Other Than My Appearance Indicates': Sex-Gender Representation in Women's Nineteenth-Century Civil War Reminiscences." *Over Here* 17.2 (1997): 161-83. Print.

Lee, Matthew. "Edmonds, Emma." *Women in World History: A Biographical Encyclopedia* Vol. 5. Detroit: Gale, 1999. 55-61. Print.

Leonard, Elizabeth D. *Yankee Women: Gender Battles in the Civil War*. New York: Norton, 1994. Print.

---. *All the Daring of the Soldier*. New York: Norton, 1999. Print.

Massey, Mary Elizabeth. *Bonnet Brigades: American Women and the Civil War*. New York: Knopf, 1966. Print.

Nelson, Randy F. *The Almanac of American Letters*. Ann Arbor: U of Michigan P, 1981. 152. Print.

Pratt, Mary Louise. "Arts of the Contact Zone." *Profession* 91 (1991): 33-40. Print.

Quigley, David. *Second Founding: New York City, Reconstruction, and the Making of American Democracy*. New York: Hill and Wang, 2004. Print.

Ropes, Hannah. *Civil War Nurse: The Diary and Letters of Hannah Ropes*. Ed. John R. Brumgardt. Knoxville: U of Tennessee P, 1980. Print.

Schultz, Jane E. "Performing Genres: Sarah Emma Edmonds' *Nurse and Spy* and the Case of the Cross-Dressed Text." *Dressing Up for War: Transformations of Gender and Genre in the Discourse and Literature of War*. Ed. Aránzazu Usandizaga and Andrew Monnickendam. Amsterdam: Rodopi, 2001. 73-92. Print.

---. *Women at the Front: Hospital Workers in Civil War America*. Chapel Hill: U of North Carolina P, 2004. Print.

Silber, Nina. *Daughters of the Union: Northern Women Fight the Civil War*. Cambridge: Harvard UP, 2005. Print.

Sizer, Lyde Cullen. "Acting Her Part: Narratives of Union Women Spies." *Divided Houses: Gender and the Civil War*. Ed. Catherine Clinton and Nina Silber. New York: Oxford UP, 1992. 114-33. Print.

Stowe, Harriet Beecher. *Uncle Tom's Cabin*. 1852. Repr. Hertfordshire: Wordsworth Editions, 1995. Print.

Twelbeck, Kirsten. "Bible Seller and Cross-Dressed Spy: Sarah Emma Edmonds and the Debate over Authenticity." *Religion in the United States*. Ed. Jeanne Cortiel et al. Heidelberg: Winter, 2011. 41-57. Print.

Young, Elizabeth. *Disarming the Nation: Women's Writing and the American Civil War*. Chicago: U of Chicago P, 1999. Print.

Whites, LeeAnn. *The Civil War as a Crisis in Gender: Augusta, Georgia, 1860-1890*. Athens: U of Georgia P, 1995. Print.

KATJA SCHMIEDER

"Do Not Cross"—TV Women Doctors Trespassing on Male Territory

Fictions centering on female doctors have always provided a site where a combination of ideas about gender and science could be provocatively narrated—provocatively because the medical profession with its privileged access to the human body was and still is conceived of as a male dominion in Western culture. Women who sought entry to this scientific dominion have since been regarded as violators and transgressors, even more so when they as scientists have aided in criminal investigations, since law enforcement agreeably belongs to male territory, too.

From the 1990s onward, especially due to Patricia Cornwell's bestselling Kay Scarpetta series,[1] fictional female doctors have entered the scene as scientists-*cum*-investigators. Other women writers and their protagonists took their chances and engaged in the procedures of law enforcement more visibly, and crime fiction's new subcategory— forensic fiction[2]—anticipated and perpetuated this development. Forensic fictions soon became a tradition, whether on the page or on the

---

[1]   Scholars agree that Patricia Cornwell is the most influential author of a new subgenre that fuses a crime plot with elements of the police procedural, scientific prose, and detailed descriptions of mutilated bodies. The story is told by a forensic heroine (cf. Palmer; Horsley and Horsley).

[2]   Since I do not plan on engaging in an in-depth genre discussion, I shall use the umbrella term forensic fiction whenever a text focuses explicitly on the activities involved in forensic science. Other scholars have used different labels in order to identify further subcategories, such as "forensic detective fiction" (Palmer), "forensic pathology novel" (Horsley and Horsley), etc.

screen. Yet while the history of science, as Ludmilla Jordanova argues, "render[s] Woman as the very 'personification of nature'" and is "marked by a drive to penetrate, uncover, and know this nature, rendering it visible under the probing scrutiny of the masculine gaze" (Palmer 56), most forensic heroines have regularly failed to address and make use of the contradictions inherent in this crucial aspect of science.

Crossing Jordan and Bones

Two particularly successful TV series, *Crossing Jordan* (2001-2007) and *Bones* (first aired 2005) have taken this subgenre to the twenty-first century, when female doctors who help solve crimes had already become icons of American popular culture.[3] Both series portray women doctors as pioneering in the field of scientific crime investigation, because examining and reading the body and its remains as a site which accommodates all necessary evidence to elucidate a narrative on what was done and *whodunnit* has largely been a male prerogative. Being aware of the masculine foundations of science and its preoccupation with vision, the characters of forensic pathologist Dr. Jordan Cavanaugh, M.D., and forensic anthropologist Dr. Temperance "Bones" Brennan, Ph.D., self-confidently withstand the voyeuristic gaze of their male colleagues as well as that of millions of viewers in front of the small screen. As transgressor figures, both enter male ground as they violate and cross boundaries while dismissing their predecessors' emotional pathos and professional conceit.

In "Wound Culture," Mark Seltzer famously pinpoints both the "excitations of the torn and opened body, the torn and exposed individual, as public spectacle" (4), and, accordingly, the medium of television, which depends on the activities of seeing and watching—visualizing what readers of forensic fiction had formerly only been able to imagine—namely, the seemingly actual activities involved in forensic science. Accordingly, the graphic gore of cutting up dead bodies is

---

[3] Along with Patricia Cornwell and Kathy Reichs, authors like Beverly Connor, Tess Gerritsen, or Lisa Black, to name but a few, have probably created the best-known forensic heroines.

displayed in all its viscerality, so viewers can participate in the spectacle by watching their television screens. Invited to align their view—and their perspective—with those of the protagonists, spectators at the same time gage the spatial and virtual hierarchies that propel and control the action.

Pioneers?

Given the almost regular appearance of the female doctor in recent crime fiction, I still refer to the forensic TV heroines on *Crossing Jordan* and *Bones* as trailblazers.[4] In the following, I will exemplify my assumption about the doubly pioneering function of both series and their forensic heroines in their roles as women, scientists, and investigators as they expose and deconstruct ideas of gaze and space in science, which are traditionally perceived as masculine. I suggest that Jordan and "Bones" appropriate the privileged and authoritative gaze their profession vests them with, as a vantage point from which they unravel the synthesis of the voyeuristic male gaze and the empirical-medical gaze. While thus unveiling the gender conservatism at work in their daily practice, they implement their very distinctive ideas of scientific truth.

Moreover, both TV shows have changed the widely accepted depiction of forensic pathology as the "royal" forensic discipline: While Jordan, the pathologist with a doctoral degree, started her career as a heart surgeon, "Bones," who holds a Ph.D., works in the field of physical anthropology. Based on their historical roles, "physicians did not touch the body, whether living or dead; that lowly charge was left to the surgeons" (Klaver 11), and while Jordan is the one putting her hands inside the body, actually anatomizing it, "Bones" never touches the soft tissue or flesh that makes for its corporeality, but only its skeletal

---

[4] Other than famous TV shows that deal with forensic science, such as *CSI, Profiler,* or *Law and Order,* both *Crossing Jordan* and *Bones* focus exclusively on the scientific practice of their female protagonists, which in spite of their involvement in criminal investigations is decidedly differentiated from detective work in the sense of law enforcement.

remains. Thus, this novel distinction between the meaning and impact of such forensic disciplines as pathology and anthropology, both of which have until recently been subsumed under forensic pathology (cf. Horsley and Horsley), is carefully developed throughout both series.

Gaze and Space

The recent fictionalization of forensic science has problematized the integration of the male medical gaze, a viewing pattern which discloses the gender dichotomy inherent in masculine science and its object, the dead, feminized body. Such traditional forensic fictions as mentioned above have moreover drawn their enormous popularity from the fact that the series' central protagonists are women scientists who seek entrance to the all-male law enforcement machinery. However, the indiscriminating and unreflected adoption of a masculine profession in the field of forensic investigation, along with its gazing habits, have almost exclusively degraded forensic heroines to what feminist scholars such as Joy Palmer call "patriarchy's patsies" (57). Hence, she suggests a productive examination of "how the gaze of the female doctor may signal a potential subversion or shift in those gendered viewing paradigms" (55).

Accordingly, I claim that the female protagonists of *Crossing Jordan* and *Bones* unravel and deconstruct the synthesis of the medical gaze and the male gaze when implementing their individual viewing patterns and perspectives: Jordan's anticipatory gaze and Tempe's reflective gaze. They thus illustrate the assumptions of Bracha L. Ettinger, who famously suspends the subject-object dichotomy prevalent in the male gaze, as conceptualized by Jacques Lacan and modified by Laura Mulvey, and in the Foucauldian medical gaze, by introducing her idea of a "matrixial trans-subjectivity," derived from the psychoanalytical concept of countertransference and the image of an inclusive, feminine matrix/womb which would engender "co-emergence," "distance-in-proximity," and "relations-without-relating" (218). This approach allows for a substitution of the process inherent in the objectifying gaze with subjectivization, or "trans-subjectivity." The female protagonists of both *Crossing Jordan* and *Bones* seem to consciously apply this dialogic viewing paradigm to the corpses as well as to the people they get in contact with, similarly trying to elicit coherent narratives.

In order to challenge the professional, quasi-militaristic office hierarchy as prescribed by law enforcement and implemented in the investigation process, in which both women get involved, they use their individual views to re-conceptualize a workspace that has been encoded as unequivocally masculine throughout history: the scientific laboratory. While Jordan's and Bones's daily routine includes dissecting corpses or skeletons with the help of phallic tools and the medical gaze, they implement their individual perspectives and subvert distinctly male hierarchies, and I argue that both series have thus re-established the lab as a feminine and private space, as opposed to the actual crime scene or the FBI office. In order to illustrate the feminization of spaces that accommodate science and technology, *Crossing Jordan* implies and embraces a psychoanalytical reading, thus sustaining Ettinger's assumptions, while *Bones* deliberately addresses another Foucauldian idea, namely that of heterotopia, which allows for this spatial reconfiguration to undermine masculine hierarchies as manifest in the investigation process.

The Transition: Dr. Jordan Cavanaugh, M.D.

The TV show *Crossing Jordan*, which aired on NBC prime time from 2001 to 2007, represents a crucial transition, epitomized by its protagonist: a transition from the 1990s forensic detective fiction heroine to the twenty-first century's TV woman doctor who combines scientific knowledge, medical skills, and investigative talent. Accordingly, the title of the show itself implies such a passage or turning point, with its specific biblical allusion to the Hebrews crossing the river Jordan in order to find the Promised Land. In further emphasizing this passage, the character of Dr. Jordan Cavanaugh takes a decisive step and radically breaks with the traditions of the female forensic scientist as established by Patricia Cornwell and her followers. Where Kay Scarpetta obediently plays by and incorporates the rules of the patriarchal order, Jordan addresses and challenges masculine authorities, especially those who deliberately pull rank. Hence, Jordan simultaneously crosses places and people while often feeling "crossed" herself.

The very first scene of *Crossing Jordan* introduces Jordan as a participant in an anger management class, a drop-dead beautiful young woman wearing a conspicuously short skirt and a tank top with a "Cherry Bomb" print on it. All eyes in the room zoom in on her after the revelation that her boss remanded her to this course as a punishment for her "kicking him in the *cojones*," which Jordan felt was the appropriate thing to do because of his "patronizing questions" ("Pilot" 0:27). The camera's and the group's voyeuristic looks intertwine with a medical gaze when ogling the eye candy in front of them with suspicion about her mental state. Yet Jordan instantly returns this view, forcing the camera to oscillate between her and the class, and thus creating an equilibrium. When Jordan further admits to "cut[ting] up dead people for a living" which would also be "a great way to manage . . . anger," the psychotherapist asks: "And just what exactly are you angry at, Dr. Cavanaugh?" ("Pilot" 0:41-0:53). Jordan verbally underscores her resistance to being objectified and snaps back with questions in return:

> You mean besides inane questions? . . . The designated hitter always ticked me off. Then, of course, there's all the crap I see in my line of work. People killed by drunk drivers, psychos who murder innocent people for no reason. Injustice. Yeah, that pisses me off pretty good. Or how about a ten-year-old girl who has to hear from her fourth-grade teacher at recess that her mom was murdered? Her dad left alone to raise her without a mom, without a wife, on a cop's salary. Does that work for you? ("Pilot" 0:54-1:24)

As a figure not only dangerous to other characters but also to conventional viewing and listening habits, most of which she off-handedly breaks down, Jordan's childhood trauma, the unsolved murder of her mother to which she refers here, seems to have instilled this anger that enables her fearless questioning and confronting of authority.

Jordan's appearance sparks attention and renders her prone to the male gaze as imposed on her by other characters and the audience alike. Simultaneously she becomes an object of constant, authoritative, even "medical" scrutiny that seeks to contain her potential dangerousness: Her employers at the Office of the Chief Medical Examiner (OCME), her partners at the FBI and the police, and her father all keep telling her to stay "under the radar," exactly because of the threat she constitutes by crossing boundaries and, thus, eluding control. As a medical examiner, Jordan's actual job is to determine cause of death by examining bodies brought to the Boston OCME in order to prepare the corpses for burial and sign them out. Since she cannot help but routinely mess with detective work, most of her partners perceive Jordan as a trespasser on their turf. The police and FBI defend what they feel belongs to the male territory of law enforcement and ask Jordan to back off from investigations, at the same time conceding, "[y]ou think like a cop!" ("Pilot" 19:32), because she is usually the one with the correct line of reasoning and with the right clues in place. Jordan not only crosses people, but she also crosses the territory of science, crime investigation, and law enforcement formerly reserved for men.

Deconstruction: Seeing and Being Seen

As illustrated by the pilot's opening scene, Jordan attracts people's looks and reactions, especially those of people professionally involved, and she feels easily annoyed by them. However, she returns their gazes not merely through reversion, as the camera angle might indicate, but by further exposing their insulting nature through instantly addressing them and talking back. Being notorious for both her quick temper and her explicit language, she respects people who share her obsession for an unconditional truth while rejecting any authority established through position, rank, or office. In this vein, she verbally attacks the interim boss, Jack Slokum, in a very outspoken way for his newly implemented control and surveillance measures at the OCME:

> I watched you turn this morgue from a place we all loved into an anal retentive dictatorship. You're an obsessive compulsive android with a Napoleon complex, and I actually live for the day when someone takes that bonsai tree of yours and shoves it so far up your ass, you'll have pine needles coming out your nose. ("There's No Place like Home" 14:50-15:11)

Along similar lines, *Crossing Jordan* promotes the stereotype of the masculine, ruthless, and ignorant FBI. With few exceptions, the arrogant and prejudiced approach of FBI agents and other government officials to crimes unequivocally leads them along trodden paths, thus missing important clues and thoughts. In the episode "One Twelve," an open critique of the investigation of the 9/11 explosions, the FBI immediately arrests a foreign-looking man for allegedly bombing a multi-story office building, accusing him of political motivation, only to find out that one of the office guards was the actual killer, with a highly personal agenda. The series and its protagonist ridicule federal authorities such as the FBI, the NSA, or the Department of Homeland Security, whose reputations were apparently to be redeemed by late 1990s and early twenty-first-century fictions linked to the "rising tide of conservatism in the US" (Valverde 100).[5] The gaze Jordan imposes as a female scientist facilitates the dissection of the integrated gaze into its male and medical parts, and as the viewer's gaze is aligned with hers, so is the dismissive perspective with regard to powerful authorities.

Accordingly, the series's pioneering work is the visualization of the male gaze's synthesis with the medical gaze, a visualization which Jordan effects and appropriates. As previously argued, she anticipates the male gaze by addressing and verbalizing it, as she responds to a colleague in a strip club: "A girl can look, can't she?" ("Born To Run" 1:18). While Cornwell's Kay Scarpetta would have been seriously stunned and frightened, Jordan lets her gaze linger on the female stripper's toned body. In the same way she stares at her colleague Trey's sweaty biceps, thus returning his look and making him feel uncomfortable when he enters the locker room and catches her stark naked. Here the viewer is invited to join Jordan reappropriating the voyeuristic gaze. At the same time, this alignment happens when Jordan is at work dissecting bodies with an array of instruments, where again the conflation of the male and medical gaze becomes visible. While viewers watch her unfold this synthesis, they "trans-subjectively" enmesh their male gaze as spectators with a medical perspective, e.g., when they attune their viewpoint with hers in doing an autopsy.

Along similar lines, viewers observe how the male gaze as exploited by Jordan backfires on her job: She dates a colleague from the police

---

[5]   Towards the end of the twentieth century, the re-introduction of the motiveless serial killer as a genuinely American threat emphasized the need for science-aided crime investigation and redeemed the FBI's reputation.

department whom she suspects of being a murderer. By integrating the voyeuristic with the medical/clinical gaze, she stares at the cop's forearm and demands "roll up your sleeves" ("Pilot" 35:22). After she detects the concealer he used to hide a bite mark, she handcuffs him to his bed, thus exploiting the productivity of her anticipatory view to catch the killer. The audience is strongly made aware of the visual implications originated by Dr. Jordan Cavanaugh, especially where the male gaze merges—or even "co-emerges"—with the medical gaze.

"I want the truth" is a phrase we hear Jordan voicing over and over again, and, in order to find the truth, she uses visualizing technology that engenders the medical gaze: stereo-microscope, UV light, databases, cameras, x-rays. Espousing her very individual approach to truth closely connects to her own integrated, anticipatory gaze: Jordan employs her visual capacities, including the male gaze, for the sake of the victims and the re-establishing of their identity. Her crusade for truth reveals the unison of scientific truth and ethical values: Other than the FBI or the police with their exclusive truth claims backed by patriarchal law and order, Jordan uses truth precisely against power and authority because, for her, truth combines science with morality and ethics.

Spaces: Home Turf, Crime Scene, and Workplace

As intensely as Jordan despises other masculine authorities, she just as intensely respects her father, who was the one who introduced her to the realm of crime investigation. Personifying the first and decisive moral authority in Jordan's life, Max Cavanaugh contributes the ethical aspect of her understanding of truth by frequently stressing that "[w]hat is right isn't necessarily the truth." Since her mother's murderer has never been found, turning the crime into a cold case, her father has become her sole "family" and, while shifting his focus from his job "on the force" to his child, he assumes a role as father, educator, trainer, and partner for Jordan. Throughout their quasi-Freudian relationship, Max provides Jordan with spiritual and professional guidance, thus figuring as a link between her private life and her career, her past and her present. His own professional path strongly affected their private past as a family and instills in her the decision to help people and solve crimes.

The paternal influence on Jordan's life is underscored in pictures of the *Crossing Jordan* team, where he always occupies a central position.

As a nine-year-old child, Jordan watched her father "stare at evidence" ("Pilot" 19:38-20:00), and this replacement of the primal scene is followed by a substituted sex education: For her, the rite of passage into adult life is her initiation into the world of crime. Soon after this incident she started joining him on a regular basis, applying a gaze of her own, while, later on, her father joins her in looking at evidence. Whenever one of her cases becomes gridlocked, Jordan turns to her father and re-stages the circumstances of the crime with him by performing a role play. Even though her father often opposes both her insistence on science's omnipotence as well as her zealous quest for truth, she depends on his combined perspective as a man, for he mostly assumes the role of the male perpetrator, and as an empirical detective who relies on hard evidence, morals, and intuition alike, always uttering discomfort when something does not "feel" right. In order to imagine the progress of events and to solve the crime, this game of mixed perspectives turns out to be decisive in investigations: Through reasoning back and by creating a parallel time and space, they simultaneously revisit the crime scene while sitting at a table. Hence the *Crossing Jordan* pilot indicates from the start that a perpetrator can be tracked down precisely because this father-daughter entity is capable of re-enacting the crime.

After Max's disappearance at the end of the third season, Jordan's boss, Garret Macy, is foregrounded as a surrogate father and, with his almost anti-authoritarian attitude, he fits smoothly into the core team,[6] whose members seem to spend their lives in the rooms of the OCME. In the series, the Forensic Department as a part of the Office of the Chief Medical Examiner is located on the upper floor of a multi-story building. In this somewhat claustrophobic enclosure, many separate and locked diverse rooms—from offices to autopsy rooms—form an organic entity, an arrangement reflected by its occupants. Likewise the forensic

---

[6]   Commenting on the ongoing fight for leadership, Macy frequently points toward his unstable position as an ME, indicating that office hierarchy is independent of sex, knowledge, or skills: "She [Yakura, leading CME] outmaneuvered me for the job, thereby ensuring my slow death in the middle rung of this place forever" ("Pilot" 3:31).

team, with Jordan the pathologist as its center, consists of diverse personalities: the burned-out and cynical Macy, a nerdy forensic entomologist of Bangladeshi background, a Holmesian criminologist from the UK, and an esoteric girl as grief counselor, each of whom is allotted sufficient space throughout the series in order to develop an individual perspective. While the team members reject succumbing to any hierarchical order other than the one based on knowledge and skills, they appropriate these dimly lit rooms, passages, nooks, and hallways, which are hidden from the public view and which strongly suggest a Freudian interpretation as a feminine sphere. This space is thus portrayed as unruly and impenetrable as Jordan's entire team, who value ethics, friendship, and mutual support over artificial hierarchies engendered by the patriarchal authority of law enforcement.

Jordan and her team embody equality, as humans and co-workers, for they act, move, and work literally on the same level. As soon as intruders threaten this equilibrium, they close ranks and expect Jordan to "lead the revolution" (Lily in "There's No Place like Home" 6:29). Jordan's emotional hardships have apparently made her fearless and irreverent of people in higher places. Comments such as "[t]ruth is, I don't care if I die" ("Pilot" 39:03) render her extremely dangerous to the masculine authorities she is not afraid to mess with. The labyrinth-like organization of the OCME, moreover, emphasizes the unruliness and elusiveness both of the forensic team and the space they occupy, at the same time defying control and hierarchy. Subsequently, their space cannot evade being consumed by and placed squarely within the hierarchy of the patriarchal order, as Jordan's colleague Trey wryly insinuates that they are all "low men on the totem pole" ("Pilot" 33:38).

The Accomplishment: Dr. Temperance Brennan, Ph.D.

While *Crossing Jordan* pioneered in its attempt to lay bare and exploit the synthesis of the male and the medical gaze, leading to an overall questioning of truth and authority, the series flinched from completing the transition from traditional forensic fictions: While Jordan became ever more anxious and sentimental throughout the series, traits that have rendered her utterly harmless, her team became deeply involved in their personal issues while complaining about being incapable of climbing the career ladder. Therefore, from 2005 onward, the new TV show *Bones* has picked up where *Crossing Jordan* got stuck. *Bones*, which has been aired on FOX ever since, and its protagonist Dr. Temperance "Bones" Brennan, took one more decisive step toward the new woman doctor: Tempe accomplishes what Jordan started, but instead of further undermining traditional viewing patterns, she represents their reconstruction. Whereas the final suturing of a corpse usually indicates some sort of closure, *Crossing Jordan* never depicts this important final act of an autopsy, and Jordan more or less leaves the bodies open for Bones's further inspection of the remains. This is exactly where the character Bones takes over: With the soft tissue removed, what is left seems to be the core of a human being's existence.

Most importantly, *Bones* has the science taking place in one big space rather than in an ensemble of various small rooms. Attached to the fictional Jeffersonian Museum in D.C., the forensic lab is located at the center of a steel-and-glass construction, a spacious building with mostly artificial skylights that bathe the scenes in a bluish tinge. Here, a physical separation as provided by walls and doors does not exist, and office desks are placed next to autopsy tables, thus "juxtaposing in a single real place several spaces, several sites that are in themselves incompatible" (Foucault, "Of Other Spaces" 4). Hence a heterotopia is established in more than one way: The team examines warriors and mummies next to freshly decomposed human remains, and sometimes the two are even connected by one and the same crime. The Jeffersonian museum which allows for the existence of the annexed lab in the first place virtually embraces the "idea of constituting a place of all times that is itself outside of time and inaccessible to its ravages," since "[h]eterotopias ... open onto ... heterochronies ... heterotopias and heterochronies are structured and distributed in a relatively complex fashion. [T]here are heterotopias of indefinitely accumulating time, for example museums and libraries" (Foucault, "Of Other Spaces" 5).

The forensic unit where Tempe and her team perform their examinations rests in the center of the building on a stage-like mezzanine with overhead passageways hovering above. This constellation symbolizes a reversed panopticon and, as the scientists gaze at their objects, they can be observed from every possible angle. When Tempe frequently refers to her team as "lab rats," she indicates the visual confinement of this space where scientists employ the medical gaze and themselves become objectified and prone to this very same gaze—like experimental rats in a labyrinth. Tempe furthermore considers the laboratory her home, whereby in every episode the famous phrase "bring it[7] back to the lab" is uttered at least once. Even though visible to outsiders, the lab figures as a distinctly private, feminine sphere, comparable to a kitchen, and more so because its bottleneck entrance renders it impenetrable to intruders: "Heterotopias always presuppose a system of opening and closing that both isolates them and makes them penetrable" (Foucault, "Of Other Spaces" 5). The small staircase, leading to the inner sanctum, thus functions as a threshold and is guarded by an automatic ID checking device.

The members of the forensic team—including Tempe's current intern prodigy, a forensic artist, and a forensic entomologist—appear to spend their lives in the lab, while forming an almost utopian, egalitarian community. They share complete mutual loyalty and equality, and—as in Jordan's team—their positions in the group are based on scientific knowledge and skills. In order to undermine their closeness and to contain their unruliness, authorities from the FBI and the Jeffersonian administrative staff frequently patronize and intimidate Bones and her team, always emphasizing the permeable borders of the lab and its low rank in the hierarchy of authorities. Accordingly, Bones is treated as an "asset" of the Jeffersonian and "given" to the FBI ("Pilot" 8:07). However, as soon as she demands full participation in a case and, thus, enters the traditionally male territory of crime investigation, law enforcement, and politics, FBI Deputy Director Cullen tells her to "get back to your lab and get used to being there" ("Pilot" 25:10), because "[scientists] don't solve murders. Cops do" ("Pilot" 30:47). Yet throughout the series, it becomes clear that, since office-based hierarchy cannot be proven scientifically, Tempe's disobedience and impoliteness form an inextricable link with her scientific persona, which in turn is needed by the FBI to solve their cases. Hence the group of forensic co-workers-*cum*-friends headed by Bones encounters and subverts the hierarchic order of male law enforcement by a quasi-anarchistic

---

[7]   Alternatively, bodies, skeletons, soil, and even cars and trees are brought "back to the lab," as if they belonged there.

arrangement based on science, even though the spatial configuration of the lab seems to suggest otherwise.

Reflection and Reconstruction

One remarkable part of the spatial configuration mentioned earlier are the overhead passageways that look down upon the lab and are joined by an elevated lounge from which the team can watch itself and its own workspace, thus self-referentially objectifying science itself to the medical gaze, and joining the spectators on the passageways and the small screen alike. On account of this, the viewer is made aware of the unusually high level of self-referentiality, intertextuality, and even metafiction on the series, something entirely absent from most recent forensic novels, films, and TV shows. There are various obvious and more implicit examples of these fictional strategies, such as recurring casts, character names, and references to popular crime and horror fiction icons.[8] The screenplay of the TV show itself uses as its intertext the famous novel series by Kathy Reichs, featuring a forensic anthropologist called Dr. Temperance Brennan.[9]

Other than Kay Scarpetta or even Jordan Cavanaugh, the protagonist Tempe problematizes and underpins the self-reflexive dynamics of metafiction and intertextuality even further: On the show, she writes forensic fiction, including the bestselling debut novel *Bred in the Bone*, about a forensic anthropologist named Kathy Reichs and her team. Very

---

[8]   Various actors from *Crossing Jordan* reappear in similar roles in *Bones*: forensic interns, victims, and even names recur. For example, a police officer in *Crossing Jordan* shares his last name, "Seel(e)y," with Booth's first name, while Jordan's and Tempe's fathers are both called Max. In the episode "Wrong Place, Wrong Time" Jordan calls Macy "Bones." On a further intertextual level, the serial killer Epps is modeled after Thomas Harris's Hannibal Lecter, while Robert Englund appears as a creepy janitor in "The Death of the Queen Bee," where Freddy Krueger is explicitly mentioned.

[9]   Kathy Reichs, who has a cameo appearance in "Judas on a Pole" (0:40-1:42), and Emily Deschanel as well as David Boreanaz, both leading actors in *Bones*, are producers and co-producers of the show, sometimes even directors.

often, Tempe's team on the series discusses the appearance of the individual characters in the novel, and suddenly the fictional dimensions are confused to the point where the viewer is made unsure whether the characters are talking about the series or about the novel's reality. While Tempe writes novels in whose stories she self-referentially fictionalizes her work as a scientist, this meta-level reflects back on her actual job: It seems the new woman doctor interconnects the authority of a scientific expert with authorship—of books and identities.

Yet while the series's plot moves safely in the web of popular cultural allusions, Tempe herself seems to be strangely and conspicuously cut off from contemporary cultural contexts and conventions, and one could arguably call her an ahistorical phenomenon, simultaneously adhering to and contradicting Foucault's idea of heterochrony. Therefore, whenever her colleagues mention something from popular culture, such as the series *The X-Files* and its protagonists Scully and Mulder (cf. "Pilot" 4:21), she famously admits: "I don't know what that means" (e.g., "Pilot"; "The Woman at the Airport"). By similarly ignoring all topics on Western contemporary cultural agendas like gender, class, "race," and pop culture itself, she eludes being contextualized and focuses on science instead, unhampered by cultural influences. Like Jordan, Tempe seeks the truth precisely by asking how and who instead of why, claiming that "motive does not matter" ("Pilot" 38:06). This de-contextualizing of the scientific approach denies all feminist revisions of science—as, e.g., summarized by Linda Jean Shepherd (cf. *Lifting the Veil*), yet Tempe pursues an anti-causal path, never asking why, even though science is built upon the masculine causal principle. She thus implements a distinctly individual perspective on science and truth that is neither feminine nor masculine, deeming traditional thinking patterns irrelevant.

As the whole series is naturally preoccupied with aspects of vision and perspective, so is its heroine, Tempe, as she is simultaneously the receiver and sender of the male and the medical gaze. As a beautiful young woman who often displays a notoriously low neckline under her masculine clothes, she attracts male attention—yet her conspicuous behavior and awkward language make her the object of multiple medical gazes. She thereby neither conforms to typical notions of female behavior, nor to the traditional image of a scientist, and her frequent and sometimes even violent clashes with authorities coupled with her good looks invite the male as well as the medical gaze of masculine representatives of law and order. On another level, Bones virtually embodies the dissecting gaze as made visible by her bright, staring, crystal-clear eyes. Rather than talking back, she stares back, thus, consciously reflecting and returning the look while being at the same time receiver and applier of the gaze.

While gluing together the bone fragments captured by her empiricist vision, Bones gathers the pieces of a synthesized male-medical gaze and reconstructs an integrated gaze arising from a female viewing matrix (cf. Ettinger 219-20). In the same vein, her friend and colleague Angela provides Tempe with the necessary details of the respective crimes. To accomplish this, Angela developed the "Angelator," a computer program which, similar to Jordan's role plays, creates a three-dimensional holographic simultaneity displaying the events of the crime and including present time of the viewer on the small screen, present time of the forensic team, actual time of the crime, and supposed time of the crime. Since "angel" is a slang synonym for "image," the Angelator was designed to integrate state-of-the-art imaging technology with scientific theory, with Angela figuring as (re)constructer and interpreter of the crime scene pictures.

Placed in the heterotopia of the lab, Bones herself personifies its heterochronies, not least through turning the present pieces of a skeleton into a past human being. Similarly, she neglects and questions contemporary contexts: She uses an awkward, outdated language while misunderstanding the mechanisms of irony and metaphor. However, even if she seems to be utterly outlandish and "out of time," making people ask Booth: "Where did you find her?" and him answering: "Museum" ("The Man in the Wall" 33:42), she is ultimately pioneering in her reconstructive approach to science. Along these lines, Bones rids the scientific gaze of its traditional masculine heritage; she re-frames disinterestedness and objectivity as gender-independent. Hence, the series picked up on further deconstructing the rigid framework that *Crossing Jordan* had begun to break up by attuning the integrated gaze with gender-independent individual perspectives.

The Fictional Anthropologist

According to Jeremy MacClancy, all of Tempe's characteristics would be typical of literary or fictional anthropologists: "Usually, these images of anthropologists are Anglocentric, fundamentally atemporal, gender-blind, and apolitical" (MacClancy 549). He differentiates between two types, one of which he claims would be

> an emotional inadequate, sheltering within objective procedures in order to keep passions at bay. These psychologically stunted individuals prefer analysing things to feeling them. . . . they study people but fail to engage with them. . . . Emotionally lopsided and usually deeply alienated, these anthropologists are often portrayed as marginalized or rootless, without significant kin or home. (MacClancy 551-52)

The character of Dr. Temperance Brennan, physical anthropologist and author, seems to consciously stick to these conventions, to reflect and ironize them; for example, when she claims "I'm not a sociopath, I'm an anthropologist" ("Pilot" 2:15).

While thus verbally sticking to this fictional image, she obviously contradicts it by her actions. Whenever she responds to circumstances outside of the realm of science, she starts off with the catchphrase "anthropologically speaking," seemingly revealing the fact that science serves as her emotional armor and joker, to be drawn when necessary, while providing her with a surplus of composure and restraint. In playing this role, she scientifically dissects her environment and— verbally and physically—attacks politicians and other authorities, such as U.S. senators, church ministers, federal judges, and her new boss, Camille, a forensic pathologist. When Tempe, for example, regularly calls religion a childish myth and the FBI a "paramilitaristic organization" ("The Parts in the Sum of the Whole" 20:18), she applies science to the extreme and de-contextualizes traditions and conventions, rendering them utterly irrelevant.

Realms within which Tempe feels obviously uncomfortable are mostly the ones that include human emotions, and this dynamic unfolds in the single most important relationship of the series. Her partner, FBI special agent Seeley Booth, was a sniper with the U.S. Army Rangers and tries to compensate for these killings by catching murderers, and while Tempe's family also has an issue with a murder from the past, both have very personal reasons for their quest for truth. Even though Tempe immediately attests to Booth's "alpha male attributes" ("The Man in the SUV" 13:59), he is the one who contributes the emotional, intuitive tone to their professional relationship. He first tests her skills in a cold case; then both negotiate their shared and individual participation in the investigation process, and soon they finally team up as equal partners. While Booth is the one who enjoys the privilege of carrying a gun, he accepts Tempe's mantra: "I'm a brain person, you're a heart person" ("Pilot" 25:22).[10] He generously grants her public success and triumph, but when Bones one too many times actively reflects on and ridicules his ostensible shortcomings and remarks, "I am the one with a doctorate," he snaps back, "I am the one with the badge and the gun" ("Pilot" 4:05).

However, their relationship is intensely gazed at by other characters as a surrogate audience, to the extent that the D.A. even blackmails Bones into kissing Booth in return for letting the former be with her family at Christmas. Despite the strong erotic undercurrents in their relationship, both Tempe and Booth resist contextual traps, such as traditional gender roles, for they rather complement each other and divvy up ratio and emotion in equal parts, as illustrated by the many talking-cure-like conversations they hold in Booth's car. On the basis of "transference" and "countertransference," they reflect, return, and switch their feminine and masculine perspectives along with the (fe)male gaze. From time to time they actually address this switching and even try to imagine that Bones is the guy and Booth is the woman. Since the car is hermetically sealed from its environment, as visualized by decidedly artificial props rushing by, their relationship seems to exist beyond time and space, de-contextualized, and, thus, untainted.

---

[10] Special thanks to my students of the MA Entering Class of 2010 at the Institute for American Studies at Leipzig University for making me aware that, in the *Bones* scene at the shooting range ("Pilot"), Bones is the one who shoots at the dummy's heart while Booth aims at the brain.

Consequences

Both texts, *Crossing Jordan* and *Bones*, deploy female protagonists who trespass on male territory by complicating the gendered dynamics at work in the epistemological foundations of science itself, in scientific practice, and in law enforcement in general. In addition, even though forensic crime fiction featuring the female scientist-*cum*-investigator has become a persisting phenomenon American popular culture of the twenty-first century, the figures Dr. Jordan Cavanaugh and Dr. Temperance Brennan can still be called pioneers because they recognize and subvert such traditional perspectives and hierarchies located at the heart of scientific crime investigation. Even though Jordan anticipates the male gaze, she voices it and returns it verbally. Bones, on the other hand, reflects and eludes the male and medical gaze by applying a reciprocal gaze of her own. However, Jordan and Tempe furthermore exploit both the male and the medical gaze, and, by extension, impose their individual perspectives—on men and masculinity in general. Moreover, subjectivity is neither lost nor simply exchanged, but rather oscillates between the protagonists and the body or skeleton—they work together to mutually fix identity.

Yet—unfortunately—from Jordan's "Cherry Bomb" T-shirt to Bones being prohibited to carry a gun or go out alone in the field, both heroines are depicted as a potential threat, to be kept in check or at least to be watched out for, in order not to endanger society. In this way, both characters are punished and silenced in the course of the series. While Jordan is metaphorically and actually tamed, Bones's agency is diminished. Hence, Jordan gradually changes from a loudmouth in flashy clothes, "poking everyone but God in the eye" ("Pilot" 11:12), to a decently dressed working woman who is not only punished with a position on the lower end of the career ladder but also with brain cancer. Bones, on the other hand, starts wearing make-up and the latest hairdo, stressing her female stature, while her importance in the scientific investigation decreases the same way her private involvement with Booth is given more airtime. Both women scientists are punished by being stuck under the glass ceiling, even if they are the "best in the world." Both are moreover punished for appropriating and verbalizing the very practices men (ab)use and, thus, both expose the hypocrisy of today's retributive justice. In their search for truth, they resist the power claims of law enforcement and of patriarchal order. Still, even though both series openly challenge masculine perspectives as derived from the empiricist and the male gaze, they complicate this project by the introduction of male father figures and partners upon whose approval both female protagonists seem to ultimately depend.

Works Cited

Bones. DVD. Twentieth Century Fox, Sept. 2005-.

Crossing Jordan. DVD. Universal Studios, Sept. 2001-May 2007.

Crossland, Zoë. "Of Clues and Signs: The Dead Body and Its Evidential Traces." *American Anthropologist* 111.1 (2009): 69-80. Print.

Ettinger, Bracha L. "Matrixial Trans-subjectivity." *Theory, Culture, Society.* 23.2-3 (2006): 218-22. Print.

Foucault, Michel. *The Birth of the Clinic: An Archaeology of Medical Perception.* 1963. Trans. A.M. Sheridan Smith. New York: Vintage, 1994. Print.

---. "Of Other Spaces (1967), Heterotopias." Trans. Jay Miskowiec. *foucault.info.* Web. 29 July 2011. Trans. of "Des espaces autres." *Architecture/Mouvement/Continuité* Oct. 1984. Print.

Horsley, Katherine, and Lee Horsley. "Body Language: Reading the Corpse in Forensic Crime Fiction." *Paradoxa: Terrain Vagues* 20 (2006): 7-32. Print.

Keller, Evelyn Fox. *Reflections on Gender and Science.* New Haven: Yale UP, 1985. Print.

Klaver, Elizabeth. *Sites of Autopsy in Contemporary Culture.* Albany: State U of New York P, 2005. Print.

Kruse, Corinna. "Producing Absolute Truth: *CSI* Science as Wishful Thinking." *American Anthropologist* 112.1 (2010): 79-91. Print.

Le Doeuff, Michèle. *The Sex of Knowing.* Trans. Kathryn Hamer and Lorraine Code. New York: Routledge, 2003. Print.

MacClancy, Jeremy. "The Literary Image of Anthropologists." *Journal of the Royal Anthropological Institute* 11.3 (2005): 549-75. Print.

Mizejewski, Linda. "Dressed to Kill: Postfeminist Noir." *Cinema Journal* 44.2 (2005): 121-27. Print.

Palmer, Joy. "Tracing Bodies: Gender, Genre, and Forensic Detective Fiction." *South Central Review* 18.3-4 (2001): 54-71. Print.

Seltzer, Mark. "Wound Culture: Trauma in the Pathological Public Sphere." *October* 80 (1997): 3-26. Print.

Shepherd, Linda Jean. *Lifting the Veil: The Feminine Face of Science*. Boston: Shambhala, 1993. Print.

Valverde, Mariana. *Law and Order: Images, Meanings, Myths*. New Brunswick: Rutgers UP, 2006. Print.

PART III:

TRANSMITTING

DISEASE

Imke Kimpel

"Like Hermits in Holes and Caves": Isolation as a Narrative Mode for Writing the Plague in Daniel Defoe's *A Journal of the Plague Year 1665*

Writing the Plague

Modern times know virtually no limits to detecting—though not necessarily always successfully medically treating—human diseases and their agents. The news media provide an ever-increasing amount of information about communicable disease, spurring research into the conditions that favor the eruption of plagues today. "Plague" thereby becomes a term attributed to various kinds of communicable outbreaks, since the "technical term *epidemic* . . . tends to homogenize, erase, and belie the diversity of experiences of people who are suffering or have suffered through what we call epidemics" (Herring and Swedlund 4).

Pestilential epidemic plague has largely vanished as a global phenomenon and certainly has completely vanished in Europe since its last major visitation of Marseilles, southern France, in 1720. Even today, however, pestilence remains a certifiable disease to be put under quarantine upon detection, and has never truly been outmaneuvered. A verified case of bubonic plague occurred as recently as 2010 in the state of Oregon, in the U.S.A., and there is evidence of epidemic in the Indian city Surat in 1994, in the African Congo in 2005 and 2006, and single cases in Madagascar in 2008. And although the plague as a highly contagious bacterial disease has been superseded by other major diseases—tuberculosis, cancer, and AIDS, to name just a few—its literary representation will presumably always remain volatile. The "plague continues to insist" (Cooke 15) on its literary reproduction as much as on its implementation in communal memory. By comparison, the influenza pandemic of 1918-19 that claimed more than twenty million lives is surprisingly underrepresented in literature (cf. Gordon 69). Modern and postmodern thinking about epidemics, including pestilence, is deeply rooted in past experiences and can in turn be re-evaluated through the imaginative power of the present (cf. Herring and Swedlund 3).

This partially "imaginative power" surfaces most prominently in Susan Sontag's seminal study *Illness as Metaphor* (1978), in which she ascribes to illnesses the ability to become metaphors for not only social and political but also moral and even cultural crises. In her study, Sontag contextualizes this phenomenon with tuberculosis and cancer—two illnesses that she considers, regardless of the masses of victims they claim, to be visited upon individuals, as ill persons are visually marked by the disease and thus set apart from the rest of the community. Sontag understands the diseases she examines as moral tests of character, whereas epidemics are more likely to be perceived as community afflictions: "moral corruption made manifest by the disease's spread" (Sontag 41). Whereas tuberculosis as much as cancer is essentially not contagious—although the linguistic power of the metaphor may eventually suggest a literal contagion with the disease—this is not true for the plague that Daniel Defoe engages in his *A Journal of the Plague Year 1665* (1722).[1] Nevertheless, the plague that is placed at center stage in Defoe's narrative also has a strong influence on language: It becomes incommunicable through contagion, for "the Sick cou'd infect none but those that came within reach of the sick Person" (Defoe 154).

> Just as plague inscribes itself upon the body of its victims, it produces textual, thematic, and stylistic symptoms upon an author's corpus. Despite the deaths plague texts inevitably recount, there is a surprising creativity bequeathed by the disease to the writer. Plague's relationship with language and its creative possibilities [are] addressed; so too is the plague witness, the one who survives to tell the tale. (Cooke 12)

---

[1]   For simplicity's sake, Defoe's *A Journal of the Plague Year 1665* will subsequently be abbreviated as *Journal*.

Defoe's *Journal* and the Tradition of Plague Writing

Defoe's *Journal* traces the last plague epidemic in England. The Great Plague of London diminished the city's population by more than 100,000 inhabitants and ranks among the last major European visitations, which include Seville in 1649, London in 1665, Vienna in 1679, East Prussia from 1711 to 1713, and Marseilles in 1720. The outbreak in Marseilles, due to its temporal proximity, prompts Defoe to publish his *Journal* alongside his shorter writings on the *Due Preparations for the Plague* and *Well for Soul and Body* out of mainly propagandistic reasons in 1722. Defoe's writings follow the introduction of the Quarantine Act of 1721 by only one year and as people's anxiety rises, his work is more and more favorably received.

The Quarantine Act succeeds *An Act to Oblige Ships Coming from Places Infected, More Effectually to Perform their Quarantine* (1710) and mostly affects incoming ships and vessels, which are obliged to provide information on the particulars of the name of the ship and its commander; the place where cargo came on board; any further stops or contact with other ships; whether or not there have been any cases of diseases on board; and how many deaths occurred during the time at sea. In the event of signs of the plague, ships would be forcefully hindered from entering the harbor. By declaring that

> [w]hereas Marseilles, and other Places in the Southern Parts of France, have, for some time past, been visited with the Plague, which occasioned just Apprehensions lest the Infection might be brought into this Kingdom from the Places so infected, or other Places trading or corresponding therewith, unless timely Care were taken to prevent the same (Defoe 225-26),

the Quarantine Act thus became a means to more or less effectively seal off the city's trade from the rest of the world, particularly France, which had posed a great threat to London's population ever since its last outbreak two years.

H.F., most likely a reference to Defoe's uncle Henry Foe, is the autodiegetic narrator and seeming survivor of the plague of 1665. Most of Defoe's fictional narrators—Robinson Crusoe is the exception—share the concealment of their true names while telling their stories to the reader. Homer O. Brown even argues that "Defoe's novels are [thus] based on a notion of radical egocentricity" (Brown 565; cf. also 562). While most of Defoe's narrators receive their names within the narrative through some rite of passage, H.F. remains anonymous to the very end. He seemingly provides the reader with an eyewitness testimony sketched from his memoranda of these years—a reconstruction of historical modules, considering that Defoe himself was only five years old when the Great Plague ravaged the city. Just as a doctor might collect data about his or her patient, H.F. collects data about the anamnesis of London: He not only maps the point of entry to the city but also statistically—albeit amateurishly—sketches its progress, finally noting its ceasing and, thus, engages in writing an "episodemic" narrative.[2]

This assumption is very vividly expressed in the various body metaphors found in the *Journal* (cf. Brandwein 340): e.g., entering the city as "an armed man" (99); or, London has a "strangely alter'd face . . . all in Tears" (17-18). H.F., therefore, critically evaluates the city's bodily symptoms and the stories he either remembers or hears. In *Plagues and Epidemics: Infected Spaces Past and Present*, D. Ann Herring and Alan C. Swedlund consider plague epidemics as anthropological entities and thus argue that "the authoritative and seemingly neutral statistical language of *counting*, so fundamental to the definition of 'epidemic,' often overwhelms *accounts* of direct and indirect human encounters with epidemics" (4). This might also explain H.F.'s affinity with the *Bills of Mortality* statistical counting in the *Journal*: Statistical figures can express what he himself lacks the expressive language for.

Carefully distinguishing between fact and fiction, H.F. provides the reader with what he believes to be a factual testimony, notwithstanding that in isolation he himself becomes the disease's symptomatic emblem (and thus its meta-fictional reference). The symptoms and effects that gradually unfold in his story are carefully woven into the narratological fabric; as Jennifer Cooke rightly suggests: "[T]he way the disease affects bodies is, indeed, suggestive of new approaches to reading texts"

---

[2] Jennifer Cooke coins the term "episodemic" (23) in order to describe a narrative style that employs a witness as narrator.

(Cooke 18). As narrator, however, H.F. remains the only possible medium to communicate the contagious subject to the reader.

Defoe's H.F. lends the seventeenth- and eighteenth-century plague an individual voice, and his experiences and statistical logbook of the city are singled out among many. In sharing the emotional horizon of the people he observes, he eventually grants the reader the very same perspective. Individual voices in the *Journal*, thus, never add up to a choir that might provide the reader with a communally shared experience—the narration is always tied to H.F. In this sense, Defoe's *Journal* aligns very closely with his most popular novels, *Robinson Crusoe* and *Moll Flanders*, and to a lesser extent *Colonel Jack*: Each of these texts is intrinsically concerned with what it means to survive in a hostile environment. To be stranded on a desert island, to be left at the mercy of the law of the street of London's criminal subculture, or to be imprisoned in a city infected with a disease of inexpressible extent eventually all boil down to one common agenda: survival. As one critic has remarked about Defoe's "'autobiographers'":

> Near the beginnings of their stories, . . . they . . . are all bereft of family and protection and are thrown into a harsh and dangerous world of deceptive appearances, whose inhabitants are indifferent, conniving, menacing. (Brown 566)

All of Defoe's narrators seem to obsessively become islands within the island of a dysfunctional or non-existent community around them (cf. Brown 567). In the end, Defoe's *Journal* may not so much be about coming to terms with life, but with death.

Defoe's plague narrative provides a literary discourse on a historical event. It tells the stories of the infected as outcasts marked in most cases by darkly protruding inflammations, or so-called "tokens," of enlarged lymph glands in the neck, armpit, and groin. If such an inflammation was not "digested," that is, opened up by force or breaking open of its own accord—perceived as one of the only possible remedies for and treatments of the plague, as it eventually at least caused a release of the unbearable pressure—it forced sufferers into unnatural and almost grotesque postures in order to relieve the tension of their swellings. Judging from H.F.'s observations of the "tokens," most cases of the plague in Defoe's *Journal* can be attributed to the bubonic variant; however, he also notes fatal cases in which the apparently infected do not show any of the primary symptoms. Hence, London's "most formidable enemy" must have been airborne when the infection reached its climax in August and early September 1665, as indicated in H.F.'s employment of the statistics of the city's mortality rates. Although this assumption is never verified in the text by medical evidence (too little is known as yet about the disease), people also fear a possible contamination via the breath of others. It seems likely that the bubonic plague developed into the more dangerous and even more infectious pneumonic variant.[3]

Isolation as a Narrative Mode

The essay at hand attempts to trace the observations of these symptoms that the narrator H.F. makes and almost relives in the *Journal* and whose writing exercise eventually isolates him not only from the community he lives in but also from the reader. The way the disease is or is not and can or cannot be communicated is crucial to an understanding of the text and the subject it examines. H.F. claims right at the beginning of his account that "no such thing as printed News Papers" existed during the time of the plague, "so that things did not spread instantly over the whole nation, as they do now" (Defoe 5), referencing the publication of Defoe's novel in 1722. Charles L. Briggs points out that nowadays

> the news media play crucial roles in deciding when research findings will be transformed into widespread changes in biopolitical perspectives or when reports on pens of infected chickens, handfuls of patients in rural hospitals, and accounts of new influenza, most recently H1N1, will set off global alarms. (40)

---

[3] "Pest" is defined by the *Pschyrembel* dictionary of clinical terms as a highly contagious bacterial disease, caused by *yersinia pestis* and transmitted by rodent fleas, has four variants: bubonic, pneumonic, septicamic, and abortive. Modern medical studies consider the airborne (pneumonic) variant of the plague to have played a crucial role in all known epidemic outbreaks since the fourteenth century.

In this argument, Defoe's *yersinia pestis* is a clear example of the connection between the means of communication and contagion via a bacterial disease. The pest spreads over London almost instantaneously, leaving people faced with their inability to match the rapidity and intensity of the threat with the communication means at hand. The plague demonstrates characteristics of "linguistic infectiousness" (Cooke 3), and Peter DeGabriele therefore rightly proposes that "the plague becomes a deadly metaphor for a universal communication which moves rapidly across all regional boundaries" (DeGabriele 9). This, however, only holds true within the frame of the fiction, as the disease easily outmatches literal transmission by mere touching. The plague itself is restrictive in its communicative means through contagion and the only question that seems crucial is who or what ultimately survives the plague?

On the assumption that Defoe's narrative unfolds a dual perspective that juxtaposes a time of great distress and desperation and a time of relief and re-establishment of community, critics such as Maximillian E. Novak have argued in favor of the survival of the community and the collective, with a particular focus on H.F.'s engagement with the city oscillating between order and disorder (cf. Novak). Others, however, have proposed that the only survivor of the plague is the individual, embodied by the narrator of the text, H.F. (cf. Zimmerman; Bastian). In a more recent attempt to avoid these two major approaches, DeGabriele's study considers an "intimate bond which is resistant to inscription in either the public or private spheres" (9) as the answer to the question of who or what survives the plague; ultimately, however, DeGabriele's approach also frames the question in terms of individuality and community.

I will argue that neither the collective nor the individual survive London's Great Plague and that H.F. only seemingly offers his survival to the reader for the sake of the re-establishment of social order:

> [I]n writing down my Memorandums of what occurred to me every Day, and out of which, afterwards, I for most of this Work as it relates to my Observations without Doors: What I wrote of my private Meditations I reserve for private Use, and desire it may not be made publick in any Account whatever. (Defoe 65-66)

His meditations are just one means for H.F. to retreat within his narrative, which after all appears to him to hold the only lasting value and remedy against contagion. Defoe's representation of the plague evokes an encoded separation of people into those infected (sick) and those not infected (sound), determined by visual (their tokens), auditory (their screams and outcries), and tangible (their fever and buboes/ inflammation) signs; he refrains, however, from creating a vision of the integration and unification of a new community with a distinct identity, just as he refrains from pinpointing the causes of the epidemic's spread. "[A]s a disease besetting a whole town, province or area, it threatened the cohesion of the social bond and called for action and containment upon a mass scale" (Cooke 2). However, the directive H.F. attempts to provide to his readers is undermined by his own narratological restrictions.

I would like to propose analyzing H.F.'s narrative in the following stages, mirroring the plague's development from December 1664 to November 1665:

1) origin and outbreak;
2) reaction, progress, and preventive measures;
3) culmination and cessation; and
4) outcome and conclusion.

Origin and Outbreak

H.F. begins his record by carefully delineating where the plague came from, where exactly it entered the country, and how it reached London. The general assumption was that the plague swept from Holland to Britain and entered London at the westward end of Drury Lane in November 1664, leaving the city untouched over the harsh winter before the next cases steadily increased the death rates in *St Giles* and *St Andrews* in February 1665 and the plague thus slowly but constantly moved eastward into the inner center of London. H.F. gathers this information from the monthly and weekly *Bills of Mortality*, which statistically sketch the death rates in all London's parishes by numbers and further break the rates down into the corresponding causes of death, as the following example illustrates:

From the 1st to the 8th of *Aug.* to the 15th to the 22. to the 29.

Fever	314	353	348	383
Spotted fever*	174	190	166	165
Surfeit	85	87	74	99
Teeth	90	113	111	133

*Any of a group of infectious diseases, including typhus, that are spread by ticks and mites and characterized by skin eruptions.

(Defoe 161)

Extracts from the *Bills*, such as the one provided above, are directly transferred into the narrative, potentially misleading the reader about their historical correctness, as H.F. at a later point in his story admits the probability of faked entries on account of doctors who were simply blackmailed in order to assign a different category to what actually was the plague. As Nicholas Seager points out in an essay, "Defoe is also aware that circumstances do not necessarily add up to facts, just as recorded plague cases do not add up to facts in the *Bills of Mortality*" (Seager 652). The insertion of the *Bills of Mortality* and their statistics nevertheless complicate the reader's engagement with the text as a historical account of the epidemic and position Defoe's "autobiographical" *Journal* at the borderline of historical novel and fictional narrative.

Reaction, Progress, and Preventive Measures

The common reaction to the outbreak that H.F. observes and recollects stresses a common belief in a self-inflicted misery: a disease that purges the sinners in a divine, all-powerful blow that appears even more powerful due to its invisibility:

> I went home indeed, griev'd and afflicted in my Mind, at the Abominable Wickedness of those Men [who would openly insult religious practice], not doubting, however, that they would be made dreadful Examples of God's Justice; for I look'd upon this dismal Time to be a particular Season of Divine Vengeance, and that God would, on this Occasion, single out the proper Objects, of his Displeasure, in a more especial and remarkable Manner, than at another Time; and that,

> tho' I did believe that many good People would, and did, fall in the
> common Calamity, and that it was no certain Rule to judge of the eternal
> State of any one, by their being distinguish'd in such a Time of general
> Destruction, neither one Way or other; yet I say, it could not but seem
> reasonable to believe, that God would not think fit to spare by his Mercy
> such open declared Enemies, that should insult his Name and Being,
> defy his Vengeance, and mock at his Worship and Worshipers, at such a
> Time, no not tho' his Mercy had thought fit to bear with, and spare them
> at other Times: That this was a Day of Visitation; a Day of God's Anger;
> and those Words came into my Thought. Jer. v. 9. Shall I not visit for
> these things, saith the Lord, and shall not my Soul be avenged [on] such
> a Nation as this? (Defoe 59)

As indicated by H.F.'s allusion to Jeremiah 9, the perception of the
plague epidemic as a divine punishment originates in biblical allusions.
The plague appears as early as Genesis 12.17, through the major part of
Exodus as the Egyptian plagues, probably most fitting to the context of
the *Journal* in Deuteronomy 28.61 as "also every sickness, and every
plague, which [is] not written in the book of this law, them will the Lord
bring upon thee, until thou be destroyed" (*King James Bible*) and as late
as Mark 5.34 with varying intensities and denotations. All early word
forms of "plague" seem to carry the rather transient connotation of
affliction—the Latin *plangere* can be translated as "(to) strike," Late
Latin *plaga* as "blow, wound," and Middle English *plage*—whereas the
common understanding of "epidemic" does not necessarily imply a
temporal limit.

Only when the first "tokens" are detected does the potentially divine
punishment receive an actual face. The increased interest among the
poor in visionaries and necromancy gives proof of the incipient
desperation spreading simultaneously with the progressive contagion of
London's population. Possible explanations of the plague's occurrence
and infectious properties ranged from those who "ascribed the plague to
the malignant conjunction of planets or to the influence of the stars, or
even to an overabundance of fruit" to other completely hypothetical
causes, suggesting "just how little was known about the epidemiology of
the plague and consequently how rhetorically powerful such
undifferentiated accounts of the plague could be when translated into
other . . . contexts" (Lund 49). The rich, either having already fled from
London or being about to do so, most likely carried the disease with

them, unknowingly spreading it beyond the city's boundaries. The increasing numbers of cases that H.F. carefully observes in the *Bills* rapidly prompt the city officials to act, and mass regulations are readily formulated.

Due measures to prevent further contagion are already in place: Family heads are required to notify the city officials of any infection in their households within two hours; infected houses are shut and remain shut for a minimum of four weeks' time until no further indication of the disease is given; the infected can either be shut among their family in houses or voluntarily join one of the many pest-houses in and around the city; examiners and wards guard the marked houses and supply the families with food and healthcare; the dead are collected from the houses and/or streets and are taken by the death carts to mass graves on the burial grounds; public fires are set in order to purify the air; maritime trade is closed and inland trade partially reduced; and those who wish to leave London are required to obtain a certificate of health prior to their departure. In short, "London, in metaphorical terms, becomes a human body with its limbs, or roads and ports, cut off from interaction with the outside world" (Brandwein 340). Assemblies of any kind are to be handled with utmost care and are to be initially isolated. Inofficial measures included the use of plague water, perfumes, smoke, and various other preventive measures.

Shortly before his own planned departure, to which he is prompted by his brother, H.F. decides not to leave London after all. Considering that H.F. does not miss out on providing his readers with statistics drawn in abundance from the *Bills of Mortality* and the published orders by the Lord Mayor, it seems rather odd that he does not or possibly cannot provide the reader with his own health certificate, which he would have had to show in order to be able to pass through the city gates. The lack of this document seems even more surprising if one considers that in the early phases of the infection these certificates were issued without any difficulty, as H.F. points out on many occasions.

Admittedly, as easily as doctors could be blackmailed into assigning different causes to what they clearly must have detected as cases of the plague, obtaining a certificate of health could not possibly have proven to be any more difficult. It seems even more surprising that H.F. does not acquire one—if not as proof of his health conditions then out of journalistic curiosity. Seeing the masses of people fleeing from London at that point, H.F. must acknowledge the "unhappy Condition of those that would be left in it [London, that is]" (11). The passive construction of this avowal not only anticipates his manifold future regret and the repentance of his decision but possibly also that his decision to stay may not have been voluntary. Taking into account that his family has already fled from the city, his occupation as a local saddler with some concern about his affiliated shop thus appears to be a rather dubious and above all trivial reason to stay in face of "a most dreadful Plague, which should lay the whole City, and even the Kingdom waste; and should destroy almost all the Nation, both Man and Beast" (25). The only valid reason, it seems, is—undoubtedly next to his journalistic curiosity—his inability to leave the city.

The reader soon learns that H.F. himself shows signs of an illness he cannot sufficiently diagnose, from which he recovers in only three days and thereby abandons the thought of being infected himself. H.F. quickly sets out a new agenda, for his stay may serve rather as a "Direction to themselves [that is, readers] to act by, than a History of my Actings" (11). His propagandistic means are obvious at this point and he carefully builds up his directive by delineating story after story of the infected (in the) city. H.F. thus leaps into the position of a critic—and that of a doctor respectively—evaluating the stories (and symptoms) he collects by sorting them into fact and fiction, carefully pondering which to pass on to the reader, and thus drifts away from his readers on an external level, as much as from the people surrounding him, on an internal level. Not only does H.F. abandon his position as the witnessing narrator but he also jeopardizes his credibility by staying in a city which, at this stage void of all remedy, seems very likely to be subsumed by the disease as a consequence.

All his orders and recommendations seem suspended when H.F. pursues his self-imposed agenda. In one of his nightly endeavors intended to satisfy his curiosity he leaves his house and follows one of the death carts to the mass graves of the burial grounds. The man also following the cart has just, so the reader learns, lost his wife and many of his children. Wishing now to set them at peace, the man is utterly disturbed by the sight of the bearers merely dumping the bodies in a hole and barely covering them with soil (cf. Defoe 53-59). At this point in the narrative, H.F. aligns himself with a man who has literarily lost everything and who is more than willing to face death upon burying his dear ones. Although "there was a strict Order to prevent People coming to those pits [that is, the burial grounds with the mass graves], and that was only to prevent Infection" (53), this is exactly the place where H.F. encounters the man. All orders and regulations formulated by London's authorities to contain the infection do not seem to apply to H.F., who easily transcends all boundaries. In his study on *The Impact of Plague in Tudor and Stuart England*, Paul Slack establishes a close connection between the plague and criminal activities, as pestilence, being a contagious illness, not only poses a threat to one's own health but also to the health conditions of others (cf. 309). Thus, the usually clear-cut boundaries between the two categories begin to blur—even for H.F.

The burial of the bodies that some critics (cf. here, for instance, Juengel) view as the unmistakable sign of a social service that is still intact at times of great peril is thus degraded to a necessity of order. H.F. strictly refrains from rumors such as that in London "the living were not sufficient to bury the dead" (Juengel 168); however, the altered burial ritual makes a powerful impression on him:

> This was a mournful Scene indeed, and affected me almost as much as the rest; but the other was awful, and full of Terror, the Cart had in it sixteen or seventeen Bodies, some were wrapt in Linen Sheets, some in Rugs, some little other than naked, or so loose, that what Covering they had, fell from them, in the shooting out of the Cart, and they fell quite naked among the rest; but the Matter was not much to them, or the Indecency much to any one else, seeing they were all dead, and were to be huddled together into the common Grave of Mankind, as we may call it, for here was no Difference made, but Poor and Rich went together; there was no other way of Burials, neither was it possible there should, for Coffins were not to be had for the prodigious Numbers that fell in such a Calamity as this. (Defoe 55)

Expressions such as "terror," "shooting," and "fell" all invoke the vocabulary of war and once again highlight the linguistic impact of the plague on the narrative.

The story of the man, in particular, accentuates H.F.'s isolation—a man who has only a family of servants, paid for their solicitousness. Once the reader is granted an insight into the recollection of his London, Defoe's narrator comes to epitomize the plague visitation that bans nearly all communication: Characters are isolated, mostly unaffected, and restricted to a private, strictly non-public realm that H.F. leaves regularly except for his meditations, which, on the one hand, constitute his innermost private experience and, on the other hand, separate him from the reader. The man whom H.F. encounters at the burial grounds, though seemingly not infected by the disease, merely "walk'd about, but two or three times groaned very deeply, and loud, and sighed as he would break his Heart" (54) and thus further illustrates the linguistic incommunicability of the disease. As much as H.F. has to face his own inability to communicate parts of his narrative and parts of the disease that besets his narrative, the disease itself, together with its imagery, remains a spectacle in which he cannot resist taking part:

> Defoe's narrators seem obsessed with concealing themselves, but the impulse leading them towards exposure appears equally strong. Complete concealment is impossible, perhaps not even desirable. On the one hand there is the insistence on building a faceless shelter around the self, but, on the other, a recurring compulsion to move out into the open. (Brown 569)

Culmination and Cessation

The retreat to a private space within the narrative is exemplified when the infection culminates in August and September 1665 in countless victims and the highest rates of new infections in the death *Bills*. All of London's inhabitants seem trapped within the city walls and are strictly surveilled by city authorities.[4]

> Within these discourses, plague is used to identify, label and advocate the removal of a "poisonous" or "dangerous" outsider group, usually a minority believed to threaten (the "health" of) society and whose extermination or containment is supposed to have a curative or restorative function. (Cooke 3)

---

[4]   Cf. Foucault, esp. Lecture 2, on the particular containment of the individual during plague epidemics and the subsequent surveillance of the population's health conditions.

H.F. transcends all implicit boundaries at the core of his own narrative and departs London for the first and only time in order to tell the story of three men: a biscuit baker, a sail-maker, and a joiner, who leave London together and live as nomads in tents or huts before being joined by more followers. For the account of the three men, the narrative voice changes to reported and partly direct speech, thus designating the narrator's retreat in the text.

H.F., ever so keen on differentiating fact and fiction, unfolds in the story of the three men an allegorical vision of an integrated, self-sustaining community that serves as a model of modest, and in the most literal sense, natural way of life in times of plague. Interestingly enough, he is not able to physically leave London at the beginning of his story but is only able to escape from it through his narrative. The unique feature of his storytelling hence becomes the way in which H.F. isolates and positions himself as an outsider. The apparent lack of communication—that is, the inability to interact with one another—is a London symptom of the plague epidemic that H.F. collects and above all inscribes into his narrative. One of Defoe's contemporaries, Richard Mead, argues in one of his pamphlets, *A Short Discourse Concerning Pestilential Contagion*, that

> whatever else be the Cause: certain it is, that at such Times, when it should be expected to see all Men unite in one common Endeavour, to moderate the publick Misery; quite otherwise, they grow regardless of each other, and Barbarities are often practised, unknown at other Times. (Mead 17-18)

The plague has a strong fracturing power, bringing about "economic disruption, political anarchy and a progressive deterioration of manners" (Steel 90-91) so that the only possible resort for H.F. remains his allegorical narrative. H.F. observes families, which are torn apart by the disease, and eventually has to acknowledge his own disintegration in the non-existent community, which elicits in him the wish for the re-establishment of social order. This social order, however, cannot be achieved in London: a city that is completely permeated by the disruptive and destructive power of a disease for which no remedy seems to exist. Daniel Gordon posits that "for Defoe, the plague shows that there are times when the whole city is nothing but human fragility writ large. The city, far from being an escape from our mortality, may only accelerate it" (76).

The internal retreat from the city to nature as much as the vision of an integrated community therefore anticipate a turning point in Defoe's *Journal*. Almost miraculously, death rates decline even though the numbers of the infected were never higher in the course of the year—the plague finally leaves London and while it travels to other English cities, the majority of people slowly return to their home.

The vision of a new and most likely more civil and even modern community—which is one of the keys to the text according to some critics (cf. Novak 248)—seems almost tangible when London's gates re-open.

H.F.'s vision coincides with the ceasing of the plague. The community that H.F. envisions in his allegorical story of the three men is only possible due to the fact that this community claims a new, inviolately pure space for itself, while the returning population of London, by contrast, eventually re-builds its community on the essentially diseased remains; that is, mass graves, burial grounds, abandoned and marked houses carrying the signs of the enforced isolation of its inhabitants on them. H.F. condemns the fact that those who already died and were only provisionally buried cannot rest undisturbed—an unusually strong judgment that barely finds an equivalent in the narrative.

Outcome and Conclusion

> ... after the ceasing of the Plague in *London*, when any one that had seen the Condition which the People had been in, and how they caress'd one another at that time, promis'd to have more Charity for the future, and to raise no more Reproaches: I say, any one that had seen them then, would have thought they would have come together with another Spirit at last. (Defoe 183)

People never change; they only adapt to the circumstances, and the belief in a universal punishment for their sins had most likely spurred their longing for company: Church services were frequented even at times of greatest peril and those who could afford it appeared more benevolent toward the poor. Nevertheless, once the external enemy vanishes, the inner solidarity likewise subsides, and H.F.'s vision has no more validity—either for the narrator or for any other member of the community.

Before the end of the narrative, in an almost casual remark while discussing five burial grounds and how these areas were used after the epidemic had left and most of the residents had returned, H.F. includes the following information on the fourth burial ground, called *Moorfields*:

> The Author of this Journal, lyes buried in that very Ground, being at his own Desire, his Sister having been buried there a few years before. (Defoe 181)

H.F.'s ongoing subliminal examination of the value of fact and fiction for his story suggests that he most likely understood himself as the author of the *Journal*. He not only retreats within his text, finding solace in his private writings and meditations, but also abandons it, just as the plague suddenly and surprisingly abandons London. The fact that the narrator/author is already dead (one might say de-constructed in the most literal sense) before the end of the novel, makes his final lines

> A dreadful Plague in London was,
> In the Year Sixty Five
> Which swept an Hundred Thousand Souls
> Away, yet I alive!
> H.F. (Defoe 193)

appear hollow and merely visionary, prompting due preparations for the plague. And these preparations are the directive that H.F. initially intended—so that his *Journal* ultimately remains the only permanent value, the only value that is "yet alive." The community can neither rebuild itself upon the essentially contaminated remains of the plague within the restrictive frame of the narrative, nor can the individual be successfully integrated into the community.

Works Cited

Bastian, F[rank]. "Defoe's *Journal of the Plague Year* Reconsidered." *Review of English Studies* ns 16.62 (1965): 151-73. Print.

Brandwein, Michelle. "Formation, Process, and Transition in *A Journal of the Plague Year*." *A Journal of the Plague Year*. By Daniel Defoe. Ed. Paula R. Backscheider. New York: Norton, 1992. 336-55. Print.

Briggs, Charles L. "Pressing Plagues: On the Mediated Communicability of Virtual Epidemics." *Plagues and Epidemics: Infected Spaces Past and Present*. Ed. D. Ann Herring and Alan C. Swedlund. Oxford: Berg, 2010. 39-59. Print.

Brown, Homer O. "The Displaced Self in the Novels of Daniel Defoe." *English Literary History* 38.4 (1971): 562-90. Print.

Cooke, Jennifer. *Legacies of Plague in Literature, Theory and Film*. Basingstoke: Palgrave, 2009. Print.

Defoe, Daniel. *A Journal of the Plague Year*. 1722. Ed. Paula R. Backscheider. New York: Norton, 1992. Print.

DeGabriele, Peter. "Intimacy, Survival, and Resistance: Daniel Defoe's *A Journal of the Plague Year*." *English Literary History* 77.1 (2010): 1-23. Print.

Foucault, Michel. *Abnormal: Lectures at the Collège de France, 1974-1975*. Trans. Graham Burchell. New York: Picador, 1999. Print.

Gordon, Daniel. "The City and the Plague in the Age of Enlightenment." *Yale French Studies* 92 (1997): 67-87. Print.

Herring, D. Ann, and Alan C. Swedlund, eds. *Plagues and Epidemics: Infected Spaces Past and Present*. Oxford: Berg, 2010. Print.

---. "Plagues and Epidemics in Anthropological Perspective." *Plagues and Epidemics: Infected Spaces Past and Present*. Ed. D. Ann Herring and Alan C. Swedlund. Oxford: Berg, 2010. 1-19. Print.

Juengel, Scott. "Writing Decomposition: Defoe and the Corpse." *Journal of Narrative Technique* 25.2 (1995): 139-53. Print.

The King James Bible. Ed. Project Gutenberg. 2nd version, 10th ed. University of Oxford Text Archive. 1992. Web. 14 March 2012.

Lund, Roger D. "Infectious Wit: Metaphor, Atheism, and the Plague in Eighteenth-Century London." *Literature and Medicine* 22.1 (2003): 45-64. Print.

Mead, Richard. *A Short Discourse on Pestilential Contagion, and the Methods to Be Used to Prevent It.* London: Sam Buckley, 1722. Print.

Novak, Maximillian E. "Defoe and the Disordered City." *PMLA* 92.2 (1977): 241-52. Print.

"Pest." *Pschyrembel Online Premium.* 2010. *Pschyrembel Klinisches Wörterbuch.* Vienna University of Technology. Web. 24 Feb 2012.

Seager, Nicholas. "Lies, Damned Lies, and Statistics: Epistemology and Fiction in Defoe's *A Journal of the Plague Year.*" *Modern Language Review* 103.3 (2008): 639-53. Print.

Slack, Paul. *The Impact of Plague in Tudor and Stuart England.* London: Routledge, 1985. Print.

Sontag, Susan. *Illness as Metaphor and AIDS and Its Metaphors.* New York: Picador, 2001. Print.

Steel, David. "Plague Writing: From Boccaccio to Camus." *Journal of European Studies* 11.2 (1981): 88-110. Print.

Zimmerman, Everett. "H.F.'s Meditations: *A Journal of the Plague Year.*" *PMLA* 87.3 (1972): 417-23. Print.

INGRID GESSNER

Contagion, Crisis, and Control: Tracing Yellow Fever in Nineteenth-Century American Literature and Culture

Introducing Epidemics of Fear

The history of North America and the United States has always been accompanied by the presence of diseases, from smallpox in the colonial period to HIV/AIDS and swine flu today. Bacteria and viruses are incredibly mobile, and their mobility links what is otherwise kept apart by means of social or ideological constructions (people and nations). Diseases, as Rüdiger Kunow has argued, are inherently transgressive phenomena (24). This holds equally true for concepts related to disease, such as contact, (im)migration, infection, and transmission, or more precisely the fear or risk of transmission and spread of panic accompanying the appearance of epidemic diseases. Besides a transgressive quality, communicable diseases also display a "transnational" quality, as they are capable of traveling clandestinely from host to host across national borders (sometimes with the help of a non-human carrier), which also feeds into a culture of fear and evokes panic. The concept of contagion in its figurative and literal usage may link the history of epidemics and panic (cf. Pernick, "Contagion" 861).[1]

---

[1] Although *contagious* has been replaced in medical dictionaries by *communicable*, in the sense of "capable of being transmitted," the concept of contagion remains important with respect to speculations about the cause of diseases. Contagion is entangled with politics and ethics: The assumption

As Martin S. Pernick points out, "[r]eferences to contagious fear were not necessarily or wholly metaphorical," since fear was seen as a direct cause of disease. In this line of argument, "[p]anic could literally be seen as both an epidemic of fear and as the agent by which . . . epidemics spread" ("Contagion" 861). A double helix of health (and emphasis on the purity of the body) and fear (or anxiety about losing health) seems to have been ingrained in U.S. society and culture from colonial times. This culture of fear (to borrow Barry Glassner's contemporary term) has been fed through various real and perceived threats, from smallpox-infected blankets, through "undetected" immigrant carriers of disease such as Typhoid Mary, to the post-9/11 anthrax scare. Throughout the nineteenth century, when waves of mass immigration fostered an ethnic and cultural diversification of society, America anxiously sought to define itself through and against threats to the national body. Notions of disease and health crises were figuratively linked to the period's experience of a highly complex layering of several social and political crises such as federalism, slavery, immigration, democratization, industrialization, and urbanization. The crisis experiences were woven into discourses of progress and nation-building, since the construction, confirmation, and assurance of a national identity seemed imperative for the social and political advancement of American nationhood during this period.

Between 1793 and 1905 the most severe epidemic outbreaks of disease in the U.S. accompanied by serious panics were due to yellow fever and cholera. In 1793, between four and five thousand Philadelphia residents, or eight to nine percent of the population, died from yellow fever. During the 1832 cholera epidemic, 3,000 people died in New York (July-August) and more than 4,000 died in New Orleans (October). The 1853 yellow fever epidemic in New Orleans claimed the lives of eight to nine thousand people or nine percent of the population.

"that another person is the source of disease [makes] the links between contagion and personal blame . . . especially close and visible. When 'other people' have been seen as the source, contagion has been used to blame outsiders and outcasts, especially immigrants and minorities" (Pernick, "Contagion" 862). Pernick also cautions researchers not to reduce contagionist medicine to politics or morality alone, but also to see it in its relations and the dependencies of its specific time and place.

Several outbreaks of yellow fever during the 1870s culminated in the devastating 1878 epidemic during which 13,000 to 20,000 people, or ten percent of the population, died in the lower Mississippi Valley (Patterson 857–58; "Major U.S. Epidemics"). With mortality rates of eight to ten percent during these major epidemics, a certain congruence of perceived and actual threat can be asserted. However, not every yellow fever epidemic was equally devastating, whereas the perceived threat remained. The last major outbreak of yellow fever in the U.S. occurred in New Orleans in 1905.

This essay explores the ideological, sociopolitical, and cultural productivity of yellow fever epidemics in the formative nineteenth century of U.S.-American history and culture. It reads yellow fever texts as representations of crisis phenomena and experiences of crisis.[2] How is the disease represented, aestheticized, and explained as meaningful? Which forms of control are suggested in times of perceived danger to minimize health risks, contain diseases or their outbreak, and to regulate human action? Do these narratives suggest a subversion of hegemonic structures which the general panic and the fear of health risks otherwise prevented or contained in society?[3] Taking up these questions in a "fiction as symbolic action" approach (Kenneth Burke), this essay examines two contemporary narrative representations of two major yellow fever epidemics: the 1793 Philadelphia epidemic with Charles Brockden Brown's *Arthur Mervyn, or, Memoirs of the Year 1793* (1799/ 1800), and the 1873 Shreveport epidemic with Wesley Bradshaw's popular sentimental novella *Angel Agnes or, The Heroine of the Yellow Fever Plague in Shreveport* (1873). I aim to show how both authors, who use yellow fever epidemics to construct narrative cultures of fear, offer different ways of interpreting and controlling what seems incomprehensible by potentially subverting or redefining existing social power structures such as slavery and patriarchy, or at least by putting

---

[2] Concepts and cultural constructs of health, invasion, contact, crisis, contagion, fear, anxiety, panic (and how to control panic narratively, for instance) frame my angle of research.

[3] With a nod to Stephen Greenblatt (21-65), I am proposing a subversion-containment dialectic of narrative cultures of fear here.

forward alternative visions for a nation eagerly trying to define itself against threats from within and without.

Tracing Yellow Fever Epidemics

> The yellow fever will discourage the growth of great cities in our nation & I view great cities as pestilential to the morals, the health and the liberties of man. True, they nourish some of the elegant arts, but the useful ones can thrive elsewhere, and less perfection in the others, with more health, virtue & freedom, would be my choice.
> (Jefferson 147)
>
> Thomas Jefferson to Benjamin Rush, 1800

Yellow fever or "yellow jack" has a long and notorious history in the United States and has been called "West-India or American yellow fever" (Rush 156) and categorized as one of "our epidemics" in the late eighteenth century by the editors of the *Medical Repository* (Caldwell, *A Reply* 16). Among them were Benjamin Rush and Charles Caldwell, a former student of Rush, both of whom corresponded and collaborated with Noah Webster. The *Medical Repository* was founded in 1797 as "a venue for many medical and natural historical topics; the editors made the disease a primary subject" (Arner 453). The emphasis on a distinct American identity vis-à-vis yellow fever and an American interpretational sovereignty regarding the disease's origin became part of a trans-Atlantic debate that was instantaneously politicized.[4] For example, Noah Webster, in his *Brief History of Epidemic and*

---

[4]   Arner cites a 1799 oration by Charles Caldwell (*A Semi-Annual Oration, on the Origin of Pestilential Diseases*), in which he identifies the cause of a late Philadelphia outbreak as of local origin, thus countering the college's assertion of importation (454).

Pestilential Diseases "fashioned his History as a domestic source by an American about American environs and most applicable to interpretations of what he and others thought to be an American disease" (Webster, *Brief History* 26-27). American scientists who believed in the non-contagionist nature of the disease presented yellow fever not only as something that originated in America, but also claimed it as their domain of research, invoking an "American intellectual independence." Charles Caldwell wrote: "As well might the parliament of Great Britain, in their present ignorance of our circumstances as a nation, attempt to legislate for all our emergencies, as her faculty to decide for us with regard to the nature, prevention, or cure of *our* epidemics" (*A Reply* 10-11; my emphasis).[5]

In her 2006 book, Molly Caldwell Crosby juxtaposes the late eighteenth-century European with an American understanding of yellow fever when she refers (also in her book title) to "[t]he American Plague ... that shaped *our* history" and that created panic and fear incomparable to other diseases (11; my emphasis). Today we know that the disease was not indigenous to America, but vector and virus originated in Africa and entered the New World through the slave trade (Patterson 856); yellow fever probably first occurred in Spanish Florida in 1649-1650 (Dobyns and Swagerty 279). In 1693, Boston and other towns were infected when ships from the West Indies brought it to then British North America (Krieg 49). The disease struck irregularly. Sometimes communities were afflicted yearly by epidemics in the summer and early fall, after which yellow fever might completely disappear and not come back for decades. Yellow fever's symptoms include jaundice, bleeding from nose and mouth, stools stained dark with blood, and copious black vomit. Yellow fever has a high case fatality rate of 15 to 50 percent and higher, whereas very high mortality rates may indicate that milder cases were not recognized as yellow fever. Survivors of yellow fever gain lifetime immunity (Patterson 855).

---

[5] It needs to be noted that the picture of American identity politics is complicated by the West Indies, which Arner describes as "a peripheral setting that presented another set of epistemological, as well as cultural and political relations to the new nation" (459).

Yellow fever was also often referred to as "strangers' disease" in the nineteenth-century United States. This corresponds to contemporary descriptions as well as modern studies that point toward a greater vulnerability of new residents and temporary visitors from Northern states, interior Southern states, and Europe (Patterson 861). Furthermore, the fatality rate of men was higher than that of women; and "adults were more likely to contract fatal cases than children. Poor people seemed to be singled out in some epidemics . . . partly because they lived near the docks, where . . . infected ships would bring the disease first, and partly because many of the poor were immunologically naïve newcomers" (Patterson 860).

It was not until 1881 that a Cuban physician, Carlos Juan Finlay, suggested that mosquitoes might actually be the culprits in the transmission of the disease.[6] And even after Finlay's proposal in 1881, scientists struggled to reconcile the geographical and the bacteriological-contagionist perspective of yellow fever—until Finlay's hypothesis was confirmed by Major Walter Reed and James Carroll in 1900.[7] Yellow fever is an acute viral disease transmitted to humans by the bite of the female *Aedes aegypti* mosquito; unspreadable through human contact and noncontagious (Patterson 855).

---

[6] As early as 1848, Josiah Clark Nott published papers in which he proposed some connection between insects and disease. Writing at a time when the term "insect" was loosely used, and before the germ theory of disease had taken hold, Nott made no clear distinction between insects as pathogens and as vectors of pathogens (cf. also Humphreys 20) and thus cannot be credited as the originator of the mosquito theory.

[7] Walter Reed headed the commission that demonstrated the correctness of Finlay's hypothesis that mosquitoes were vectors of yellow fever. This was the first of many viral diseases shown to be arthropod-borne. With the emergence and growing acceptance of Pasteurian germ theory and other microbiological findings and medical innovations by the 1870s and 1880s (Pasteur gave his famous lecture at the Sorbonne on April 7, 1864), a new era of medical history and understanding of medicine had set in. For an investigation of the influence of medicine in American literature (1845-1915) in light of the emerging germ theory, cf. Davis.

Infecting the Nation: Charles Brockden Brown's *Arthur Mervyn, or, Memoirs of the Year 1793* (1799/1800)

> The Evils of pestilence by which this city has lately been afflicted will probably form an era in its history.
> (*Arthur Mervyn* 3)

These facts were unknown to Charles Brockden Brown when he wrote *Arthur Mervyn*, a gothic novel in the true vein of social critique in 1799/1800. In what he calls a "brief but faithful sketch," his observations provide an "instructive" model of "benevolence" and "virtue" for his readers to copy (*AM* 3).[8] In *Arthur Mervyn*, yellow fever, which had befallen the new nation in 1793 after a hiatus of some 30 years, provides a dramatic setting and represents the complex experience of crisis and transformation the young nation was facing.[9] Instead of interpreting the epidemic outbreak of yellow fever in Philadelphia with a Puritan lens as God's punishment and as a transgression of the perceived purity of the body, Brown fictionally explores the epidemic from the perspective of the Enlightenment. In his preface he states that he "has ventured to methodize his own reflections" upon the "medical and political discussions which are now afloat in the community" (*AM* 3), referring to a wealth of written and spoken material, of which his novel is only a part (cf. Waterman 216). Brown proposes engaging the discussions in a twofold manner: first, to present a moral tale that is, second, informed by medical knowledge and political discourse in order to offer a means of control in the face of a medical but also sociopolitical crisis of the 1790s.

Without concrete medical evidence, medical technologies, or the Pasteurian germ theory that emerged more than half a century later, the

---

[8]   In the following, for simplicity's sake, I will use *AM* for *Arthur Mervyn, or, Memoirs of the Year 1793*.

[9]   Gesa Mackenthun similarly argues, "the disease becomes symbolic of a society out of joint"; "a fitting metaphor for expressing this state of flux and this fear" (61; 63).

debates around the origin of the fever were almost instantaneously politicized: A xenophobic contagionist school believed in the communicability of the fever via infected products imported to the city and saw ship passengers of French and African origins as a source of the fever.[10] Federalists in particular used this interpretation of the disease to express anti-Republican ideas and to blame the epidemic on the French. They called for a need to isolate America from the revolutionary "contagions" that had passed from France to the West Indies and were about to spread to the United States. A miasmatic, environmentalist school argued against the fever's communicability and believed in the domestic origin of the disease due to poor urban sanitation and hygiene. The latter theory served a Jeffersonian Democratic Republican rhetoric of separation of city vs. country.[11] It should, however, be pointed out that the correlation of contagionists and non-contagionists to a specific partisan affiliation is more complicated than Pernick's model. Physicians of the "Friendly Club" with whom Brown was associated supported the, at the time, more progressive view of non-contagionism.[12] Although Brown's friend Benjamin Rush was a Jeffersonian Democratic Republican, not all members of the club and Brown's circle shared this affiliation.

Arthur Mervyn includes both speculations that the disease was of domestic miasmatic origin, as Brown's circle, including his friend Rush,

---

[10] Cf. Pernick, "Politics, Parties, and Pestilence" 568; Powell 16. Referring to Pernick, Gesa Mackenthun equally points to the rhetorical purpose within the debates. Mackenthun writes: "Thus, the 1793 yellow fever . . . acquired the status of a powerful metaphor . . . . It provided Jeffersonians with arguments in favor of a healthy agrarian republic and Federalists with rhetorical fodder for their antidemocratic and Francophobic sentiments" (54). Cf. also Arner.

[11] Cf. Jefferson, who discourages the "growth of great cities in our nation" (147). Jefferson believed that social health required a rural lifestyle. In like fashion, William Penn warns his wife, "of Citys and towns of concourse beware. ... A country life and estate I like best for my children" (qtd. in Clarkson 316-17). And Noah Webster asks: "Why should cities be erected, if they are only to be the tombs of men?" (*A Collection of Papers* 208).

[12] Cf. also Waterman 219-20. Today we know that contrary to the widely held medical opinion of the time, the Philadelphia epidemic was most probably introduced by French refugees from Haiti/Saint-Domingue (Patterson 856).

proposed, and that it was a menace from abroad. Vincentio Lodi brings both money and fever from Guadaloupe. The villain Welbeck meets Lodi, who has contracted "a violent disease . . . in the tropical islands" (72) in chapter 10. This is also the first time "Yellow or Malignant Fever" (72) is identified by name. When the title figure of the novel, young Quaker Arthur Mervyn, is driven out of his family's country home by his father's widow and sets out for Philadelphia in pursuit of education and wealth that he hopes to find in the city, he encounters wagons traveling from the city, only to learn upon his arrival that yellow fever has struck there. He subsequently develops a theory of an outside origin of the disease, which is later contradicted by the enlightened Quaker and physician Medlicote:

> He combated an opinion I had casually formed respecting the origin of the epidemic, and imputed it not to infected substances imported from east or west, but to a morbid constitution of the atmosphere, owing wholly or in part to filthy streets, airless habitations, and squalid persons. (123)

In chapter 8, the "sultry" atmosphere and unbearable heat already serve to foreshadow the fever scenes and hint at environmental causes of the disease: "The air was remarkably sultry. Lifted sashes and lofty ceilings were insufficient to attemper it. The perturbation of my thoughts affected my body, and the heat which oppressed me was aggravated, by my restlessness, almost into fever" (58). The "contagious atmosphere" (153) or "an atmosphere so contagious and deadly" (133) remains a theme throughout the fever section in the first part of the novel.

Although Brown includes contagionist and non-contagionist speculations about the fever's origin, he primarily constructs yellow fever as "a symbol for social crisis" (Grabo 103): Yellow fever along with commercial corruption and the slave trade are spreading from within.[13] The symbolic reading of fever as social allegory has been put forward by several critics[14] who "have pointed to ways in which 'contagion' . . . seems to speak to contemporary discussions about the

---

[13] In this sense, I follow symbolic–figurative interpretations of the disease that entail consequences for the treatment of the real and the figurative disease(s).

[14] Cf. Levine; Tompkins; Samuels; Stern; and Gould.

French Revolution, . . . the Alien and Sedition Acts, the rise of a market economy, patriarchal anxieties, and a breakdown of fellow feeling in the highly partisan Federal era" (Waterman 219). Through the events that unfold in the novel, commercial corruption as the result of an unhealthy social environment is tied to the disease's origin; the fever, as Bill Christophersen calls it, is the "social toll of America's money ethic" (113). For example, the morally corrupt Thetford, who falls into a lunatic panic when his servant becomes sick, dies together with his whole family.[15] Wallace, in pursuit of financial independence under Thetford's corrupt stewardship, ignores his loved one's plea to leave the infected city, contracts the disease, and dies. And even Mervyn's infected body could be read as a result of his earlier involvement in Welbeck's moral corruption. Further examples include Welbeck, who returns to the fever-ridden city to secure the money he suspects within the pages of Lodi's notebook. At Bush Hill hospital, the attendants are described as putting their health at risk for the sake of monetary compensation. Here Brown relied on Mathew Carey's problematic and biased account regarding the hospital attendants.[16] The social disease that structurally underlies the narrative is the violence associated with the slave trade, which Brown does not attribute to Africans, who remain largely disembodied and speechless,[17] but to the merchants who prosper from slavery's benefits and a nation that allows this. In Medlicote's words, the fever is not attributed "to infected substances imported from East or West, but to a morbid constitution of the atmosphere" (123), that is, an American "constitutional defect."[18] The threat of black revolution

---

[15] This is, of course, also a further instance of criticism of the contagionist stance.

[16] See Griffith; and Lapsansky for an analysis of Carey's account and an assessment of the role of African Americans during the epidemic.

[17] This is in contrast to John Edgar Wideman's "Fever" (1989) and *The Cattle Killing* (1996); these fictional narratives are based on Richard Allen and Absalom Jones's *Narrative of the Proceedings of the Black People, during the Late Awful Calamity* (1794).

[18] Cf. Christophersen 108. This defect is mirrored by a literal "constitutional" defect Arthur is assumed to harbor in his body: "The seeds of an early and lingering death are sown in my constitution" (*AM* 104).

spreading to the U.S. as a direct result of slavery's aberrations is also broadly associated with a "fever."[19]

Yellow fever is primarily represented in chapters 15-23 of the novel's first part and is first introduced in chapter 1 when the fever-stricken Arthur Mervyn is picked up by Dr. Stevens (whose name is not provided until chapter 4 of the second part). Returning to his house in the evening, Dr. Stevens quite literally stumbles over the sick Arthur Mervyn, and immediately infers "that [Arthur's] disease was pestilential, [which] did not deter [him] from approaching and examining him more closely" (5). Stevens diagnoses Mervyn on the basis of observation. The enlightened physician's stance represents a sanitationist view in light of a disease he believes to be non-contagious and of local origin; Dr. Stevens advocates "cleanliness, reasonable exercise, and a wholesome diet" and argues against popular measures, such as "filling the house with exhalations of gunpowder, vinegar, or tar" (5). After his recovery in the Stevens household, Mervyn is prompted to relate his tale to defend himself against accusations. His account makes up the whole first part of the novel. Mervyn first gives a longer introduction to and description of the fever in the form of a fever rumor in chapter 13. The rumor that "gradually swelled to formidable dimensions" reaches Mervyn during his retreat in a Quaker farmhouse: "The city, we were told, was involved in confusion and panic, for a pestilential disease had begun its destructive progress. Magistrates and citizens were flying to the country. . . . The numbers of the sick multiplied beyond all example; . . . . The malady was malignant and unsparing" (99). A vivid and horrifying account follows, with wives deserted by husbands, children by parents, people dying isolated in their houses or being "seized by the disease in the streets" and perishing "in the public ways." A lack of nurses and undertakers produces "air with deadly exhalations" that adds "tenfold to the devastation" (99). The "epidemic of fear" (to use Martin S. Pernick's phrase), the rumors and tales Mervyn recalls having picked up, "distorted and diversified a thousand ways by the credulity and exaggeration of the tellers" (*AM* 99),

---

[19] Brown's abolitionist stance is even more emphatically expressed in his non-fiction writings, e.g., *An Address to the Government* (1803) (cf. Christophersen 108).

precedes his actual firsthand experience of the epidemic. Contagion not only serves as metaphor, but contagious fear has reached the countryside, which is also reflected in the employment of disease-related terminology: The nearest neighbor of the Hadwins (where Mervyn resides), "though not un*infected* by the general panic persisted to visit the city daily with his *market-cart*" (102; first emphasis mine). In the first part of the novel, the city remains, structurally, a space of corruption: Two main sections describe Mervyn's two ventures into the city; he first experiences commercial corruption (chaps. 2-12), and then physical corruption during the yellow fever epidemic (chaps. 13-23). At the end of chapter 16, when Mervyn senses that he "had received this corrosive poison," he succinctly expresses the spatial dichotomy: "I wondered at the contrariety that exists between the scenes of the city and the country; and fostered with more zeal than ever, the resolution to avoid those seats of depravity and danger" (118).

The symbolic employment of the disease and contagion does not necessarily rule out newer readings of the fever as a medical crisis widely discussed in information networks of the time (cf. Waterman; Arner). Brown, with the help of the medical knowledge available to him—through his friends and his involvement in contemporary medical discourses—assumes authority in *Arthur Mervyn* to interpret the disease, its origin, and its possible treatment in a literal, medical sense. Like the writings of his "scientific friends," Brown's "novelistic enterprise" was based on "observational practices" (Waterman 241) and generated a wide audience, thus inevitably also informing the formation of identity in the new nation. Bryan Waterman cites as evidence the words of narrator-physician Stevens, who, at the beginning of the second part of the novel, recognizes that "[d]uring this season of pestilence, [his] opportunities of observation had been numerous, and [he] had not suffered them to pass unimproved" (*AM* 167). Furthermore, "Mervyn's ability to read his diseased environment transforms unself-consciously into a desire to classify his diverse surroundings; self-government leads to social authority as his authoritative narrative drowns out competing voices" (Waterman 243). Mervyn's character development, especially in the second part of the novel, where a recovered Mervyn sets out to clean up the city's moral corruption and thus provides the means of the epidemic's eradication, could easily be applied as a vision for the young nation (which not coincidentally is the same age as the novel's protagonist).

Moving South: Wesley Bradshaw's *Angel Agnes, or, The Heroine of the Yellow Fever Plague in Shreveport* (1873)

> May God protect you, reader of this book, from all manner of sickness; but above all, from that thrice dreaded pestilence, yellow fever. Of all the scourge ever sent upon poor sinful man, none equals in horror and loathsomeness yellow fever. (Bradshaw 3)

Yellow fever became, and Brown's preface can thus seem prophetic, somewhat of a constant in nineteenth-century America; with "periodical visitations of this calamity," it produced "change in manners and population . . . in the highest degree memorable" (*AM* 3). By the 1840s, yellow fever had retreated from Northern cities to the South, where its frequency and malignancy seemed to rise concurrently with almost yearly epidemics in Southern maritime cities and, by the 1870s, in cities further inland connected through a growing system of rail transportation. A "new anxiety about regional disparities" between North and South could be detected in the writings of medical Southerners, Margaret Humphreys observes (46). Yellow fever became the reason for most of the medical reform activity and public health action in the South, and quarantines the most popular measure in Southern efforts to control it (cf. Humphreys 47). This was mainly due to the fact that the "doctrine of transportability" had (re)emerged in the South after the 1840s (53). The local origin cause was seriously doubted by the majority of Southern medical authors when the earliest cases of yellow fever in East Coast cities during the 1850s "could all be traced to ships arriving from yellow fever-infested Caribbean ports" (Humphreys 24). Yellow fever's transmissibility subsequently became more and more accepted—especially in the last two decades of the nineteenth century when research on other diseases helped formulate a "germ theory of yellow fever" (25). Since the role of "filth" in the evolution of the disease remained to be proven, sanitarians often failed to convince legislators that sanitation could help eradicate the disease; sanitary reform remained secondary to quarantine management (cf. Humphreys 54; 57). The strictness and rigidity of quarantines, and sometimes even shotgun quarantines, varied with the level of public anxiety accompanying an epidemic. For example, when in 1878 yellow fever spread as far north as to affect the Midwestern states of Indiana, Illinois, and Ohio, the "dramatic images of panic and death . . . generated a nationwide sentiment in favor of federal enforcement of a strong quarantine" (Humphreys 61). Yellow fever, despite its primarily Southern manifestation, remained a national problem and affected the national economy. An increased reliance on the importance of quarantine measures dominated federal public health involvement in the late nineteenth century.[20]

Several yellow fever epidemics gripped the South in the 1870s. In 1873, the comparatively small Louisiana city Shreveport, on the Red River, was struck. The Shreveport epidemic, during which 16 to 17 percent of the city's population died, still ranks as one of the worst yellow fever outbreaks in the United States.[21] Its devastating progression was covered (not always accurately and often with a sensationalist bent) in newspapers across the nation, as well as extensively in *Frank Leslie's Illustrated News*. Several reports show that contributions to relieve the situation in the Louisiana city came from all over the nation (for example, "The Yellow Fever: . . . Subscriptions for the Aid of Shreveport"; "Yellow Fever: . . . Relief Contributions"). In this atmosphere, Wesley Bradshaw (aka Charles Wesley Alexander) wrote and published the sentimental novella *Angel Agnes, or, The*

---

[20] Humphreys contends that analogies likening yellow fever to an invading army or imported commodities rhetorically constructed the disease as a national calamity. In this line of reasoning, it was easy to argue that "protection from yellow fever should be in the hands of the federal government, just as military security and international diplomacy were constitutionally reserved for federal jurisdiction" (12).

[21] I am basing the mortality rate of 16.5 percent on Patterson, who lists 759 yellow fever deaths (cf. Patterson 858), and on the 1870 Census, which lists 4,607 Shreveport residents (*Statistics of Population* Table 3: 155).

Heroine of the Yellow Fever Plague in Shreveport. It is the story of Agnes Arnold, the adopted daughter of a wealthy Philadelphia businessman who reads about the yellow fever epidemic and decides to go to Shreveport to offer her assistance. This echoes the real presence and assistance of out-of-town volunteers, many of whom fell victim to the disease and were buried at Shreveport. Bradshaw uses the disease as a projection screen for virtue, dedication, and goodness; in other words, morality as a means to control yellow fever. The disease is also employed as a formula of danger to feed into a culture of fear.

Earlier popular historical fictions by Bradshaw also feed into this culture with themes of the Civil War (*Pauline of the Potomac, Or General McClellan's Spy* [1862]; *Maud of the Mississippi* [1863]; *General Sherman's Indian Spy* [1865]; *The Angel of the Battlefield* [1865]), or the hardships of the Mormon trek to Utah (*Brigham Young's Daughter* [1870]). This kind of sensational literature democratized the war in that it obliterated distinctions in rank, class, or between men and women by fantasizing about female heroines with access to high-ranking generals. Bradshaw's literary debut, *Pauline of the Potomac* (1862), features such a heroine, whose father has dedicated her on his deathbed to their country.[22] In *Angel Agnes*, Bradshaw employs a similar formula of an initial family disruption that leaves an orphaned female heroine destined to fight yellow fever. Analogies to the Civil War are inserted early in the narrative: "During the late war, fond fathers sent their sons to the battle-field, not that they wished to have them slaughtered, but willing that, for the sake of their cause, they should take the risk" (7). It is by the same reasoning that Mrs. Arnold approves of her adopted daughter's wish to go to the diseased city of Shreveport. The narrative addresses veteran readers directly, and even puts the female heroine's emotional strength above that of the veterans:

> Reader, if you are a man, possibly you have been in the army, and then possibly you have been in a column, to which has been assigned the task of storming a well-served battery of pieces. If so, you may remember the feelings that were within your heart as you left the last friendly cover of woods . . . . To Agnes Arnold going into Shreveport, the emotions must

---

[22] Cf. Fahs (241-45) for a brief analysis of Bradshaw's Civil War writings.

have been very much like yours in front of that battery. Yet there was no fluttering of her pulse. (Bradshaw 8)

Following up on Bradshaw's Civil War successes and feeding on the attention the fever received in the 1870s, *Angel Agnes* not unsurprisingly became a national bestseller and was reissued in 1878 during the yellow fever epidemic that affected several Southern states and cities (Memphis in particular) before it faded into obscurity. Bradshaw's novella follows the traditional formula of sentimental fiction with its focus on marginalized groups who lack power, such as mothers, children, and blacks, but who are symbolically empowered to serve as social models while true emancipation is withheld. Sentimental strategies furthermore include suffering (sick) children and infants[23]; partings (Agnes leaving her adopted mother) and reunions (with her fiancé, who then dies); domestic settings mirroring moral settings; and a hierarchy of values (of Christian piety, loyalty, and solidarity) which are also represented in the novella by the Sisters of Mercy Agnes meets on the train.

The saintlike, "angelic" Agnes[24] seems to operate on a higher moral level than her patients with regard to the disease; she is never infected by the fever.[25] This speaks of the resort to an older discourse regarding disease and character: Agnes's work ethic, her superior moral goodness—together with the scientifically inexplicable power of the treatment she administers to her patients—is offered as a means of controlling the disease. The narrative reverts to the notion of character as the main notion of redemption and control, and Agnes is "not a mere fancy nurse. Far from it. Up went her sleeves, and for the next two hours she worked with her four patients like a Trojan" (10). Agnes ignores

---

[23] In reality children were less likely to be struck by yellow fever and suffered from milder cases.

[24] Apart from the title, we learn from the sick Sister Theresa that Agnes's patients call her "Angel Agnes"; Theresa prays that "God and the saints keep [her] an angel, as [she] is now," which also foreshadows Agnes's untimely death (Bradshaw 19).

[25] Brown's contemporary and friend, Benjamin Rush, had held sympathy as essential to a physician's success "sometimes so powerful, as to predominate over the fear of death" (Rush qtd. in Haakonssen 218).

official measures to control the epidemic such as quarantine and boards a train to Shreveport despite the regulations:

> A little short of the stricken city they were all stopped, and it required the positive statement of the Sisters of Mercy that their youthful, lovely companion was really going into the place for the purpose of nursing the sick.
>
> "Miss," asked an elderly gentleman, "were you ever acclimated here? Because if you were not, we cannot let you pass, for you would only get the fever yourself, and become a care instead of a help to us. Not only that, but you would surely be a corpse inside of twenty-four hours." Agnes explained to the firm but kind gentleman, her New Orleans experience, and he relaxed and said: "In that case, Miss Arnold, I sincerely welcome you, and in the name of the sick and dying people here, pray God that you may be spared to help them. Pass through, and heaven bless your brave and noble heart!" (Bradshaw 8)

When the train is stopped and Agnes is interrogated, it is through her earlier experience in yellow fever-stricken New Orleans that she is admitted into the diseased city. The passage also refers to the medical opinion of the time that not all residents were equally vulnerable when yellow fever struck a city and that one could become "acclimatized" (Patterson 860). An 1856 report in the *New Orleans Medical Surgical Journal*, for example, noted the extreme vulnerability of—what the text referred to as—"unseasoned" newcomers to the local "climate" of New Orleans in contrast to the immunity of its native citizens (qtd. in Patterson 860). Patterson points out that "it was believed well into the 19th century that new residents could become 'acclimatized' to local fevers without a life-threatening illness and could gradually acquire the immunities conveyed by native birth" (Patterson 860).

The city's attempts to burn tar and pitch as disinfectants are dismissed by Agnes as ludicrous. At one point, she "would have laughed at the silly man . . . who had nearly choked himself by thrusting his head into the dense black fumes" (9). Her attitude seems to echo the sanitationist view of a Doctor Stevens in *Arthur Mervyn* who, as mentioned above, promotes a healthy living and diet over the burning of gunpowder or tar. Judging from her actions, Agnes seems not to believe in or rather to fear a person-to-person transportability of the disease. Her treatment of the sick Sister Theresa shows "how little she dreaded the pestilence, for, instead of going to another room, she lifted Theresa further over the bed, and laying herself down beside her, placed her arm over her" (18). Agnes strictly adheres to her own "design and method" to keep herself in "perfect health and spirits" (22) and apparently defies the risk of infection. Agnes, we are told, in her "treatment of the sick victims . . . would not interfere with the medicine they were taking" (11). However, the narrative also procures the view that "during the whole epidemic, it seemed as though mere medicine was of no avail whatever, and that really the methods and means used by the natives, independent of the doctors, did all the good that was done" (11). When the district's physician pays a visit to the house under Agnes's care (and one might add control), he is astonished in light of the recovery of the fever victims. He attributes the recoveries to Agnes's "faithful and intelligent nursing" and admits the ineffectual modes of treatment his own profession employs, failing "in nearly eighty per cent of every hundred" (14). Prompted to elaborate on the efficacy of what the physician terms "grandmother remedies," Agnes rejects this denotation and instead attributes her treatment to a Spanish gentleman from Havana:

> "This is not a grandmother's remedy, Doctor," smilingly replied Agnes. "It was told to me some years ago in New Orleans." She here concisely narrated to him the history of her experience when she helped to nurse her father in the latter city. "Who was it told you, Miss Arnold? was it Dr. Robinson? He was noted about that period for his success in treating bad cases of the fever.
>
> Once in Vera Cruz he took the vomito, and was saved by this treatment." (Bradshaw 14)

The text thus presents a treatment supposedly originating in Cuba as most successful. This is remarkable because the origin of the Shreveport yellow fever epidemic at the time was traced to Cuba, as newspapers reported ("Yellow Fever at Shreveport"). Yet the question of origin or the concept of transportability—which was most probably known to Bradshaw—never comes up in the novella, which focuses on treatment and healing. With his promise that he would not fail to try the yellow fever remedy and subsequently also recording her smallpox remedy, the physician, furthermore, remains the one to authorize Agnes's treatment and actions. In the narrative, the successful "Spanish" therapy of putting the fever patient's feet in hot and very strong mustard water and then applying salt mackerel to the patient's feet is also conveyed to a black undertaker by Agnes. By dictating the steps of her treatment to the black man, she assumes an authority that is not necessarily medical. The black man exclaims: "I knowed it was magic—somethin' like that, and not medicine at all!" (13). The hierarchical social structure of African American undertaker, female nurse, and male doctor is firmly established and confirmed in the text. In providing a potential "Spanish" colonizer's recipe for the treatment, the narrative not only suggests a non-white remedy for the disease, but also constructs "Spanish" as superior, and thus at least questions a WASP-ish identity construction that partly rests on a contrast to Catholic Spain. A critical stance toward the Protestant clergy is also expressed earlier in the narrative, when Agnes explains to her adoptive mother why she needs to go to Shreveport: "It is strange that we see no account of ministers or members of any denomination but the Roman Church volunteering to go to the stricken city. All seem to stand aloof but them. How noble are those truly Christian and devoted women, the Sisters of Mercy!" (7).

Agnes, who constantly shows courage—"a girl of steady, powerful nerves, and cool temper" (11)—and a seemingly never-ending devotion and selflessness, never contracts the fever and instead dies of a broken spine and severe internal injuries she sustains from a fall due to fatigue after caring too extensively for one of her many patients, a 12-month-old infant. She wishes to be buried next to her intended husband, George Harkness, who succumbs to the fever earlier in the novella. What makes Agnes so powerful in this scene is the fact that she is dying: It is she who dictates what is to be done, in a "most composed manner" (27). This temporary reversal of power relations, a popular strategy of sentimental fiction, is also significant in terms of my argument, since Agnes is the one in control, not only in her dying hour and when she is about to begin a new life ("I have no fear of death, I am prepared for it"; "Come, Death, O come" [27]), but also when she is caring for her patients. At one point, the doctor endorses her superiority as nurse and woman: "Miss Arnold, you are worth all our nurses; and really I'm afraid all us physicians also put together. . . . I really begin to wish I was a woman myself so that if I should get the fever I might have you to nurse me well again," to which Agnes replies: "O never mind about the being a woman, Doctor, . . . if you should be so unfortunate as to get it, I'll come and nurse you" (20). The narrative constructs Agnes as a social role model whose superior behavior is offered as remedy for the larger disease; a future female emancipation might be hinted at, but is not carried through.

In the short narrative form of *Angel Agnes*, yellow fever is not fully aestheticized into a language of disease that would represent the nation's experience of political and social crisis (as is the case in *Arthur Mervyn*). The Shreveport disaster serves as a formula setting to please a readership darkly fascinated by a fear of death and craving a tale of horror. For example, the novella opens with the exclamation of "Nothing but sickness! nothing but horror!" to be found in diseased Shreveport (4). Later, when a Sister who has fallen sick is described, we learn that the disease means the loss of one's natural self and the dethroning of reason (cf. 18). At the same time, *Angel Agnes* remains a sentimental tale of virtue, dedication, and generosity.

Concluding Remarks

My readings of *Arthur Mervyn* and *Angel Agnes* show how both texts depict narrative cultures of fear that denounce corrupt commercial practices as well as slavery (in *Arthur Mervyn*) and, at least temporarily, reverse patriarchal structures (in *Angel Agnes*). Both texts put forward alternative visions for a nation that is eagerly trying to define itself against threats to national health in the nineteenth century. With *Angel Agnes*, Bradshaw constructs a popular story which offers certain redeeming moments based on sentimental strategies of victimization and power reversal. While the male doctor remains the authority by offering approval of Agnes's treatment, Agnes also assumes that authority by lecturing others on the Spanish therapy. The novella thus at least temporarily reverses ingrained gender norms of the time as well as a prerogative of medical interpretation and treatment of diseases. By making the effective cure non-white—but Spanish colonialist—in origin and administered by a woman, *Angel Agnes* thus also puts forth a vision of a medical profession that acknowledges the role of women (nurses in this case) and an accepted co-existence of alternative cures and traditional (native) medicine as well as a critical stance against quarantine measures.

As cause of the national crisis and thus disease, *Arthur Mervyn* diagnoses American society's repression of the racial question, its economic reliance on slavery, and its denial of a growing segment of mass society with free black and hybrid Caribbean/French subjects as future equals. It can be cured by an acceptance of a more diverse makeup of U.S.-American society on its way to defining a distinct national identity. As a means to control the disease (as a symbol for the crisis within), *Arthur Mervyn* thus puts forward a vision of a "postcolonial" transformation of the U.S., which is triggered by the same process already prevalent in Caribbean societies and destined to spread to the United States (cf. Mackenthun 67). This will lead to a more hybrid societal makeup and a cultural diversity shaping a distinct national identity, or, to use Carmen Birkle's words, Brown puts forward "a vision of geographical, social, and political integration."

Works Cited

Allen, Richard, and Absalom Jones. *A Narrative of the Proceedings of the Black People, During the Late Awful Calamity in Philadelphia, in the Year 1793.* Philadelphia: William W. Woodward, 1794. Print.

Arner, Katherine. "Making Yellow Fever American: The Early American Republic, the British Empire and the Geopolitics of Disease in the Atlantic World." *Atlantic Studies* 7.4 (2010): 447-71. Print.

Birkle, Carmen. "Conference Proposal." Conference on "Literature and Medicine." Marburg, 11-13 Feb. 2011.

Bradshaw, Wesley. *Angel Agnes, or, The Heroine of the Yellow Fever Plague in Shreveport.* Philadelphia: Old Franklin, 1873. Print.

Brown, Charles Brockden. *An Address to the Government of the United States, on the Cession of Louisiana to the French and on the Late Breach of Treaty by the Spaniards Including the Translation of a Memorial, on the War of St. Domingo, and Cession of the Missisippi [i.e., Mississippi] to France, Drawn up by a French Counsellor of State.* A New Edition Revised, Corrected and Improved. Philadelphia: John Conrad; M. and J. Conrad; and Rapin, Conrad; H. Maxwell, Printer, 1803. Early American Imprints. 2nd ser. no. 3880.

---. *Arthur Mervyn, or, Memoirs of the Year 1793, with Related Texts.* Ed. Philip Barnard and Stephen Shapiro. Indianapolis: Hackett, 2008. Print.

Burke, Kenneth. *Language as Symbolic Action: Essays on Life, Literature, and Method.* Berkeley: U of California P, 1966. Print.

Caldwell, Charles. *A Reply to Dr. Haygarth's "Letter to Dr. Percival, on Infectious Fevers," and, His "Address to the College of Physicians at Philadelphia, on the Preventing of the American Pestilence," Exposing the Medical, Philosophical, and Literary Errors of that Author, and Vindicating the Right which Is the Faculty of the United States Have to Think and Decide for Themselves, Respecting the Diseases of Their Own Country, Uninfluenced by the Notions of the Physicians of Europe.* Philadelphia: Thomas and William Bradford, 1802. Early American Imprints. 2nd ser. no. 1981.

---. *A Semi-Annual Oration, on the Origin of Pestilential Diseases, Delivered before the Academy of Medicine of Philadelphia, on the 17th Day of December, 1798.* Philadelphia: Thomas and Samuel F. Bradford, 1799. Early American Imprints. 1st ser. no. 35263.

Christophersen, Bill. *The Apparition in the Glass: Charles Brockden Brown's American Gothic.* Athens: U of Georgia P, 1993. Print.

Clarkson, Thomas. *Memoirs of the Private and Public Life of William Penn.* London: R. Taylor for Longman, Hurst, Rees, Orme, and Brown, 1813. Print.

Crosby, Molly Caldwell. *The American Plague: The Untold Story of Yellow Fever, the Epidemic That Shaped Our History.* New York: Berkley, 2007. Print.

Davis, Cynthia J. *Bodily and Narrative Forms: The Influence of Medicine on American Literature, 1845-1915.* Stanford: Stanford UP, 2000. Print.

Dobyns, Henry F., and William R. Swagerty. *Their Number Become Thinned: Native American Population Dynamics in Eastern North America.* Knoxville: U of Tennessee P/Newberry Library Center for the History of the American Indian, 1983. Print.

Fahs, Alice. *The Imagined Civil War: Popular Literature of the North and South, 1861-1865.* Chapel Hill: U of North Carolina P, 2003. Print.

Glassner, Barry. *The Culture of Fear: Why Americans Are Afraid of the Wrong Things: Crime, Drugs, Minorities, Teen Moms, Killer Kids, Mutant Microbes, Plane Crashes, Road Rage, & So Much More.* New York: Basic, 2010. Print.

Gould, Philip. "Race, Commerce, and the Literature of Yellow Fever in Early National Philadelphia." *Early American Literature* 35.2 (2000): 157-86. Print.

Grabo, Norman S. *The Coincidental Art of Charles Brockden Brown*. Chapel Hill: U of North Carolina P, 1981. Print.

Greenblatt, Stephen. *Shakespearean Negotiations: The Circulation of Social Energy in Renaissance England*. Berkeley: U of California P, 1988. Print. New Historicism 4.

Griffith, Sally F. "'A Total Dissolution of the Bonds of Society': Community Death and Regeneration in Matthew Carey's *Short Account of the Malignant Fever*." *A Melancholy Scene of Devastation: The Public Response to the 1793 Philadelphia Yellow Fever Epidemic*. Ed. J. Worth Estes and Billy G. Smith. Canton: Science History, 1997. 45-59. Print.

Haakonssen, Lisbeth. *Medicine and Morals in the Enlightenment: John Gregory, Thomas Percival and Benjamin Rush*. Amsterdam: Rodopi, 1997. Print.

Humphreys, Margaret. *Yellow Fever and the South*. Baltimore: Johns Hopkins UP, 1999. Print.

Jefferson, Thomas. *The Works of Thomas Jefferson*. Ed. Paul Leicester Ford. Vol. 9. 12 vols. New York: Cosimo, 2009. Print.

Krieg, Joann P. *Epidemics in the Modern World*. New York: Twayne, 1992. Print.

Kunow, Rüdiger. "In Sickness and in Health: Transnationalism Reconsidered." *Virtually American? Denationalizing North American Studies*. Ed. Mita Banerjee. Heidelberg: Winter, 2009. 23-36. Print.

Lapsansky, Philip. "'Abigail, a Negress': The Role and the Legacy of African Americans in the Yellow Fever Epidemic." *A Melancholy Scene of Devastation: The Public Response to the 1793 Philadelphia Yellow Fever Epidemic*. Ed. J. Worth Estes and Billy G. Smith. Canton: Science History, 1997. 61-78. Print.

Levine, Robert S. *Conspiracy and Romance: Studies in Brockden Brown, Cooper, Hawthorne, and Melville*. Cambridge: Cambridge UP, 1989. Print.

Mackenthun, Gesa. *Fictions of the Black Atlantic in American Foundational Literature*. London: Routledge, 2004. Print.

"Major U.S. Epidemics." *Information Please Database*. Pearson Education. 2007. Web. 29 Sept. 2011.

Patterson, K. David. "Yellow Fever Epidemics and Mortality in the United States, 1693-1905." *Social Science and Medicine* 34.8 (1992): 855-65. Print.

Pernick, Martin S. "Contagion and Culture." *American Literary History* 14.4 (2002): 858-65. Print.

---. "Politics, Parties, and Pestilence: Epidemic Yellow Fever in Philadelphia and the Rise of the First Party System." *William and Mary Quarterly* 3rd ser. 29.4 (1972): 559-86. Print.

Powell, J. H. *Bring Out Your Dead: The Great Plague of Yellow Fever in Philadelphia in 1793*. 1949. Philadelphia: U of Pennsylvania P, 1993. Print.

Rush, Benjamin. "Facts Intended to Prove the Yellow Fever Not Be Contagious, and Instances of Its Supposed Contagion Explained upon other Principles." *Medical Repository* 6.2 (1803): 155-71. Print.

Samuels, Shirley. *Romances of the Republic: Women, the Family, and Violence in the Literature of the Early American Nation*. New York: Oxford UP, 1996. Print.

Statistics of Population, Tables I-VIII Inclusive. Washington: GPO, 1872. Print.

Stern, Julia A. *The Plight of Feeling: Sympathy and Dissent in the Early American Novel*. Chicago: U of Chicago P, 1997. Print.

"The Yellow Fever: No Cases in Little Rock—Subscriptions for the Aid of Shreveport and Memphis—The Quarantine on the Railroads." *Daily Arkansas Gazette* 7 Oct. 1873: Col. D. Print.

Tompkins, Jane. *Sensational Designs: The Cultural Work of American Fiction, 1790-1860*. New York: Oxford UP, 1985. Print.

Waterman, Bryan. "*Arthur Mervyn*'s Medical Repository and the Early Republic's Knowledge Industries." *American Literary History* 15.2 (2003): 213-47. Print.

Webster, Noah. *A Brief History of Epidemic and Pestilential Diseases with the Principal Phenomena of the Physical World, which Precede and Accompany them, and Observations Deduced from the Facts Stated, in Two Volumes*. Hartford: Hudson and Goodwin, 1799. Early American Imprints. Print. 1st ser. no. 36687.

---. *A Collection of Papers on the Subject of Bilious Fevers, Prevalent in the United-States for a Few Years Past*. New York: Hopkins, Webb, 1796. Print.

Wideman, John Edgar. "Fever." *The Stories of John Edgar Wideman*. New York: Pantheon, 1992. 239-66. Print.

---. *The Cattle Killing*. Boston: Houghton, 1996. Print.

"Yellow Fever at Shreveport." *Daily Evening Bulletin* 30 Sept. 1873: Col. D. Print.

"Yellow Fever: The Plague at Memphis and Shreveport—Relief Contributions." *Milwaukee Daily Sentinel* 25 Oct. 1873: Col. D. Print.

ASTRID HAAS

Remedial Laughter:
American Stage Comedy about AIDS

> "You've had the disease! You've been to the demonstration! Now see the musical!"
> —Promotional slogan for *AIDS! The Musical!* (qtd. in Jones xiii)

Can one, may one, really laugh about AIDS? Is it acceptable to make fun of a lethal pandemic that has carried away millions of people in the past three decades? While AIDS (Acquired Immune Deficiency Syndrome) is a fairly recent phenomenon, the issue at stake—the social (in)acceptability of humor, and in particular of stage comedy as an artistic form of expression, in dealing with serious subjects such as natural disasters, human-caused calamities, or social and religious taboos—is a very old one and will probably never cease to cause controversy. However, this matter would never have come up, if, indeed, people had not been recurring to comic forms of expression to respond to disasters, calamities, and taboos in the first place. In the following essay I will analyze the phenomenon of U.S.-American stage comedies about the AIDS epidemic against the backdrop of the social and psychological functions of the comic as well as the relation between Western stage comedy and controversial subjects.

Stage Comedy and the Controversial Subject

Peter L. Berger has differentiated among several forms and functions of the comic: "The comic as diversion" includes all forms of benign humor that are "intended to evoke pleasure, relaxation, and good will" (99). "The comic as a game of intellect" (135), appearing especially in wit and language games, provides one with the satisfaction of demonstrating one's cognitive abilities (61-62). "The comic as consolation" most prominently takes the shape of tragicomedy or black humor. It "provokes laughter through tears" (117) and consoles, as it acknowledges the presence of the tragic yet momentarily suspends and thereby symbolically defies it (58, 117). Irony, parody, and satire are the predominant forms of "the comic as weapon" (157). They "deliberate[ly] use . . . the comic for purposes of attack" by "belittling, humiliating, or debunking" their targets (157, 51). Commonly directed against ideas, institutions, social groups, and their respective representatives or against individuals of high status, these forms of the comic provide an outlet for anxieties whose expression in other forms may be subject to socio-cultural taboo or political repression (51-53, 157). The various forms of the comic always had a place in society, illuminating a civilization by holding up a mirror to it. While they may either scrutinize a given social order or, contrarily, affirm it, all forms of humor and the comic tend to create social group cohesion and distinction from other groups, as well as to offer (temporary) relief from social constraints (66-72, 78).

As Mathias Mayer argues, literature provides a particularly fruitful forum for articulating ethical concerns, because works of literature, and especially epic and dramatic fiction, present multiple options of human action and problematize them and their evaluation within a given context (13). Western theater has employed comic forms of expression since antiquity to entertain audiences, voice popular anxieties, or scrutinize prevailing social mores and political power structures (cf. Weitz). Nonetheless, especially owing to the danger—inherent in any form of comic expression—that "laughing along with" the target of ridicule turns into "laughing about" it (Jauß 281-83; my translation), playwrights have time and again been forced to justify their use of comic forms, in particular when addressing (potentially) controversial subjects. In the preface to his comedy *Le Tartuffe* (1669), for instance, the French playwright Molière prominently defends his artistic right to unmask and thereby criticize religious hypocrisy, as he invokes the support of high-standing members of society, among them the French king, as well as voicing his own respect for true believers who—unlike the titular character of *Le Tartuffe*—do not (ab)use faith to pursue other, non-religious goals. Molière further refers to the widely accepted social function and value of comic theater as an educational tool: By unmasking human flaws and follies in an entertaining and benign manner, he argues, comedy reaches out to people more successfully than conventional moral instruction (33-40).

While *Le Tartuffe* has long become a staple of the Western theatrical repertoire, current dramatic responses to topical controversial issues often remain reluctant to approach their subject matter in a comic format. The most famous case in the West unquestionably includes comedies about the Holocaust. The large scale of the atrocities committed has raised concerns and fueled debates about the possibilities and adequate forms of literary representation that last to this day (Rohr), and it has long rendered comic approaches to the Shoah a particular taboo. Following similar and slightly earlier developments in film and the novel,[1] the first theatrical satires, comedies, and farces addressing the Holocaust found their way to theater stages in the mid-1990s. What distinguishes these from the other, mostly documentary and commemorative dramatic formats is a shift away from the claim to an "authentic" representation of the historical events to focusing on the construction of memory and the role of discourses and representations therein (Rohr 163-68, 173). As the issue has remained controversial, playwrights of Holocaust comedies often feel the need to justify their work. The British playwright Roy Kift, for example, defends his comic take on life in a concentration camp, *Camp Comedy* (1999), by invoking the psychosocial function and educational value of humor:

---

[1]   The early 1940s saw a first wave of screen and stage satires about the Nazi regime, but once the full dimension of the Holocaust became known, comic takes on the subject were considered inappropriate. A revival of the earlier satirical tradition, now with a critical eye to the medialization of history and the developing "Holocaust industry," has taken place since the 1970s and in particular since the 1990s (Rohr 160-61, 166, 170, 173, 175-76).

At first sight, the juxtaposition of comedy and concentration camp seems to be not only impossible but also morally indefensible, how much more grotesque must it seem that comedy, songs and laughter in the form of cabaret were almost a daily experience in the Theresianstadt camp. But since the inmates themselves considered laughter to be a perfectly acceptable response to their predicament, there may be valuable lessons here to be learnt for modern writers trying to find an appropriate formal approach to tackling the Holocaust in performance. (147-49)

In a similar vein, U.S.-American and British theater has responded to the terrorist attacks of September 11, 2001 in several waves, moving from a theater of testimony and mourning via plays that historically contextualize the attacks or address problems of artistic representation to a new political theater that critically engages with U.S.-American politics at large (Esch-van Kan). According to Anneka Esch-van Kan, it was not until 2006 that the first play with a somewhat ludic approach to 9/11, Kirk Lynn's *Major Bang—Or, How I Learned to Stop Worrying and Love the Dirty Bomb*, emerged (136-37).

American AIDS Theater: From Testimony to Comedy

The path Anglo-American 9/11 plays have taken to date strikingly echoes (with the final steps not yet taken) the development during the 1980s and 90s of U.S.-American theater—and narrative literature in general (Haas 61-63)—about AIDS.[2] The fact that AIDS was quickly perceived as an epidemic and an STD (sexually transmitted disease) that over-proportionally affects already socially marginal(ized) groups has fundamentally shaped patterns of response and representation. Owing to a set of interconnected circumstances, gay and bisexual men have always made up the largest segment of HIV (the virus that causes AIDS) and AIDS patients in the United States to this day, followed by intravenous drug users and different groups of people of color (Haas 37). The predominant societal discourses about HIV/AIDS in the United

---

[2]   There are further parallels between the discourses about 9/11 and AIDS in the United States (Haas 294-95). For a detailed analysis of U.S.-American AIDS theater, including the plays mentioned here, cf. Haas.

States tend to frame the syndrome as both consequence and indicator of socio-sexual deviance, whose otherness it renders visible. Building upon the paradox-laden perception of the socio-cultural other as "both abject weakness and powerful threat" (Kruger 41), popular and even some scientific discourses often portray the main "risk groups" for HIV/AIDS not only as being responsible for their own condition but also as a menace to public health and national values. They commonly pit these "guilty AIDS carriers" against the implicitly "innocent victims" of HIV infection such as children, hemophiliacs, and heterosexual partners of bisexuals or drug injectors (Haas 40).

Emerging in particular "out of the already politicized lesbian and gay movement" (Román, *Acts* 69), the first AIDS plays produced in the U.S. were profoundly shaped by and concerned with "educational messages, behavioral models, and social practices designed to ensure and enhance the physical, emotional, spiritual, and political survival of the gay community" (Jones x; also Saal 1-2, 9-10) and that transcended artistic concerns. Plays written and first produced during the 1980s were often explicitly didactic: They testified to individual and collective experiences; provided a public forum to express anger and grief; and educated audiences about available prevention and treatment measures; as well as raising the political consciousness necessary to confront alarmingly reactionary local and national AIDS policies (Haas 69-71).

From the earliest plays onwards, elements of the comic have run through U.S.-American AIDS theater, functioning in particular as a strategy of consolation that could help come to terms with terminal illness and death, on the one hand, and to counter tendencies of either victimizing or vilifying HIV/AIDS patients, on the other (Haas 69-70, 78). For instance, William M. Hoffman's 1985 play *As Is* (Haas 76-96), the first AIDS play produced on a mainstream stage in the United States, abounds with elements of the comic: humorous depictions of gay life in the time of AIDS; witty, sometimes cynical dialogues; and a set of gay, ethnic, and hospital jokes that circulated in the United States during the mid-1980s characterize the atmosphere of the play (Hoffman 3-7, 12, 19-20, 23-33, 42, 55-56, 77-80, 91-92). Akin to Molière's and Roy Kift's defenses of *Le Tartuffe* and *Camp Comedy*, respectively, Hoffman justifies his use of the comedic in a work addressing as serious a subject as AIDS in his foreword: Not only does he claim that the humor had entered *As Is* against his intention; he also invokes his own involvement in gay AIDS activism as well as the approval he received for his play from his dying father and from different people living with HIV/AIDS as the factors that reconciled him with the comic side of his play.[3]

Even though many plays continued to explicitly emerge out of a political consciousness and as a contribution to AIDS activism, a second wave of U.S.-American AIDS literature—including plays—written since the late 1980s, according to Lawrence Howe, was "much better equipped to go beyond the initial shock, disbelief, and grief that distinguishes the first wave's representations of AIDS as an emerging, mysterious crisis" (404). In drawing upon devices of defamiliarization, including many elements of the comic such as humor, irony, satire, or the grotesque, AIDS plays of the 1990s provide readers with new strategies of dealing with an epidemic not to be soon conquered (Haas 71-72). Nonetheless, even as daring a project as the alternative theatrical project *AIDS! The Musical!* (1991) was consciously placed in an AIDS activist context to legitimize its use of a fierce humor to approach its deadly subject matter. Not only does the above-cited promotional slogan allude to a political demonstration, but the creators of the show, Wendell Jones, David Stanley, and Robert Berg, explicitly characterize their work as "'an all-singing, all dancing, all queer voyage into a world of AIDS activism, new age gatherings, sleazy sex clubs, radical faeries, lesbian love, and fags bashing back!'" (qtd. in Jones xiii). At the same time, however, the self-confident approach of *AIDS! The Musical!* to address HIV/AIDS in form of a musical comedy points to the new direction U.S.-American AIDS theater has taken during the 1990s, a direction I will now analyze in greater detail, using two of the most prominent AIDS comedies as examples: Paula Vogel's *The Baltimore Waltz* (1991) and Paul Rudnick's *Jeffrey* (1992).[4]

---

[3]   Hoffman xiv-xv; also Boccardi 129-32. Similar to William M. Hoffman, Roy Kift has dedicated his essay about the historical cabarets in the Theresienstadt concentration camp to a friend and Holocaust survivor (168).

[4]   The most prominent U.S.-American AIDS play that features various comic scenes is, of course, Tony Kushner's two-part play *Angels in America: A Gay Fantasia on National Themes* (1991/92). However, as this play is more complex in style (cf. Haas 191-98), it will not be discussed here.

Satirical Reverse Transcription: Paula Vogel's *The Baltimore Waltz*

Paula Vogel's 1991 play *The Baltimore Waltz* (cf. Haas 174-90) stands out among U.S.-American AIDS plays for its indirect, highly stylized treatment of its subject that defies an easy formal categorization. According to Tish Dace, "Vogel creates simultaneously a compassionate comedy about death, a bedroom farce, and a satire on American AIDS policy" (597). The play blends together various cultural forms, among them the travel account, the thriller movie, and the public service announcement. With its often illogical plot, use of repetition as a key element of the dialogue, and grotesque characters, it recalls Martin Esslin's conceptualization of the Theatre of the Absurd. *The Baltimore Waltz* deals with a strange European journey the schoolteacher Anna undertakes with her brother Carl after being diagnosed with a lethal illness. Their final destination is Vienna, where Anna is to seek treatment unavailable in the United States. However, the play is interspersed with hints that Anna made up her illness and the journey as a strategy of coping with the AIDS death of her brother, which is revealed at the end of the play.

As Paula Vogel states in a note on her play, the work is based on autobiographical experience: "In 1986, my brother Carl invited me to join him in a joint excursion to Europe. Due to pressures of time and money, I declined, never dreaming that he was HIV-positive. . . . *The Baltimore Waltz* [is] a journey with Carl to Europe that exists only in the imagination" (2). Presenting her fictional journey as a camp version of the never-made trip with her own brother, the playwright pays tribute to her sibling. The written dedication of *The Baltimore Waltz*, "to the memory of Carl—because I cannot sew" (3), explicitly turns the play into a specific form of public commemoration: a substitute for a panel of the Names Project AIDS Memorial Quilt (Dace 598; Schultz 225-26; on the quilt, cf. Haas 117). In addition to anchoring the play in the experience of personal loss, Anna's mourning and the presence of Carl Vogel in *The Baltimore Waltz* align the play with the acts of testimony and commemoration that characterize especially U.S.-American AIDS plays of the 1980s. Beyond its function of preserving and sharing memory, the claim of the testimonial text to discursive authority and truth-telling endows *The Baltimore Waltz*—like *As Is* earlier—with the artistic and political license to treat its serious subject satirically (Shepard and Lamb 205).

The humor that runs through *The Baltimore Waltz* is strikingly more ludic and less desperate than the comic elements in *As Is* and other earlier AIDS theater. This becomes particularly manifest in the way Vogel's play satirically displaces AIDS with a fictive disease that ironizes cultural stereotypes (Vogel 12, 19-25, 36-39, 44-55; also Schultz 242-43) alongside criticizing the hegemonic U.S.-American AIDS discourses: Acquired Toilet Disease (ATD)—a pun on both "AIDS" and "STD"—a lethal affliction of single schoolteachers caused by children's urine and transmitted via toilet seats, parodically reworks the biomedical and socio-political framing of HIV/AIDS in the United States (Vogel 10-11, 18; also Schultz 14-15, 225-30). The principle of replacing AIDS with ATD strikingly recalls the biochemical process of reverse transcription. Metaphorically similar to the way retroviruses like HIV "transcribe" their single-stranded RNA template into a double-stranded DNA molecule they can incorporate into the human host DNA (Mahy 279), Anna first "transcribes" her brother, deceased from AIDS, into an ATD-afflicted version of herself in *The Baltimore Waltz*, a transcription process that is once again reversed at the end of the play (Vogel 55-57). This strategy urges audiences, who have followed the sympathetically drawn heterosexual woman with compassion on her journey with an "elementary school illness," to recognize the role of their preconceived notions about HIV/AIDS and those it afflicts (Boccardi 267, 275; Schultz 232-33, 240-41; Watkins 177-78).

As it reverses the major risk groups and modes of transmission of AIDS in its depiction of ATD, *The Baltimore Waltz* questions the popular associations between AIDS and socio-sexual "deviance." In not presenting sexual activity but children's urine as a serious health threat (Vogel 9-12, 17), the play signifies upon the popular fears surrounding body fluids and sexual acts in the time of AIDS, and it interrogates the common ascriptions of innocence and guilt, safety and risk, victim and perpetrator, according to a person's socio-sexual status (Román, *"Baltimore Waltz"* 520; Schultz 238, 241-42; Watkins 177-78). The key arguments put forth to counter social ostracism in the play, however, are taken from the verbal strategy real AIDS activists employed to defend the civil liberties of people with HIV/AIDS in the 1980s, the claim "It's not a crime. It's an illness" (Vogel 17; also Shepard and Lamb 205). *The*

Baltimore Waltz particularly foregrounds how closely notions of otherness are tied to questions of political power and representation. In a humorous manner, the play exposes the historical disregard of the U.S.-American political elite and mainstream media to the spread of AIDS unless the health of prominent citizens was at stake (Haas 43-46, 50-54). As Carl argues poignantly in the play: "If Sandra Day O'Connor sat on just one infected potty, the media would be clamoring to do articles on ATD. If just one grandchild of George Bush caught this thing during toilet training, that would be the last we'd hear about the space program" (12; also Schultz 234).

The lack of political commitment to fight ATD/AIDS in the United States manifests itself especially in a scene of *The Baltimore Waltz* that signifies upon the setting of public health priorities. Announcing a campaign called "Operation Squat," a public health official states:

> There is no known cure for ATD right now, and we are acknowledging the urgency of this dread disease by recognizing it as our 82nd national health priority. Right now, ATD is the fourth major cause of death of single schoolteachers, ages twenty-four to forty . . . . If you are in the high-risk category—single elementary schoolteachers, classroom aides, custodians and playground drug pushers—follow these simple guides. (18)

The behavioral rules the fictional "Operation Squat" subsequently advises—washing one's hands after using the toilet, never sitting on a public toilet seat, or avoiding public restrooms altogether (18-19; also Boccardi 275-76; Schultz 233)—rework the guidelines the United States Health Service issued in 1983 to respond to the speculation of medical researchers that HIV could be transmitted through regular household contacts (Haas 51-52, 54). In evoking this moment in the history of AIDS in the United States, *The Baltimore Waltz* further points out the helplessness of a medico-political establishment in the face of a serious health threat it has not mastered.

Employing the style of public health information campaigns, "Operation Squat" more specifically scrutinizes the political controversies that have repeatedly surrounded public AIDS education and prevention measures in the United States. As a result of the strict federal regulations established for providing information on sexual and drug-using practices, government-sponsored AIDS education programs to this day are severely limited in their outreach capacities and tend to primarily cater to the needs of the comparatively low-risk populace of the white heterosexual middle class (Haas 43-46). The ATD prevention campaign in *The Baltimore Waltz* signifies upon the limits and faults of such programs by ridiculing the targeting practices of public health initiatives in general and AIDS education guidelines in particular (Schultz 234; Shepard and Lamb 205). "Operation Squat" gains its satirical quality from dressing a matter of low priority and rare occurrence in the warning rhetoric of public health promotion initiatives and from its ridiculous-sounding name that underlines the discrepancy between style and content of the campaign. By including "playground drug pushers" in the list of potential ATD victims—and thus reversing the trajectory of death usually brought forth by the dealers to their juvenile customers—the play undermines the claim of public health education to objectivity and political neutrality and raises the crucial question of whose health is truly endangered.

The Baltimore Waltz further dismantles the deep involvement of medical science in the political power structures that determine the public handling of health matters. Language and discourse signify the gap between the medico-political establishment and society at large. The almost unintelligible, medical jargon-ridden speech of the two doctors in the play especially generates anxieties in face of an inexplicable, incurable illness that neither political nor medical authorities appear to fight efficiently. When asked to elucidate Anna's medical condition, her Baltimore physician replies with a cascade of medical terms: "There are exudative and proliferative inflammatory alterations of the endocardium, consisting of necrotic debris, fibrinoid material and disintegrating fibroblastic cells" (9; also 10-12, 52, 55; Schultz 230-32). And the same doctor's explanation of the political implications of ATD tellingly makes no mention of the sick:

> Well, first of all, the Center for Disease Control doesn't wish to inspire an all-out panic in communities. Secondly, we think education on this topic is the responsibility of the NEA, not the government. And if word of this pestilence gets out inappropriately, the PTA is going to be all over the school system demanding mandatory testing of every toilet seat in every lavatory. It's kindling for a political disaster. (11)

The doctor's unintelligible statement creates a sense of a medical establishment, itself lacking knowledge of ATD, alienated from the powerless and confused population, whose needs the doctor considers an annoyance at best (the Parent-Teacher Association, PTA) and irrelevant at worst (the infected persons). In its comical exaggeration of mass testing, this statement scrutinizes the public debates in the United States during the mid-1980s about mandatory mass screenings of AIDS risk groups (Boccardi 271-72; on this debate cf. Haas 44). Referring to ATD as a "pestilence," the physician in *The Baltimore Waltz* further evokes long-standing societal fears of almost inevitable, large-scale painful suffering associated with bubonic plague and similar epidemics in Western history (Haas 22, 42-43). Not the disease in question but public discourses about it and the political interventions they inform are what appears to be the "real" danger to the medical authorities in the play.

The motif of medical disregard for the patient also informs the character of Dr. Todesrocheln in *The Baltimore Waltz*, a mysterious Viennese urologist whose urine therapy Anna seeks in desperate hope of a cure. His telling name ("death rattle"), paired with his strange looks; solitary status as someone who is "somewhat unorthodox, outside the medical community" (Vogel 12); uncommon methods; and dubious medical credentials (cf. Vogel 12, 15, 52-55; also Schultz 235-36) make him a picture-book embodiment of the mad-scientist stereotype. Since the early nineteenth century, the unscrupulous researcher whose Promethean drive often leads to conducting ethically illicit experiments has been a typological figure in Western culture that powerfully captures popular anxieties about the growing distance between scientific and general knowledge as well as the rising popular fears of the consequences of uncontrolled scientific development (Haynes 3-5, 187-210). Wearing "one sinister black glove" (52) and engaging in a struggle of his hands for a urine flask (52-53), Dr. Todesrocheln explicitly evokes Dr. Strangelove, the titular scientist and government military advisor in Stanley Kubrick's 1964 screen satire on United States Cold War paranoia, *Dr. Strangelove—Or, How I Learned to Stop Worrying and Love the Bomb* (Kubrick). As a quack sibling of apparently similarly sinister political persuasion to Dr. Strangelove, Dr. Todesrocheln blends the mad-scientist cliché with the equally popular image of the foolish investigator obsessed with trivial yet strange research projects, a figure that signifies both upon the popular cult of science and its inability to tackle many pressing problems (Haynes 3, 35-49, 66-73).

As a foolish and mad scientist, Dr. Todesrocheln articulates societal uneasiness about a medical establishment that has shown little will or ability to fight AIDS (Vogel 12, 15, 52-53). The threatening aspect of this establishment becomes visible in Dr. Todesrocheln's apparent endorsement of the medical experiments that were performed on concentration camp inmates in Nazi Germany, as he boasts that "thanks to the advancement of medical science, there are no limits to our thirst for knowledge. ... So much data has been needlessly, carelessly destroyed in the past—the medical collections of Ravensbruck senselessly annihilated" (53). Carefully avoiding an untenable one-to-one analogy between the AIDS-era United States and Nazi Germany, *The Baltimore Waltz* nonetheless employs these references to scrutinize U.S.-American AIDS anxieties and policies as being part of a larger history of political atrocities in which medical science has been complicit time and again (Shepard and Lamb 205, 212-13).

While it is Anna's brother Carl who is revealed to have died from AIDS at the end of the play, by displacing Carl's AIDS with Anna's ATD for most of the narrative, *The Baltimore Waltz* addresses women as patients of a serious illness. In its parodic health education campaign, the play scrutinizes the low priority both AIDS and health threats to women are given in U.S.-American health politics. Anna, whom her doctor reproaches for having used a classroom toilet, forces audiences to confront a woman's affliction with HIV/AIDS beyond the two major modes of framing female patients in mainstream U.S.-American societal discourse, the vilification of the socio-sexually "deviant" and the victimization of "mainstream" (white middle-class) women (Haas 41-42, 54-55). As Anna is a single woman without children, *The Baltimore Waltz* precludes a reductive reading of the affliction of its female protagonist in light of how she might threaten the health of a husband or child (Vogel 18-19; also Boccardi 273-76).

Anna's attempt to come to terms with her own mortality scrutinizes the schematization of people's response to terminal illness. In a parodic scene, *The Baltimore Waltz* shows her pass through the six archetypal stages of human confrontation with terminal illness identified by Elisabeth Kübler-Ross (Haas 82) within a single, sleepless night. The play even allows Anna to talk back to the classification scheme: "What does she know about what it feels like to die?! Kübler-Ross can sit on my face!" (29; also 26-29; Schultz 236; Watkins 178). The play further claims that "unbeknownst to Elizabeth Kübler-Ross, there is a Seventh Stage . . . : Lust" (29). In adding this final stage to the standard model, and in having the previously sexually "tame" Anna embark on her journey in search of casual sex as well as medical treatment, *The Baltimore Waltz* refutes the popular assumption that a serious illness, especially among women, commands celibacy and puts an end to sexual desire (Vogel 26, 31-33, 40-41, 44-46; also Boccardi 277; Schultz 236; Watkins 178-79).

Consisting entirely of lovingly mocked cultural stereotypes and Hollywood images of the continent, Carl and Anna's journey satirizes the European grand tour popular among travelers from the United States. Anna's numerous sexual adventures with male service personnel on her trip in *The Baltimore Waltz* explore the erotic potential of women in defiance of traditional codes of female decency. The drama's playful signifying upon traditional gendered connections of travel and sex subverts the notion of the educational value of the grand tour (Stowe). While Anna's promiscuity poses no health threat within the epidemiology of ATD, it generates anxieties with regard to her standing in for her AIDS-afflicted brother, especially as the actor who is to play all of Anna's male sex partners also embodies a mysterious male stranger who pursues Carl throughout the journey. Thus, the way *The Baltimore Waltz* validates sexuality challenges societal notions of gender and sexual conduct in the context of AIDS (Boccardi 277-78, 283; Schultz 237, 240; Watkins 178-79).

Romantic Comedy of Serodiscordance: Paul Rudnick's *Jeffrey*

Alberto Sandoval points out that, "AIDS theatre entered a new phase when *Jeffrey* opened off-Broadway. The message now is that AIDS has become a part of life and all that can be done is accept it, move on and laugh about it" (52). Called by the playwright himself "a blend of the highest farce and the most devastating tragedy, laced with the gay style that has allowed a ravaged community to survive with its wisecracks and wardrobes intact" (qtd. in Eads 248), Paul Rudnick's 1992 play *Jeffrey* chronicles the struggle of the gay actor and waiter Jeffrey Calloway with his fear of AIDS and complications in life in a series of short, comic vignettes (Haas 237-51). To avoid the compromises of safer sex, Jeffrey vows sexual abstinence, a decision that is not only scrutinized by his friends but also challenged when he falls in love with the HIV-positive Steve. After an erroneous journey through the gay scene of New York, he finally comes to embrace a relationship with Steve.

Following a strategy already employed in *The Baltimore Waltz*, *Jeffrey* employs elements of the comic to critique the homophobic societal framing of gay men as threats to society in mainstream U.S.-American discourses and validates gay men's multiple struggles against the AIDS epidemic. Rudnick argues accordingly that he considered the time ready for a comic exploration of AIDS. Nonetheless, echoing William M. Hoffman and Paula Vogel, he underlines the legitimacy of a humorous take on the serious matter of AIDS by anchoring his fictional work in personal testimony to the epidemic: In several interviews, he cites the approval he received from both his terminally ill father and several HIV-positive friends (Baker 206), and he has dedicated his play to his father (Rudnick 3). In his introduction, Rudnick moreover invokes the comic as a strategy to cope with the presence of AIDS and death: "Audiences often imagine that a comedy about AIDS is impossible; *Jeffrey* is a tribute to people who battle disease and fear with passion, humor and style" (5).

Jeffrey blends together and reworks a number of literary and cinematographic styles and genres to create a panorama of AIDS-era gay Manhattan that is both socially assertive and politically critical. A strong element of parody mingles with the self-referentiality and flamboyance of gay camp performance in the play's portrayal of the New York gay community, as the protagonist Jeffrey passes through a host of (stereo)typical places and situations. The witty dialogue and fast pace of the play, its featuring a number of burlesque scenes, and the fact that as few as eight actors are to embody the 42 roles draw upon the U.S.-American screwball comedy, with its typological characters, slapstick elements, and sexual themes (Baker 206; on the screwball comedy, cf. Sennett 54-73, 110-29). Presenting a lovingly mocking look at gay life in New York in the early 1990s, *Jeffrey* shows how profoundly the AIDS epidemic informs gay sexuality and culture. Through the parodies of a lecherous gay priest who promotes safer sex measures and of a New Age self-help guru (27-30, 47-52), the play scrutinizes the failure of both organized religion and alternative spiritual movements in dealing with AIDS, namely the homophobic sexual principles of the Catholic Church and the conservative societal agenda of a New Age movement that explicitly blames diseases on non-committed relationships (Haas 44-45).

Jeffrey depicts AIDS awareness as transcending, yet prominently including, the gay experience, for instance in scenes set at an AIDS fund-raiser ball or a memorial service. With its "Western" theme and camp performances of the gay caterers in their "Cowboy/Indian" attire (18-23), the ball signifies upon the Western's ideology of rugged white masculinity and its often erotically charged male bonds as well as the gay cultural offspring of the Western hero, the masculine-coded type of the "cowboy" popular in gay sex culture of the 1980s (Haas 240). The ball in *Jeffrey* humorously mocks the normative white masculinity of the Western and the gay assimilationist striving for social privilege without scrutinizing either American heterosexual society or gay culture per se. The fact that the Western ball serves as a fund-raiser for an AIDS charity at the same time raises spectatorial consciousness of the ongoing necessity to fight the epidemic. In a similar vein as the ball, the fictive television quiz show "It's Just Sex" is based on and promotes basic AIDS awareness. The show's quiz about sex and AIDS alludes to the "Just Say No" campaign of AIDS and drug education headed by Nancy Reagan during the mid-1980s (15-17; cf. Haas 240). As it parodistically reworks the exclusive promotion of sexual abstinence and the rejection of homosexuality that characterized Reagan's campaign, *Jeffrey* stakes a claim for a pragmatic, gay- and sex-positive approach to AIDS prevention that targets health risks rather than identity categories and informs people instead of policing them.

Jeffrey prominently interrogates popular assumptions about HIV/AIDS through the character of the HIV-positive Steve, especially in a scene depicting a chance meeting of Steve and Jeffrey in a hospital lounge. Here, Steve dons protective medical garb in a camp performance of a fashion show and cynically comments upon the gown's having been "sterilized over five thousand times" (43) and about the necessity of wearing gloves (44). With this scene, the play follows American AIDS plays of the 1980s, such as *As Is*, signifying upon popular fears in the United States concerning physical contact with AIDS patients to scrutinize the ways U.S.-American culture often limits people with

HIV/AIDS to their medical condition, treats them with fear, and excludes them from social life.

As this defiant gay spirit shown by Steve in the hospital scene manifests itself in *Jeffrey* primarily through the appraisal of safer sex, Jeffrey's vow of abstinence puts his environment into a crisis that triggers the comic plot. His in itself legitimate choice—based on his view that "sex wasn't meant to be safe or negotiated, or fatal" (11)—is considered socially disruptive by the gay community, and the play solves the sexual crisis by having Jeffrey finally renounce abstinence and embrace a relationship and safer sex practices (13-14, 26-27, 45-46, 61-63; also Román, *Acts* 247). The narrative of *Jeffrey* powerfully signifies upon the suspicious attitude of heterosexual U.S.-American society toward the celebration of sex in gay culture in the age of AIDS. Yet, the play only substitutes one oppressive discourse with another. In an environment governed by the ideology of safer sex as primary means of HIV prevention, the play equates abstinence with subjugation to the epidemic and suggests that only a sexually active man can be an asset to the gay world. As it is not people's HIV status that matters here but their ideological conformity, the normative voice of the gay community polices socio-sexual behavior rather than the medical condition it claims to fight (14-15, 24-25, 60, 62-63; also Román, *Acts* 244, 247-48).

The tendency of comedy to privilege "the renewal of community over the triumph of the individual" (Román, "Negative" 205), articulated in the play's dealing with the sexual choice of its protagonist, also characterizes the depiction of gay effeminacy in *Jeffrey*. Widely criticized especially from within the gay community as fostering anti-gay societal bias by confirming the traditional stereotype of gay "unmanliness," effeminacy is celebrated in the play as a legitimate way of gay life and as clearly superior to the assimilative drive to normative masculinity. As the protagonist puts it: "I hate that gay role models are supposed to be just like straight people. As if straight people were ever like that" (24). The play represents gay effeminacy and flamboyance through the figures of Jeffrey's friends, the interior designer Sterling and his lover Darius, a chorus singer/dancer in the musical *Cats*. Functioning as a gay mirror image of Middle America at the same time—they are even likened to "an advertisement for connubial bliss" (25)—, Sterling and Darius signify upon the exclusion of gay men from the popular understanding of bourgeois U.S.-American society and committed relationships. *Jeffrey* thus defies gay social pressure to present only images of the gay experience likely to generate mainstream societal sympathy. However, as it carefully balances the stereotypical qualities of Sterling and Darius with their model behavior, the play compromises the political potential of satire and camp performance in favor of a conciliatory tone that affirms the prevailing social order rather than challenging it.

Underlined by evocative George Gershwin tunes and slide projections of picture-book New York scenes (7, 38, 60, 63), *Jeffrey* frames the story of Jeffrey and Steve's relationship in the mold of (heterosexual) romantic comedy in which the intervention of antagonistic forces temporarily thwarts the love of the protagonists. While AIDS takes the place of the obstacle to romantic happiness in *Jeffrey*, it is Jeffrey's unwillingness to accept sexual compromises and personal loss, rather than the epidemic itself, that the play invokes as the actual source of his trouble. By shifting the cause of the dramatic tension from the all-too-real socio-medical threat of AIDS to the exaggerated anxieties of the individual protagonist, the play addresses the serious issue in a light manner familiar to audiences in the United States, educating spectators by means of an entertaining narrative and affirming the U.S.-American ideology of liberal individualism.

Reconciling the two lovers on the observation deck of an Empire State Building framed against a nocturnal skyline with a glowing full moon, the final scene of *Jeffrey* (60-63) borrows heavily from the aesthetics of urban romanticism, alluding in particular to the finale of Rob Reiner's 1989 heterosexual romantic film comedy, *When Harry Met Sally*.[5] As it reworks a genre conventionally asserting the normative ideal of heterosexual romance and marriage to depict a gay love story in the second decade of the AIDS epidemic, *Jeffrey* affirms both gay and straight experiences: The play argues that gay romantic love is worthwhile and possible despite AIDS, and the adherence of gay men to the ideal of romance makes it even more valid. Following the

---

[5]   Reiner; also Sennett 285. The screen adaptation of *Jeffrey* enforces the parallels to Reiner's movie to a much greater degree than the play, thereby underlining the film's claim to the status of mainstream-compatible romantic comedy represented by *When Harry Met Sally* (Haas 248-50).

convention of romantic comedy, the play provides narrative closure through a happy ending that asserts the mainstream U.S.-American ideology of the couple as a safe haven from personal and societal anxieties. However, as they are two serodiscordant gay men—one being HIV-negative, the other -positive—Jeffrey and Steve are at odds with the traditional connotation of the couple as signifiers of health and reproduction who will regenerate society. Even though *Jeffrey* claims a place for the gay couple as integral part of U.S.-American society, the romantic involvement of the lovers can only temporarily deflect the possibility of Jeffrey's seroconversion and the knowledge of Steve's premature death (Román, *Acts* 242, 247-48).

Conclusion

Rooted in religious ritual, the theater has since antiquity served as a forum for direct interaction and public debate; for moral, cultural, or political instruction; and for the formation of communities (Haas 3; Saal 1). Likewise, people have recurred to forms of the comic to negotiate individual or collective anxieties and grief as well as voice testimony and political critique. Both traditions merge in stage comedy as a form of artistic expression that understands (and uses) the comic as a more powerful tool for reaching out to and getting its concerns across to society. The cultural specificity of humor turns theatrical comedy about controversial subjects, from religious beliefs to instances of genocide, into a particularly sensitive matter. To justify their comic takes on such topics, playwrights have time and again invoked the societal value of their work, the therapeutic function of humor, and/or their own personal testimony to the serious issue in question.

Theater about the AIDS epidemic in the United States during the 1980s and 90s is a telling case in point. With the initial shock and anger about the epidemic gone, U.S.-American AIDS plays of the 1990s approach their subject in a formally and thematically more diverse manner that prominently includes several plays explicitly written in a comic format. Parodically reworking major popular assumptions about AIDS, Paula Vogel's satirical play *The Baltimore Waltz* exposes the prejudices and power structures implicit in the discursive rendering of the epidemic and those it affects. As it employs a fictional disease, its discourses and policies, the play defamiliarizes the subjects of AIDS, homophobia, and political disregard for the sick to challenge mainstream audiences' feeling of being personally safe from these "threats." Through its satirical "reverse transcription" of AIDS, the play questions major categories of thought such as the figure of the "innocent victim" or the sexual and gendered connotation of AIDS (also Schultz 241-42). Its avowedly anti-naturalist depiction of the epidemic links *The Baltimore Waltz* to other AIDS plays written and first performed around the same time. As Arnold Aronson observes, Vogel's play

> typified an emerging trend in the nineties toward plays of grief and rage that, by functioning on an allegorical or metaphorical level, removed themselves from the specifics of newspaper headlines and allowed audiences to place the tragedy in a larger historical and, importantly, emotional framework. (154)

While *The Baltimore Waltz* represents satire rather than the more benign format of comedy, Alberto Sandoval-Sánchez argues that "with [Paul Rudnick's play] *Jeffrey*, AIDS has entered the realm of comedy, leaving behind its lugubrious phase" (53). To this, Rudnick adds: "This play couldn't have been written earlier . . . We needed the first generation of AIDS plays . . . to get the word out. Now we can put AIDS in other contexts and we can see HIV-positive people as romantic and sexy" (qtd. in Reginato 9; cf. also Baker 206, 209). *Jeffrey*'s advocating romance and safe sex subscribes to the heterosexual bourgeois U.S.-American ideology of the couple and thus engages in a discourse of gay sameness of values to straight society beneath a façade of sexual difference. Likewise, in depicting gay Manhattan as a world of its own, quite separate from the larger heteronormative world around it, the play fails to challenge the feeling of personal safety from AIDS and social change that informs the mainstream U.S.-American discursive framing of the epidemic. However, like *The Baltimore Waltz*, *Jeffrey* is carefully grounded in the playwright's personal experience with the epidemic. As a romantic comedy, it transcends the use of humor in earlier AIDS plays as a means to console and provoke laughter to keep from crying. Instead, it makes a strong claim for a self-confident gay life in full recognition of the ongoing struggle against the epidemic.

Works Cited

Aronson, Arnold. "American Theatre in Context: 1945–Present." *The Cambridge History of American Theatre: Post-World War II to the 1990s*. Ed. Don B. Wilmeth and Christopher Bigsby. Cambridge: Cambridge UP, 2000. 87-162. Print.

Baker, Rob. *The Art of AIDS: From Stigma to Conscience*. New York: Continuum, 1994. Print.

Berger, Peter L. *Redeeming Laughter: The Comic Dimension of Human Experience*. Berlin: de Gruyter, 1997. Print.

Boccardi, Robert Francis. *An Examination of Selected American Plays Produced in New York between 1984 and 1993 Relating to the Issue of AIDS*. Diss. New York University, 1994. Ann Arbor: UMI, 1994. Microform.

Dace, Tish. "Vogel, Paula (Anne)." *Contemporary American Dramatists*. Ed. Kathryn Ann Berney and N. G. Templeton. London: St. James, 1994. 595-99. Print.

Eads, Martha Greene. "Paul Rudnick." *Dictionary of Literary Biography*. Ed. Christopher J. Wheatley. Vol. 266. Detroit: Gale, 2003. 245-54. Print.

Esch-van Kan, Anneka. "Der 11. September und das amerikanische Theater." *Nine Eleven: Ästhetische Verarbeitungen des 11. September 2001*. Ed. Ingo Irsigler and Christoph Jürgensen. Heidelberg: Winter, 2008. 127-42. Print.

Esslin, Martin. *The Theatre of the Absurd*. Rev. and updated ed. Woodstock: Overlook, 1973. Print.

Haas, Astrid. *Stages of Agency: The Contributions of American Drama to the AIDS Discourse*. Heidelberg: Winter, 2011. Print.

Haynes, Roslynn D. *From Faust to Strangelove: Representations of the Scientist in Western Literature*. Baltimore: Johns Hopkins UP, 1994. Print.

Hoffman, William M. *As Is*. New York: Vintage, 1985. Print.

Howe, Lawrence. "Critical Anthologies of the Plague Years: Responding to AIDS Literature." *Contemporary Literature* 35.2 (1994): 395-416. Print.

Jauß, Hans Robert. *Ästhetische Erfahrung und literarische Hermeneutik*. Frankfurt am Main: Suhrkamp, 1982. Print.

Jones, Therese. Introduction. *Sharing the Delirium: Second Generation AIDS Plays and Performances*. Ed. Jones. Portsmouth: Heinemann, 1994. ix-xvi. Print.

Jones, Wendell, David Stanley, and Robert Berg. "*AIDS! The Musical!*" *Sharing the Delirium: Second Generation AIDS Plays and Performances.* Ed. Therese Jones. Portsmouth: Heinemann, 1994. 207-64. Print.

Kift, Roy. "Reality and Illusion in the Theresienstadt Cabaret." *Staging the Holocaust: The Shoah in Drama and Performance.* Ed. Claude Schumacher. Cambridge: Cambridge UP, 1998. 147-68. Print.

Kruger, Steven F. *AIDS Narratives: Gender and Sexuality, Fiction and Science.* New York: Garland, 1996. Print.

Kubrick, Stanley, dir. *Dr. Strangelove, Or: How I Learned to Stop Worrying and Love the Bomb.* Writ. Stanley Kubrick, Terry Southern, and Peter George. Columbia: Hawk Films, 1963. DVD.

Mahy, Brian W. J. *A Dictionary of Virology.* 2nd ed. San Diego: Academic, 1997. Print.

Mayer, Mathias. *Der erste Weltkrieg und die literarische Ethik: Historische und systematische Perspektiven.* Munich: Fink, 2010. Print.

Molière [Jean-Baptiste Poquelin]. Preface. *Le Tartuffe, ou: L'imposteur: Comédie, 1664-1669.* By Molière. Ed. Jean-Pierre Collinet. Paris: Librairie Générale française, 1985. 33-41. Print.

Reginato, James. "'Jeffrey' Takes Manhattan." *Women's Wear Daily* 3 February 1993: 9. Print.

Reiner, Rob, dir. *When Harry Met Sally.* Writ. Nora Ephron. Palace / Castle Rock / Nelson Entertainment, 1989. DVD.

Rohr, Susanne. "'Genocide Pop:' The Holocaust as Media Event." *The Holocaust, Art, and Taboo: Transatlantic Exchanges on the Ethics and Aesthetics of Representation.* Ed. Sophia Komor and Susanne Rohr. Heidelberg: Winter, 2010. 155-78. Print.

Román, David. *Acts of Intervention: Performance, Gay Culture, and AIDS.* Bloomington: Indiana UP, 1998. Print.

---. "*The Baltimore Waltz.*" *Theatre Journal* 44.4 (December 1992): 520-22. Print.

---. "Negative Identifications: HIV-Negative Gay Men in Representation and Preformance." *Of Borders and Threshholds: Theatre History, Practice, and Theory.* Ed. Michal Kobialka. Minneapolis: U of Minnesota P, 1999. 184-213. Print.

Rudnick, Paul. *Jeffrey.* New York: Dramatists Play Service, 1994. Print.

Saal, Ilka. *Dramatizing the Disease: Responses to AIDS on the US American Stage*. Marburg: Tectum, 1997. Microform.

Sandoval, Alberto. "Staging AIDS: What's Latinos Got to Do With It?" *Negotiating Performance: Gender, Sexuality, and Theatricality in Latin/o America*. Ed. Diana Taylor and Juan Villegas. Durham: Duke UP, 1994. 49-66. Print.

Schultz, Raymond Thomas. *When the "A-Word" Is Never Spoken: The Direct and Subtle Impact of AIDS on Gay Dramatic Literature*. Diss. Wayne State University, 1999. Ann Arbor: UMI, 2000. Microform.

Sennett, Ted. *Laughing in the Dark: Movie Comedy from Groucho to Woody*. New York: St. Martin's, 1992. Print.

Shepard, Alan, and Mary Lamb. "The Memory Palace in Paula Vogel's Plays." *Southern Women Playwrights: New Essays in Literary History and Criticism*. Ed. Robert L. McDonald and Linda Rohrer Paige. Tuscaloosa: U of Alabama P, 2002. 198-217. Print.

Stowe, William W. *Going Abroad: European Travel in Nineteenth-Century American Culture*. Princeton: Princeton UP, 1994. Print.

Vogel, Paula. *The Baltimore Waltz. The Baltimore Waltz and Other Plays*. New York: Theatre Communications Group, 1996. 1-57. Print.

Watkins, Beth. "Women, AIDS, and Theatre: Representations and Resistances." *Journal of Medical Humanities* 19.2-3 (1998): 167-80. Print.

Weitz, Eric. *The Cambridge Introduction to Comedy*. Cambridge: Cambridge UP, 2009. Print.

Rüdiger Kunow

The Biology of Community:
Contagious Diseases, Old Age, Biotech, and Cultural Studies

In this article, I want to enter the ongoing debate about the public presence of human life in democratic societies of the global North, with particular emphasis on the United States. The forms this presence will take are themselves multiply determined along the axes of the individual and the collective, normative and non-normative life forms, as well as the inside and the outside of the nation state. This is especially so in moments when certain forms of human life are perceived as less valuable, as diseased, or even as endangering others. It is at such moments that the tacit assumptions governing a society's understanding of what counts as human come up for debate, when figurations of the human perform important political, social, and cultural work. Hence, a full understanding of what Carmen Birkle in her introduction to this volume describes as the links between disease, nationhood, and the dehumanization of certain life forms requires a triangulation of the perspectives offered by structures of *mobility*, *governmentality* and *disciplinarity*.

The relationships between these domains are of course varied and complicated and cannot be addressed in the compass of this article with any pretense at comprehensiveness. In this essay, I will therefore focus on how the biology of human life—especially in its bacteriological and micro-biological variants—has been presenting an authoritative and persuasive vocabulary to articulate the essence and the compass of what "we, the people" stands for at particular historical junctures, not only in the EuroAmerican world but more recently in the context of "powerful nationalist aspirations in newly affluent Asia" (Ong 5). The language of biology has proven to be so authoritative and persuasive because its pronouncements have been able to claim the prestige of the "hard sciences," as Georges Canguilhem (cf. *Ideology*) and Stephen Katz, among others, have noted: "As we well know, concepts of norms, normality, and pathology migrated from medicine to became [sic] the moral and statistical standards by which social [and, I might add, cultural] relations in general would be governed" (Katz 44). In point of fact, however, the medical understanding of the body relies on constructs no less than those circulating in the lay culture. And medical experts fall for the lure of suggestive metaphors and elegant rhetorical figures just as much as other people. Relations between the somatic and the semantic are far from being as straightforward and smooth as the prestige routinely accorded to scientific pronouncement seems to warrant. And even while it has been something like an article of faith in American and Cultural Studies that the human body is also above all else discursively constructed, that assumption has recently come under critique from the perspective of "the new critical materialisms" (19) for marginalizing "the importance of bodies in situating empirical actors within a material environment of nature, other bodies, and the socioeconomic structures that dictate where and how they find sustenance" (Coole and Frost 29). In this way, a focus on the human body takes us straight to the heart of current disciplinary controversy.

In order to discuss this complex of problems further, I will visit three interconnected sites, in which biological matter and cultural practices are mutually imbricated with crucial implications for the public presence of human life, especially in its vulnerable and liminal conditions and situations. These sites are: a) the mobility of bio-matter; b) figurations of late life in the public sphere; and c) the challenges posed by the advent of biotechnology.

The trajectory of my argument is as follows: In the opening section called "Mobility, or Bio-Based Communities" I seek to describe how mobility on the microbiotic level performs wide-ranging cultural work in the context of ethnic or social Otherness. In the next part I will offer a few thoughts on how stages and ages of life have been "govern-mentalized" (Athanasiou 145). I will call it "'Embedded Life': Age-ncy in the Public Sphere." And in the third and final part, I want to discuss how advances in biotechnology, especially the geneticization of the human body, impact on our understanding of what life is and what the future relationships of individuals and communities toward life can be. I call this concluding section: "Failed Bodies, or, The Survival of the Fairest."

Mobility, or Bio-Based Communities

Mobility is undoubtedly one of the crucial experiences of our time. In the context of what Jürgen Habermas has called an "economically fashioned global society" ("Postnationale Konstellation" 95; my translation), mobility has become an aggregate of complex individual and collective, real and imagined processes. Such processes involve the deregulated mobility of goods and capital (mobility "from above"), the regulated mobility of people (mobility "from below") as well as the simultaneously regulated and anarchic mobility of ideas, images, and information ("horizontal mobility").

The very fact that "mobility practices" exist at all levels has also refashioned the research protocols and the analytical vocabularies of the Humanities, including those of American Studies. Since "human mobility implicates *both* physical bodies moving through material landscapes *and* categorical figures moving through representational spaces" (Delaney qtd. in Cresswell 4), our discipline has organized its search for adequate conceptualizations around efforts such as those of the New, the Transnational, the Hemispheric, or Transcultural American Studies (Rowe). However, what has remained pretty much outside the purview of these critical projects is a particular type of mobility that is truly transnational, truly transcultural, and at times even hemispheric: I will call it here *biological mobility*. The term references the largely overlooked or disregarded movement of life forms such as bacteria, germs, microbes, viruses. All of these are constantly "on the move," traveling as freely, if not more freely (Markel 5), than the proverbial migrants that have captivated so much of our critical attention. In fact, biological mobility is a highly dynamic and compelling form of transnational mobility which manifests itself in contagious, often epidemic illnesses, among them the Nile and Ebola fevers, SARS, avian and pig influenzas or the whole array of sexually transmitted diseases, most prominent among them HIV-AIDS.

Mobile microbes are in biomedical parlance often called "contact communicants," and this coinage reminds us of the multiple linkages that exist between communicability and communication, linkages which are not exhausted by the common etymological root. Biological mobility is not in itself meaningful; rather, it produces effects that insistently demand to be made so. This desire for meaning and representation is nourished by the fact that the actual moment of biological communication, the moment of transmission from one person to the next that is called "infection" remains for the most part invisible to the eye of the beholder. There is thus an element of privacy, even secrecy, involved here, a secrecy which, in truly dialectic fashion, produces a desire for revelation. This is why, as "germs . . . travel from one living being to another . . . there is a narrative power" vested in them (Markel 7). This is the reason why there is an elective affinity between contagion and narration that, at certain historical junctures, has acted as a catalyst for the development of radical new modes of representation, e.g., in Thucydides's *History of the Peloponnesian War* (ca. 400 B.C.E.) or Boccaccio's *Decameron* (c. 1349-53), Defoe's *Journal of the Plague Year* (1722), and the first U.S. novel, Charles Brocken Brown's *Arthur Mervyn, or Memoirs of the Year 1793* (1799/1800) all the way down to the AIDS fiction of the 1980s and 1990s.[1] And it must be added that especially with the advent of mass media in the latter decades of the nineteenth century, narratives of disease have "constitute[d] potentially profitable forms of news and entertainment" (Tomes 627). Such practices of "disease 'sell'" (628) are by no means a thing of the past, as shown by this mini-story from a *New York Times Magazine* special section on public health issues in the context of globalization: "[A] mosquito infested with the malaria parasite . . . can be buzzing in Ghana at dawn and dining on an airport employee in Boston by cocktail hour" (qtd. in Albertini 449).

As this example of current fear with its subdued apocalyptic rhetoric shows, more is involved in thinking mobility and biology together than merely registering the unimpeded flow of pathogens. Rather, biomobility invites serious questions about the permeability and

---

[1]   For analyses of some of these texts, see Ingrid Gessner's, Astrid Haas's, and Imke Kimpel's contributions in this volume.

porousness of bodies, individual and national; in addition, it can also serve as a timely reminder of what might be called—pace Fredric Jameson—*the dialectic of externalization and internalization*, i.e., "the rhythm by which we objectify ourselves and then reinteriorize the objective results at some higher level" (*Hegel Variations* 19)—in much plainer words: what makes people rich will also make them sick. It may be questionable, though, whether the chain of mobility sustaining capitalist globalization that produces much-desired mobile bodies, only to expose these same bodies to a whole new panoply of equally mobile pathogenic material, deserves to be designed as "some higher level." However this may be, the dialectic of externalization and internalization that is unfolding itself here, reminds us in useful ways of the fact that we should not read biomobility as being just "about" itinerant bio matter; rather it deserves to be understood as involving what Agamben, Esposito or Judith Butler from various perspectives have addressed as *the problem of living-with-others*, of all those "out there"—I am quoting Butler here—"on whom my life depends, people I do not know and may never know" (*Precarious Life* xii).

I want to illustrate some of the issues involved in biological cohabitation with the help of a well-known example, that of Mary Mallon, a.k.a. "Typhoid Mary." During the 1910s, the first-generation immigrant from Ireland who worked as a cook in casual employment on Long Island, NY, was arguably one the most prominent women living in the U.S. What made her famous (or infamous) was that she was suspected of spreading typhoid among the families of her various employers (Leavitt). When first confronted with the charge in 1909, Mallon refused to be examined by public health officials. She was forcibly moved to a hospital where she tested positive for the typhoid bacillus. When Mallon filed a *habeas corpus* appeal against the quarantine subsequently imposed on her, a debate ensued which set the state's obligation to safeguard the health of the general public against the civil liberties of an individual person (for details cf. Leavitt, *Typhoid Mary*). At first, Mallon's appeal was rejected by the courts but eventually she won her release, assumed an alias, and disappeared. When she was rediscovered, years later, she immediately became a *cause célèbre* again. *The New York Times*, for example, saluted her with the headline: "'Typhoid Mary' has reappeared . . . Human Culture Tube, Herself Immune, Spreads the Disease Wherever She Goes" (qtd. in

Wald 105). Lauren Berlant's concept of "a world of public intimacy" (1), which merges in a most volatile and lacerating way the most private and the most public elements of human life, and Anthony Giddens's related idea of a relentless "transformation of intimacy" (7) into a public good, together offer a nuanced understanding of the play of interiorization and exteriorization as it unfolded in the Mallon case.

This transformation of the most intimate into the most public must also be understood in terms of gendered relations. The 1910s in the U.S. were also the time of the New Woman, i.e., "unattached" and independent young female persons from the lower and the middle classes working away from home in factories or offices. This unprecedented form of female mobility was perceived critically in many quarters of U.S. society at that time; it is the backdrop against which Theodore Dreiser's *Sister Carrie* (1900) or Stephen Crane's *Maggie: A Girl of the Streets* (1893) were written; it is also the setting for the contemporary reaction to "Typhoid Mary." Mary Mallon's was what Elisabeth Bronfen has in a different context called an "excessively present feminine body" (81). Mallon's insertion into the public space scripted the mobile female body as doubly deviant, not only morally but also medically; bacteriology and public health in this way became stand-ins for moral judgment.

Both contenders in the Mallon case were actively involved in inserting it into the public domain of the unfolding mass media. That this should happen so quickly and so easily is due in no small part to the fact that the medical sensation occurred at a critical juncture that Nancy Tomes describes as

> the convergence of two revolutions, one in the scientific world, the other in the newspaper industry. The scientific revolution was precipitated by the work of Louis Pasteur, Robert Koch, and their contemporaries, who in the late 1800s provided convincing experimental proof of what came to be known as the germ theory of disease .... The discovery of the germ coincided with the late-nineteenth-century print revolution, which both cheapened the cost of newspapers and books and quickened the pace of news reporting. The so-called penny press pioneered a new kind of print journalism that redefined the conception of newsworthiness to include regular reportage on health and disease issues. (629)

I would like to add here that print journalism could itself rely on the availability of a *cultural script*, the script of a person hiding out in the maze of the metropolis, a person whose (criminal) deviancy makes it imperative that he or she be found, possibly with the help of a kind of urban pathfinder: the detective. This urban hide-and-seek script possibly originated with Edgar Allan Poe. And the public health inspectors doubling as disease detectives on Mallon's trail were in many ways like the narrator of Poe's "Man of the Crowd" (1840): paradoxically attached to the object of his search, "firmly resolved that we should not part" and looking at Mary Mallon as "the type and the genius of deep crime" (107, 109). The irony of this medical detective story was probably this: Pursuing Mallon taught contemporary observers, experts, and the general public alike one thing above all else—that she was unreadable. Mallon was a healthy young woman, yet a carrier of disease, so the only way to find her was to follow the traces she left, traces of infection. In her case, as in many cases of communicable disease, the gaze, even the expert gaze, revealed—nothing; common knowledge, especially in the visual register, was of no help here, since her body *did* communicate (namely infection) but it was *not* expressive, or, in the closing words of Poe's story: "*es laesst sich nicht lessen*" (109; italics and German-language original). This is perhaps also the moment to note that communicable diseases and the cultural responses to them can be shown to possess a histrionics of their own, a certain *dramaturgy* which characterizes, for example, the "disease detective" genre (for more details cf. Wald 20-23, 68) with its characteristic beginnings, twists and turns, and, hopefully, a happy end.

Looking back at the Mallon case it becomes apparent that biotic mobility precipitates critical situations in which the line between the public and the private becomes blurry. Since communicable diseases are illnesses associated with the crowd, they shift the focus from the individual to the multitude (a related argument can be found in Hardt and Negri xiv), and to governmentality at large. And with regard to this realignment of the public and the private, Canguilhem's understanding of immunity as a "concept in waiting" (139) is very helpful, because in times of medical crisis it is only through the presumption of a shared immunity from contagion of social and cultural others that the nation as imagined community achieves something that might be termed "imagined immunity." This community/immunity cannot be configured without a certain representational archive, a "language of purity." As the years following the "Typhoid Mary" episode would show, narratives "of cleansing and of the fight against the invisible enemy ... again and again structured twentieth-century politics" (Sarasin et al. 42; my translation), as also in the 1980s:

> New York City [during the Bicentennial] had hosted the greatest party ever known. The guests had come from all over the world . . . . This was the part the epidemiologists would later note when they stayed up late at night and the conversation drifted toward where it had started and when. They would remember that glorious night in New York Harbor, all those sailors, and recall: From all over the world they came to New York. (Shilts 3)

Here, at the very opening of Randy Shilts's bestselling *And the Band Played On: Politics, People, and the AIDS Epidemic* (1987), biomobility figures as the "dark undercurrent" of the everyday vernacular mobility that is constantly bringing strangers into the heart of the nation, the nation understood as an *ecosystem under siege*. The relation of biomobility and governmentality is in Shilts's rendering of the evolving HIV-AIDS crisis configured as desire for the absent father-regulator, as the channels of connection that link the U.S. to the rest of the world turn out to be in truth the channels of contamination. Even more importantly, there is a delay or *deferral* at work here. The diseased stranger's "real" identity, as a spreader of a dangerous biotic material, reveals itself only later, when it is already too late. In this way his or her presence in the public space can be likened to that of a Trojan horse, carrying inside a gift that is deadly and disastrous, but deferred. And while the idea of the "Trojan stranger" is much older, going back to a 1912 article for the *New York State Journal of Medicine* (Wald 75), we all know how the underlying idea sustaining such representation of the diseased Other, as a kind of *sleeper* that will sometime later unleash his/her terrible biological weapons, has attained even greater resonance in the public mind (Mayer 20) in the aftermath of the events of September 11, 2001.

"Embedded Life": Age-ncy in the Public Sphere

As Foucault and others have shown, the progressive evolvement of biopolitics in EuroAmerican modernity has brought about what he calls an "*anatomo-politics of the human body*" (139) charged with inscribing upon the individual body the norms of governmentality. As a result, the human body became progressively "embedded" in an ever more intricate network of regulating norms and agencies. Biopolitics has intervened especially at both extreme ends of the body's life course, in reproductive rights or duties and in those pertaining to senior citizens. I will focus on the latter, reading "old age" as a name for vital connections between the private, individual body and the body politic.

The concept of "old age" entered the sphere of governmentality at a time when the nation, after its external, territorial consolidation in the course of the nineteenth century, proceeded to consolidate its internal powers as well. In making a certain stage/age of the human life course the determining criterion, the state selectively identified a group of people and positioned them as objects of governance. As more and more institutions were created to address the needs of the elderly, a historically new form of citizenship emerged, an "intimate citizenship" that was essentially not so much about rights, such as voting rights, but about entitlements through which a person's aged body became the object of state care and intervention. In the course of time, the private and the public merged in a form of *public intimacy*, which became invested with politico-symbolic functions as the "imaginative focus, . . . [and an] indicator, of a caring society and of national coherence and inclusiveness" (Biggs 308).

In the United States, this process occurred much later than in the other capitalist societies of the global North. New Deal and Great Society programs attempted to circumscribe the civic identity of "senior citizens" and did so by establishing various government-sponsored entitlement programs (social security, Medicaid). Here, as elsewhere, the affable address "senior citizens" came to project a publicly mandated age identity, an identity whose most salient component was its effective public effacement. People identified by that term were regarded as having "bowed out" (or having been "bowed out") of active participation in the routines of the rest of the community. This process was also reflected in the creating of specific age-related heterotopias: the retirement home as institutionalization and symbolic representation of a particular Western-style form of aging.

Mandatory retirement (officially extinct since 1978) is a showcase example of the ambivalences of the civic identity of late life. Originally developed as an act of public benevolence, even munificence, toward deserving elders, it soon became a norm which defined a compulsory socio-cultural role for people who had reached "a certain age," a norm which required their non-presence in the public domain. They were, as the saying goes, sent "to the pastures."

Since the collapse of state-sponsored Communism, we can observe a paradigm shift from welfare capitalism to neo-liberalism with profound effects on many areas of life, and also on late life. The particular civic identity termed "old age" has in recent years come under attack, as the power of definition over senescence and its place in the public sphere is increasingly moving from the nation states and their institutions to the financial sector, and here especially to IGOs like the World Bank or the IMF or various expert groups.

A milestone in this direction was the 1994 World Bank paper "Averting the Old Age Crisis" (supplemented in 2005 with a statement on "Old Age Income Support in the Twenty-First Century"). This policy statement is ostensibly a description of the status quo. However, it is saturated with rhetoric, using metaphor, simile, and a host of tropes that we would rather expect to find in literary texts. With regard to such genres of governmental writing, there is no reason why the skills of our discipline in the critical reading of texts could not and should not be brought to bear on these discourses that have effectively re-defined the key terms in which human life in its later stages came to be viewed in the public sphere. These terms are essentially economic in nature, and they reflect neo-liberalism's overall tendency to regard human beings merely "as a source of inefficiency" (Korten 23).

In accordance with such a premise, the presence of elderly populations has come to be viewed first and foremost as a problem, the World Bank even calls it a crisis, and a "pressure on a country's resources and government budgets [which] increases exponentially as populations age" and which "hinder[s] economic growth" (2; cf. also xiii). In a kind of "trickle down" effect, the World Bank statement (including its 2005 amendment), plus other "expert predictions" (the 1999 Human Development Report, the 2002 Valencia Forum/Second World Assembly on Ageing, etc.) has been extremely effective in re-conceptualizing the public identity of human beings in the later phases of their life: from rights (human rights, citizenship rights) to risks—risks related to the economic future of the country; fiscal viability; the international competitiveness of the United States; and most of all a risk for future generations. In related fashion, the Peterson Institute sees demographic change in terms of "a massive iceberg, [that] looms ahead in the future of the largest and most affluent economies of the world" (Peterson 3).

Such predictions derive their critical momentum from the way in which statistics on life expectancy are becoming an effective and powerful representational strategy (representation here understood in both its semiotic and political senses): Human life is being understood in terms of economic effectiveness. In other words, human life becomes human capital. Measured by these standards and failing, "old age" can then be used to ground forms of comparative biopolitics and can in this way become a key factor in the theoretical scaffolding of globalization processes (Kunow 300-08; Magnus 219-39). This has happened in the context of the "War against Terror": In his comparative sketch of the rise and fall of civilizations, the late Samuel P. Huntington makes reference to what he calls the "demographic bulge" (118), i.e., the relative youthfulness of some Muslim nations, to suggest that, in the coming clash of civilizations, the EuroAmerican sphere will be seriously disadvantaged because its population is older, hence less likely to withstand the assault from a supposedly youthful and aggressive Islam.

"Boomerangst" (Magnus 295) or, in more sober terms, the "'public burden of aging' scenario" (Polivka 233) has highlighted the ambivalence underlying the insertion of human life into key areas of governmentality: On the one hand, and for the first time in U.S. history, the social imaginary came to include a sense of voluntarily incurred obligations toward a cross-sectional group of people, independent of social, ethnic, or cultural background, simply on the basis of perceived impairments of the human body. On the other hand, understanding elderly people primarily as clients of the government had the (unintended?) effect of (re-)presenting them in the public sphere, not as citizen-subjects but as objects, wards of public concern and scrutiny, producing costs while not contributing measurably to the well-being of society. In short: when it comes to the later stages of life, age has come to mean loss of age-ncy. This process has currently reached a new high point, in the ongoing debates on the future of social security.

"Old age" in all this is not just a category of governmentality, a socially mandated identity badge, but also *a critical idiom through which collectivities imagine and articulate a consciousness*" (Cohen xvii; emphasis original) of who they are and what visions of the good life they share. If late life is now increasingly reconfigured, in lay and expert discourses alike, as a burden, an economic liability, and an obstacle to political power, we might well ask what the relationship between the human body and the body politic will be like in the future. This involves not only late life, but all forms of human life, especially those that have become weak or otherwise "useless." And this brings me to my third section.

Failed Bodies, or, The Survival of the Fairest

In this section, I want to take a look at the effects of the biotechnicalization of human life. I use that expression as a blanket term to comprise a variety of activities which have emerged as a result of advances in molecular biology and medicine, such as pre-implantation diagnostics, stem-cell research, tissue grafting, etc. More than twenty years ago, Fredric Jameson argued that the emerging new stage of global capitalism would be characterized by the drive to bring under its domination two as yet uncolonized areas: nature and the unconscious (*Postmodernism* 49). Concerning nature, especially human nature, his statement has been truly prophetic: we seem to be witnessing a fundamental shift in the conception of human life—variously called "the golden age of biotechnology" (Kass 9) or "the age of 'biocybernetic reproduction'" (Mitchell 14)—in which the horizon of intelligibility of human life is expanding widely and rapidly.

This is no longer a matter merely of cosmetic surgery or assisted pregnancies: Rather, the "stupendous successes" of biotechnology (Kass 14), or, more soberly, the genome revolution, will soon make available to a growing number of people—even middle-class Americans— substantial medical and genetic interventions which are no longer merely curative or restorative but aim at an improved performativity of the human body across the various stages of its life course. Pre-implantation diagnosis can or will make it possible to eliminate defects before a baby is born while post-menopausal women or men in their 70s and 80s are enabled to parent children. Once again, as in the case of senior citizens, life is embedded, this time in a new, no longer nation-centric but "genocentric" (Keane 473; Rouvroy 99) biopolitics.

Within this larger changeover in the understanding of embodied human life from therapeutic to enhancement orientations, those who are willing to "invest" into their bodies are now given a chance to overcome, at least in part, the restraints of their biological endowment and especially those restraints deriving from increasing vulnerability to disease as the body gets old. Human life thus becomes "a series of processes that can be ... potentially re-engineered" (Novas and Rose 487). All this holds out the promise of a techno-utopia in which the ancient dream of humanity to uncover the secrets of life and to attain eternal youth, if not eternal life, is at long last coming to be realized. It may be true that, as some observers caution, "[b]io-techniques [sic] are sold in future markets and are not yet profitable" (McCallum 200). I would read such statements as reminders that human life has, in a very literal sense, become a "futures market," just like those financial instruments traded at the stock market, a commodity traded on the basis of its projected value at some point in the future.

This orientation to future body performance puts increasing pressure on people today to actually put to use all the available biomedical enhancement procedures. If, for example, the other children in your daughter's class do receive memory enhancement or other stimulant drugs (Kass 16), then withholding these from your child may feel like a form of child neglect. Or, if you are old and frail, and don't do anything about it, that may come to be seen as a person's own fault, as an individual's culpable conduct. Why did you not take an anti-aging medication or go to the body enhancement shop? This tendency toward "the survival of the fairest" (Keane 467-94) may in due time have far-reaching repercussions for insurance eligibility and entitlement programs in the future.

At this point it may be helpful—and especially so from an American Studies perspective—to entertain a hypothetical idea (presented in a slightly different form by Nikolas Rose 255), namely that the new forms of biology-based self-management may well herald the return of a culturally repressed: Weberian inner-worldly asceticism. One could thus read the emergence of the biologically enhanced person in terms of a *bio-medicalization of the Puritan work ethic*. What is more, one might even add a footnote to the Weberian thesis by saying that the ascendency of neoliberal capitalism has finally found a matching partner in a compatible personality structure: the self-enhancing performative individual. His/her ethic is no longer Puritan but perfectionist, no longer linking the other-worldly spiritual domain with the material realities of this world, but one material domain with another.

What I see emerging as a result of all this is a new cultural narrative, for which I suggest the provisional term *biographies of culpability*. Such narratives are likely themselves caught up in the "web of normalcy" (Butler and Taylor 197) in which human life has always been entangled but which is now biotechnically redesigned, and thus woven ever more tightly, and which produces an extended casuistry or risks—risks vested in so-called deviant sexual behavior (HIV-AIDS), socio-cultural idiosyncrasies (living with domestic animals produces avian influenza) or the wrong dietary tastes (obesity). The degree to which new biocultural norms are in these cases inscribed into individual bodies becomes clear when we remind ourselves that identity construction in these biographies of culpability occurs not only in moments of acute public health crises; it has by now become part of everyday life, certainly in the United States, in discourses promoting health concerns, dieting, and fitness regimes, in short, "an increasing stress on personal reconstruction through acting on the body" (Rose 26). What is more, these life stories, as the case of "Typhoid Mary" has shown, are more often than not authored, not so much by the individual himself or herself, but in and by the public.

The extent to which the geneticization of human life has already become an integral part of the cultural imaginary of U.S.-American society can perhaps be illustrated through an example from the archives of urban legend: In the year 2000, a group of Evangelical Christians presumably launched "The Second Coming Project." They no longer wanted to wait for the Second Coming of Jesus Christ but wished to precipitate it by cloning him. Their motto was: "In order to save the world from sin, we must clone Jesus to initiate the Second Coming of the Christ." They had intended to do that by taking cells from relics such as the Turin Shroud or the Veil of Veronica and then implant the zygote into the womb of a virginal young woman who had volunteered to bring the baby Jesus to term in a second Virgin birth. The Second Coming Project, with a post-office box in Berkeley, CA, even solicited and received donations for this (cf. "Clone of Contention").

How credible is that story? As it turned out, the Second Coming Project was just one of the many millennial spoofs circulating in the

U.S. around Y2K, but the idea is almost too good to be false. However, this story should not be dismissed too lightly. As W. J. T. Mitchell has recently shown, cloning has become "a symbolic condensation" in contemporary U.S. society, even an "exemplar . . . of a wide range of biopolitical phenomena" (xii), ranging from anxieties about reproductive medicine all the way to fears of terrorism based on models of biological intervention. And, adding to Mitchell's analysis, one can observe that the scenarios of biotechnical reproduction have become global.

In France, cloning served as the basis for two books by French writer Didier van Cauwelaert who in his 2005 *Cloner le Christ?* takes up and expands the Second Coming Project. He has one of the principal instigators explain the project in broad historical sweep:

> C'est la Résurrection. La fameuse Résurrection dont parlent les chrétiens. C'est un clonage, tout simple, accéléré, un peu plus sophistiqué que celui que je peux faire. . . . Les scientifiques extraterrestres ayant créé le monde auraient donc conçu, d'après elle, un prototype Jésus, refabriqué après sa mort en modèle de série, pour faire face à la demande du consommateur des siècles futures, quand même l'Église du XXIe siècle refuserait le lui délivrer son autorisation de mise sur le marché. (151)

Not surprisingly, this passage can be found in a chapter called "Messianic Park."

What Cauwelaert is envisioning here, is nothing less than the happy union of the two most powerful utopian visions currently animating the American collective imaginary: evangelical religion and cutting-edge high tech. And the Second Coming cloning project is by no means the only case in which religion and cutting-edge technology are imagined together: There is also the *Left Behind* series, jointly authored by Tim LaHaye and Jerry B. Jenkins, itself a mega-seller, with more than 40 million copies sold. *Left Behind* also takes as its *donné* the coming of Christ, and presents an imaginary apocalyptic scenario in which the Tribulation Force (a multicultural group of Evangelical Christians) is engaging the anti-Christ (a former United Nations secretary general) with the help of hi-tech gadgetry, including supersonic jets and light-speed internet communication (www.leftbehind.com).

Whatever our views on biotech and its promises for a blithe future may be—clearly, the rapid advances in biology and medicine have dramatically expanded the discretionary autonomy of human beings over their bodies. When biology is no longer destiny, this will profoundly modify what Habermas called the "ethical self-understanding of the species" (*Future* 16). Such issues are far too important to leave to the biomedical industry, which is, after all, in important ways an *industry*—and has no bones about it, as we can read on the *Human Genome Project Information* website: "[An] important feature of the HGP project was the federal government's long-standing dedication to the transfer to technology to the private sector. By licensing technologies to private companies . . . the project catalyzed the multibillion-dollar U.S. biotechnology industry and fostered the development of new medical applications." Please note what comes first, and what last, in this description. In view of this, it is indeed surprising, as Antoinette Rouvroy notes, that in some sectors of the public sphere the bio-tech sector still enjoys at least "the presumption of neutrality and inherent goodness (the logic of healing) . . . despite the huge involvement of profit-driven businesses at each stage of the project" (20-21). Maybe it is time to update President Eisenhower's notion of a military-industrial complex and speak of a biological industrial complex that is acting in important ways in U.S. society.

At this point, I want to take the discussion into yet another domain by "disciplining" it: From an American Studies perspective, and especially that version of our discipline that has drawn its inspirations from Cultural Studies, the rapid advances in biotechnologies, in tandem with the demise of the welfare state and a wide-spread fear of global epidemics, pose important questions about the relations of culture and biology, but even more importantly about the position of human life, especially in its frail, precarious, and apparently useless moments. These questions are addressed at least in part in the context of the recently proclaimed "biological turn" in American and cultural studies; yet another turn, one is tempted to say. While I share some views expounded in the "Biocultures Manifesto" of 2007, for example that "[b]iology . . . cannot exist outside culture; culture, as a practice, cannot exist outside biology" (Davis and Morris 418), I want to do a bit more than begging the biocultural obvious and propose that we need a cultural critique of the overall *biologization* of the human body in U.S. culture today.

The "grounded terrain of practices, representations, languages, and customs" (439) of which Stuart Hall has famously spoken has shifted, or perhaps, expanded, from the socio-cultural domain to the sciences, and here the most recondite, complicated but also dynamic fields. It is true, human life has always been a social and cultural form and norm, and life under the impact of the "genome revolution" is no different; in fact, it may even be more cultural than before. Why? After all, the arcane of micro-biology and the operations of anthro-technology are such that they require a lot of translation. Even a cursory look at the titles of papers by medical and biological experts will show that there is a lot of translation work going on, even in expert communication. We in our discipline would do well to look that not too much of the "human" in human life is getting lost in that translation.

What is more, the question "what are the norms that constrain our conceptions of who is human and who is not . . . whose lives are worth protecting, valuing, furthering" may indeed, as Judith Butler and Sunaura Taylor suggest, "really [get] to the heart of the issue" (213) but such questions are no longer brokered in the public sphere of democratic societies but instead in the more limited-access spaces of expert debate. The World Bank paper or the Human Development Report, or the U.S. Health and Retirement Survey, and the U.S. Longitudinal Surveys of Aging which I mentioned above, or the papers published by the National Human Genome Research Institution can claim status as expert recommendations, they produce important knowledge, coming from highly specialized experts who more often than not have been selected by other "experts," and they are often not accountable to any democratically elected body. Small wonder, therefore, that "the inscription of bodies, and of life itself, in the social and political order" by experts in the fields of science and governance has been theorized in Agambian terms, as "zones of exception" (Giorgi and Pinkus 39).

The idea that we in American Studies or Cultural Studies, for that matter, can and indeed should intervene in these inscriptions, that we do have something to say about how human life is inserted into the public sphere, is not the conceptual over-reaching of a disgruntled Americanist. In fact, when the President's Council on Bioethics was established by then president George W. Bush in 2001, it began its work with a discussion of Nathaniel Hawthorne's story "The Birthmark" (Kass 14), which tells us that the technological imaginary does not have an

exclusive monopoly over how human life is defined, nor over what is
considered a good life, worthwhile living.

Coda

At the beginning of this article, I said that I would attempt a critique
of the overall biologization of human life that seems one of the salient
features of our time. By way of conclusion, I want to argue now that
such a focus takes us to a critical point for our discipline and for the
humanities in general, a point where the epistemological obligations of
cultural critique expand into ethical obligations. This is so because
reflecting on the communicative dynamics in which human life,
especially in its weak, useless, or otherwise undesirable forms, on how
social and cultural norms are made to "reside in and find a concrete
manifestation" (Armour and St. Ville 6) in the human body, opens up a
space for reflection (and action) about the present and future status of
human life in the United States and also in capitalist societies all over
the world. I call this the *civic meaning of human life*, because social
formations do not exist in and by themselves, but, as the Frankfurt
School has shown, reproduce themselves through acts of communication
in which the contours of what passes as acceptable, even desirable forms
of human life, are negotiated and defined (Kellner, "Habermas, the
Public Sphere, and Democracy").

There is more involved here than an instance of Foucauldian
biopolitics because we are being asked to consider or reconsider "the
relationship between representation and humanization" (Butler 140). In
a figure of thought that for me has echoes of Adorno, Judith Butler
enters a plea in her post-9/11 reflections, *Precarious Life*, that the
humanities should pay more attention than they have done so far to heed
"the cry of the human within the sphere of [public] appearance . . ."
(147). What this calls for in her view is a practice of "cultural analyses
that seek to understand how best to depict the human, human grief and
suffering, and how best to admit the 'faces' of those against whom war
is waged in public representation" (xviii). Butler's reference here is
primarily to "the erasure from public representation of the names,
images, and narratives of those the US has killed" (xiv) during the Bush
administration's "War on Terror," but they are not the only ones whose

public presence is freighted with acrimonious images. Old people as greedy geezers, disabled persons as burdens on the public domain, or those who otherwise fail the standards of the enhanced body—these are areas of concern for a cultural critique that seeks to counter the public dehumanization of human suffering and weakness. For Butler, such a critique represents a move by the humanities to be true to its name and to claim political relevance: "If the humanities has a future as cultural criticism, and cultural criticism has a task at the present moment, it is no doubt to return us to the human where we do not expect to find it, in its frailty and at the limits of its capacity to make sense" (151).

Works Cited

Albertini, Bill. "Contagion and the Necessary Accident." *Discourse* 30.3 (Fall 2008): 443-67. Print.

Armour, Ellen T., and Susan M. St. Ville. "Judith Butler: In Theory." *Bodily Citations: Religion and Judith Butler.* Ed. Armour and St. Ville. New York: Columbia UP, 2006. 1-12. Print.

Athanasiou, Athena. "Technologies of Humanness, Aporias of Biopolitics, and the Cut Body of Humanity." *Differences: A Journal of Feminist Cultural Studies* 14.1 (Spring 2003): 125-62. Print.

Berlant, Lauren. *The Queen of America Goes to Washington City: Essays on Sex and Citizenship.* Durham: Duke UP, 1997. Print.

Biggs, Simon. "Toward Critical Narrativity: Stories of Aging in Contemporary Social Policy." *Journal of Aging Studies* 15.4 (2001): 303-16. Print.

Bourdain, Anthony. *Typhoid Mary: An Urban Historical.* New York: Bloomsbury, 2001. Print.

Bronfen, Elisabeth. "Pin-Ups and the Violence of Beauty." *The Body as Interface: Dialogues between the Disciplines.* Ed. Sabine Sielke and Elisabeth Schäfer-Wünsche. Heidelberg: Winter, 2007. 81-93. Print.

Butler, Judith. *Precarious Life: The Powers of Mourning and Violence.* London: Verso, 2004. Print.

---, and Sunaura Taylor. "Interdependence." *Examined Life: Excursions with Contemporary Thinkers.* Ed. Astra Taylor. New York: New Press, 2009. 185-213. Print.

Canguilhem, Georges. *Ideology and Rationality in the History of the Life Sciences*. Trans. Arthur Goldhammer. Cambridge: MIT P, 1988. Print.

Cauwelaert, Didier van. *Cloner le Christ?* Paris: Albin Michel, 2005. Print.

"Clone of Contention." Web. 28 Aug. 2011. <http://www.snopes.com>.

Cohen, Lawrence. *No Aging in India: Alzheimer's, the Bad Family, and Other Modern Things*. Berkeley: U of California P, 1998. Print.

Coole, Diana, and Samantha Frost. "Introducing the New Materialisms." *New Materialisms: Ontology, Agency, and Politics*. Ed. Coole and Frost. Durham: Duke UP, 2010. 1-43. Print.

Cresswell, Tim. *On the Move: Mobility in the Western World*. New York: Routledge, 2006. Print.

Davis, Lennard J., and David B. Morris. "Biocultures Manifesto." *New Literary History* 38.3 (2007): 411-18. Print.

Delaney, David. "Laws of Motion and Immobilization: Bodies, Figures and the Politics of Mobility." Mobilities Conference. University of Wales. Gregynog Hall, Wales, 1999. Conference paper.

Foucault, Michel. *The History of Sexuality*. Vol. 1: *An Introduction*. Trans. Robert Hurley. 1978. New York: Vintage, 1990. Print.

Galusca, Roxana. "From Fictive Ability to National Identity: Disability, Medical Inspection, and Public Health Regulations on Ellis Island." *Cultural Critique* 72 (2009): 137-63. Print.

Giddens, Anthony. *The Transformation of Intimacy: Sexuality, Love and Eroticism in Modern Societies*. Cambridge: Polity, 1992. Print.

Giorgi, Gabriel, and Karen Pinkus. "Zones of Exception: Biopolitical Territories in the Neoliberal Era." *Diacritics* 36.2 (Summer 2006): 99-108. Print.

Habermas, Jürgen. *The Future of Human Nature*. Cambridge: Polity, 2003. Print.

---. "Die postnationale Konstellation und die Zukunft der Demokratie." *Die postnationale Konstellation: Politische Essays*. By Habermas. Frankfurt am Main: Suhrkamp, 1998. 91-169. Print.

Hall, Stuart. "Gramsci's Relevance for the Study of Race and Ethnicity." 1986. Rpt. in *Stuart Hall: Critical Dialogues in Cultural Studies*. Ed. David Morley and Kuan-Hsing Chen. London: Routledge, 1996. 411-40. Print.

Hardt, Michael, and Antonio Negri. *Multitude: War and Democracy in the Age of Empire*. New York: Penguin, 2004. Print.

Hasian, Marouf A. "Power, Medical Knowledge, and the Rhetorical Invention of Typhoid Mary.'" *Journal of Medical Humanities* 21.3 (2000): 123-39. Print.

Huntington, Samuel P. *The Clash of Civilizatons and the Remaking of the World Order*. New York: Simon & Schuster, 1996. Print.

Jameson, Fredric. *The Hegel Variations: On the* Phenomenology of Spirit. New York: Verso, 2010. Print.

---. *Postmodernism, or, the Cultural Logic of Late Capitalism*. New York: Verso, 1991. Print.

Kass, Leon R. "Ageless Bodies, Happy Souls: Biotechnology and the Pursuit of Perfection." *The New Atlantis* 1 (2003): 9-28. Print.

Katz, Stephen. *Disciplining Old Age: The Formation of Gerontological Knowledge*. Charlottesville: U of Virginia P, 1996. Print.

Keane, David. "Survival of the Fairest? Evolution and the Geneticization of Human Rights." *Oxford Journal of Legal Studies* 30.3 (2010): 467-94. Print.

Kellner, Douglas. "Habermas, the Public Sphere, and Democracy: A Critical Intervention." Web. 27 August 2011.

Korten, David C. *When Corporations Rule the World*. West Hartford: Kumarian Press; San Francisco: Berrett-Koehler Publishers, 1995. Print.

Kraut, Alan M. *Silent Travelers: Germs, Genes, and the "Immigrant Menace."* Baltimore: Johns Hopkins UP, 1995. Print.

Kunow, Rüdiger. "Old Age and Globalization." *A Guide to Humanistic Studies in Aging: What Does It Mean to Grow Old?* Ed. Thomas R. Cole, Ruth E. Ray, and Robert Kastenbaum. Baltimore: Johns Hopkins UP, 2010. 293-318. Print.

LaHaye, Tim, and Jerry B. Jenkins. *Left Behind: A Novel of the Earth's Last Days*. Wheaton: Tyndale, 1995. Print.

Leavitt, Judith Walzer. "'Typhoid Mary' Strikes Back: Bacteriological Theory and Practice in Early 20th-Century Public Health." *Sickness and Health in America: Readings in the History of Medicine and Public Health*. Ed. Judith Walzer Leavitt and Ronald L. Numbers. Third rev. ed. Madison: U of Wisconsin P, 1997. 555-72. Print.

---. *Typhoid Mary: Captive to the Public's Health*. Boston: Beacon, 1996. Print.

Magnus, George. *The Age of Aging: How Demographics Are Changing the Global Economy and Our World*. Singapore: Wiley, 2009. Print.

McCallum, Cecilia. Review of *Remaking Life and Death: Towards an Anthropology of the Biosciences.* Ed. Sarah Franklin and Margaret Lock. Santa Fe: School of American American Research Press, 2003. *Anthropological Quarterly* 77.1 (2004): 197-202. Print.

Markel, Howard. *When Germs Travel: Six Major Epidemics That Have Invaded America Since 1900 and the Fears They Have Unleashed.* 2004. New York: Vintage, 2005. Print.

Mayer, Ruth. "Virus Discourse: The Rhetoric of Threat and Terrorism in the Biothriller." *Cultural Critique* 66 (2007): 1-20. Print.

Mitchell, W. J. T. *Cloning Terror: The War of Images, 9/11 to the Present.* Chicago: U of Chicago P, 2011. Print.

Novas, Carlos, and Nikolas Rose. "Genetic Risk and the Birth of the Somatic Individual." *Economy and Society* 29.4 (2000): 485-513. Print.

Ong, Aihwa. "An Analytics of Biotechnology and Ethics at Multiple Scales." Introduction. *Asian Biotech: Ethics and Communities of Fate.* Ed. Aihwa Ong and Nancy N. Chen. Durham: Duke UP, 2010. 1-51. Print.

Peterson, Peter G. *Gray Dawn: How the Coming Age Wave Will Transform America and the World.* New York: Random, 1999. Print.

Poe, Edgar Allan. "The Man of the Crowd." *Tales of Mystery and Imagination.* New York: Dutton, 1977. 101-09. Print.

Polivka, Larry. "Postmodern Aging and the Loss of Meaning." *Journal of Aging and Identity* 5.4 (2000): 225-35. Print.

Rose, Nikolas. *The Politics of Life Itself: Biomedicine, Power, and Subjectivity in the Twenty-First Century.* Princeton: Princeton UP, 2007. Print.

Rouvroy, Antoinette. *Human Genes and Neoliberal Governance: A Foucauldian Critique.* New York: Routledge, 2008. Print.

Rowe, John Carlos. "Post-Narionalism, Globalism, and the New American Studies." *Post-Nationalist American Studies.* Ed. John Carlos Rowe. Berkeley: U of California P, 2000. 23-37. Print.

Sarasin, Philipp, Silvia Berger, Marianne Hänseler, and Myriam Spörri. "Bakteriologie und Moderne: Eine Einleitung." *Bakteriologie und Moderne: Studien zur Biopolitik des Unsichtbaren, 1870-1920.* Ed. Sarasin, Berger, Hänseler, and Spörri. Frankfurt am Main: Suhrkamp, 2007. 8-43. Print.

Shilts, Randy. *And the Band Played On: Politics, People, and the AIDS Epidemic.* New York: St. Martin's, 1987. Print.

Slack, Paul. Introduction. *Epidemics and Ideas: Essays on the Historical Perception of Pestilence.* Ed. Terence Ranger and Paul Slack. Cambridge: Cambridge UP, 1992. 1-20. Print.

Tomes, Nancy. "Epidemic Entertainments: Disease and Popular Culture in Early-Twentieth-Century America." *American Literary History* 14.4 (2002): 625-52. Print.

Treichler, Paula A. *How to Have Theory in an Epidemic: Cultural Chronicles of AIDS.* Durham: Duke UP, 1999. Print.

Wald, Priscilla. *Contagious: Cultures, Carriers and the Outbreak Narrative.* Durham: Duke UP, 2008. Print.

World Bank. *Averting the Old Age Crisis.* Oxford: Oxford UP, 1994. Print.

PART IV:

HEALING NARRATIVES

CHRISTINE MARKS

Metaphors We Heal By:
Communicating Pain through
Illness Narratives

> The word enters between us and the pain
> like a pretence of silence.
> It is a silencing. It is a needle
> unpicking the stitch
> between blood and clay.
>
> The word is the first small step
> to freedom
> from oneself.
>
> In case others
> are present.
>
> Miroslav Holub, "Brief Reflection on the
> Word 'Pain'"

Introduction

The experience of pain often occurs as a caesura in the natural rhythm of life—literally a cutting, a hewing off of the self from the world. Pain, as Elaine Scarry has stated, "does not simply resist language but actively destroys it, bringing about an immediate reversion to a state anterior to language" (4). To Scarry, pain emerges as "some deep subterranean fact," "an invisible geography," "as distant as . . . interstellar events . . . of not yet detectable intergalactic screams" (3).

Yet the majority of people in pain feel an increased need to excavate the unspeakable, to share the invisible geography of pain with others, to overcome the unrepresentability intrinsically connected to the trauma of pain. Illness narratives have long served as a means to overcome the isolation of pain and to reach out across the interstellar space separating the person in pain from her environment. Anne Hunsaker Hawkins has demonstrated in *Reconstructing Illness: Studies in Pathography* that illness narratives are an attempt to reestablish a balanced sense of self through the creation of "necessary fictions out of the building blocks of metaphor, image, archetype, and myth" (18). Anatole Broyard, a *New York Times* literary critic who died of prostate cancer in 1990, wrote in his posthumously published collection of essays *Intoxicated by My Illness* that "the sick man sees everything as metaphor" (7). He suggested that metaphors may assume a particularly powerful presence in the life of an ill person. Metaphors, according to Broyard, "may be as necessary to illness as they are to literature, as comforting to the patient as his own bathrobe and slippers" (18).

While metaphors may assist in a reinscription of the body into a collective "interworld" (Merleau-Ponty 415), where "my body and the other's are one whole, two sides of one and the same phenomenon" (Merleau-Ponty 412) and where the "metaphors we live by" (Lakoff and Johnson) connect us in an intersubjective embodied realism that forms a common ground of communication, both the metaphorization of illness and the use of illness as metaphor have been and continue to be contested and divisive practices. In his *Time* magazine column of 29 December 2010, for instance, the political journalist Joe Klein compared the news on cable television to an epileptic seizure, using the disorder to convey a sense of the news' often incomprehensible jumble of sound bites, flashy images, and fragmented bits of information. In a letter to the editor, an indignant reader afterwards complained that Klein's insensitive choice of employing epilepsy as a means of giving expression to the shrillness of cable news would further heighten the stigmatization of a disorder already complicated by misunderstanding and fear.[1] In a recent contribution to the *New York Times*, writer and

---

[1]   In a critique of Lauren Slater's use of epilepsy as metaphor in *Lying: A Metaphorical Memoir* (2000), G. Thomas Couser strictly rejects Slater's

former *New Yorker* editor Daniel Menaker carefully weighs the advantages and disadvantages of a militarization of language representing cancer. While he admits the possible negative impacts of such metaphorization of cancer, he also emphasizes that "[i]t can help us feel less frightened and more composed when facing surgery. It can strengthen our resolve to stay in the best shape possible and to deal with pain when it comes" ("Cancer: Fighting Words").

These two recent examples illustrate that the cautionary tale against linking illness and metaphor as told by Susan Sontag in her seminal text *Illness as Metaphor* continues to reverberate in American society today. Sontag warned against the use of illness, in particular tuberculosis, cancer, and, in a later essay, AIDS, as metaphor, and insisted that "the most truthful way of regarding illness—and the healthiest way of being ill—is one most purified of, most resistant to, metaphoric thinking" (3). Sontag conglomerates a wealth of evidence against the use of metaphor, demonstrating, for example, the stylization of tuberculosis as the ideal romantic disease, in which the patient is consumed by his or her passions, the demonization of cancer as an insidious killer that both patients and doctors must wage war against, and the damaging equation of AIDS with pollution or the plague. While the irresponsible attachment of either glorifying or degrading images and concepts to illness can cause great damage to ill people's identities, in many cases metaphors may also serve as a source of imaginative power that can help overcome the isolation of the ill self. Indeed, Sontag herself qualified her categorical rejection of associating illness and metaphor in her essay "AIDS and Its Metaphors," granting that "one cannot think without metaphors," which, however, "does not mean there aren't some metaphors we might well abstain from or try to retire" (93). Lisa Diedrich contends in *Treatments: Language, Politics, and the Culture of Illness* that both Sontag's "de-metaphorizing idea and metaphorical language . . . might be useful to the person who is ill, and both have been crucial in transforming the way illness is spoken" (29). Patients, as Diedrich underlines, may "use metaphors to empower them to challenge the

---

exploitation of "familiarizing metaphors [to] domesticate alien or abstract entities" (125), as "her choice of a disability as a metaphor for her experience involves her in a misrepresentation of those who have this condition" (112).

conventional medical narratives of illness that emphasize the patient's passivity" (30). And, indeed, there appears to be an element of empowerment and a possibility of reconnecting with the world in the use of metaphor. On the other hand, metaphoric representation may never completely close the gap between the ill self and the world. Kathlyn Conway, in her *Illness and the Limits of Expression*, endorses the notion that "for those who are ill or disabled, writing frustrates as much as it heals" as it "allow[s] us to face the limits of the self and its expression in language" (3). Conway rejects the possibility of transcending the body through linguistic expression and criticizes the "triumph narrative" (7) that follows a rather foreseeable plot structure starting out with illness and chaos and ending with either a cure or a newfound spiritual superiority that establishes the mind as master over the body. As Conway reminds her readers, the representation of illness and pain doubtless has both its limits and dangers; yet, as I will demonstrate below, metaphor is situated at the "stitch / between blood and clay" (Holub 4-5), body and mind, and is therefore the "first small step / to freedom / from oneself" (Holub 6-8), a step toward the other.

Embodiment and Representation: Metaphors of Pain

The extensive presence of metaphors in everyday thinking has been established by George Lakoff and Mark Johnson in their text *Metaphors We Live By*, in which they claim that "metaphor is pervasive in everyday life, not just in language but in thought and action" and that "[o]ur ordinary conceptual system . . . is fundamentally metaphoric in nature" (3). They support this thesis with substantial evidence from everyday language, disclosing metaphor as a basic component of all human thought processes. In their categorization of various types of metaphors, they list, among others, conceptual metaphors (e.g., "argument is war" or "time is money"), orientational metaphors (e.g., "happy is up, sad is down" or "conscious is up, unconscious is down"), and ontological metaphors, which view nonphysical things as entities (e.g., "the mind is a machine," "I'm a little rusty today," or "My mind isn't operating today"), as well as personification as a special kind of ontological metaphor (e.g., "Inflation is backing us into a corner") and metonymy (e.g., "He likes to read the Marquis de Sade," or "He's in dance") (14-

40). Their examples of orientational metaphors, significantly, also include metaphors of health and illness that situate health on top and illness at the bottom: "He's at the peak of health. . . . He's in top shape. As to his health, he's way up there. He fell ill. . . . He came down with the flu. His health is declining" (*Metaphors* 15). Metaphors shape our understanding of the world, and they are practically never neutral or value-free. The association of illness with a decline or fall from the uplifted stage of health exemplifies the value systems conjoined to the metaphorical systems we live by.[2]

In *Philosophy in the Flesh*, Lakoff and Johnson develop their interpretation of metaphoric conceptual systems into a philosophy of embodied realism by emphasizing that "[b]ecause our conceptual systems grow out of our bodies, meaning is grounded in and through our bodies" (6), and that "our common embodiment allows for common, stable truths" (6). Our embodied perception of the world thus creates a space of shared intersubjectivity that forms the basis of mutual understanding and communication. This idea certainly shows an affinity to French philosopher Maurice Merleau-Ponty's reflections on self, body, and the "interworld" in his *Phenomenology of Perception.* Merleau-Ponty here underlines the role the body plays in shaping our intentionality: "Bodily existence," he writes, "establishes our first consonance with the world" (192). At the heart of Merleau-Ponty's philosophical enterprise lies an ontology of embodied connectedness— to exist inevitably means to be engaged in the world, and the self has no way of separating its consciousness from this lived engagement. It is always enmeshed in the very substance it may strive to appropriate: "The world is not what I think, but what I live through. I am open to the world, I have no doubt that I am in communication with it, but I do not possess it; it is inexhaustible" (Merleau-Ponty xviii-xix). To live is to be in relation with the other, and to be part of the world requires a willingness to share and respect the other's space in it: "I enter into a pact with the other, having resolved to live in an interworld in which I accord as much place to others as to myself" (Merleau-Ponty 415).

---

[2]   As I will explore below, Lynne Greenberg's memoir *The Body Broken* revolves around the association of her neck fracture with a fall into an abyss, which she contextualizes with various myths elucidating the idea of a fall.

What, then, happens to this pact between self and other, to the common ground of understanding formed by our being in the world and the metaphoric systems evolving out of our embodied presence, when illness and pain cause a rupture in the mutuality and connectedness envisioned by Merleau-Ponty and Lakoff and Johnson? Physical pain isolates, since the person in pain feels it alone and nobody else perceives the experience of this pain like he or she does. Can metaphors in this case still serve as an expression of shared corporeal experience or do they misrepresent the true experience of pain? Can metaphors provide a passageway for the other to share an understanding of the pain of the self and generate a genuine mediation of pain? Before presenting some examples of such narratives at the limit of the self, I would like to rethink the connection between metaphor and illness, and in particular between metaphor and pain, by drawing on Scarry's ideas about pain and the imagination, in order to consider metaphor anew as a potential bridge between someone in pain and the person receiving the metaphorical expression of such pain. My aim is certainly not an unconditional rehabilitation of the use of metaphor but rather a reconceptualization of the use of metaphor in communicating pain. The idea is not to theorize the use of pain *as* metaphor, as in Sontag's example of cancer, or the above-noted use of epilepsy, but to create a theoretical framework for the potential of metaphor to overcome the incommunicability of pain and to transgress the boundary between, in Susan Sontag's—ironically metaphoric—expression: "the kingdom of the well . . . the kingdom of the sick" (3).

Elaine Scarry's groundbreaking work *The Body in Pain* investigates the seemingly insurmountable barrier between pain and language. "Physical pain," according to Scarry, "has no voice" (3) and "does not simply resist language but actively destroys it, bringing about an immediate reversion to a state anterior to language" (4). Not only does pain resist language, it also brings about an "absolute split" (4) between self and other. Scarry's basic argument about the inexpressibility of pain has been quoted rather excessively, so that is has become an established tenet in academic theorizing of the body and language. Yet what has been mostly neglected is that Scarry's investigation of the separation and isolation of the body in pain is indeed filled with concessions to the human need for linguistic expression and even admissions of the potential success of certain endeavors to express pain.

We do not have direct access to the other's inner states unless these states are translated into facial expressions, body language, or linguistic representation.[3] Representing pain through language is, at best, complicated, and frequently words fail to give shape to the ungraspable. Scarry, after making the bold claim that pain has no voice, qualifies her remark by suggesting that "when ... [pain] at last finds a voice, it begins to tell a story" (3). She also emphasizes the importance of language in establishing a connection between the self and its environment, to counteract the isolation caused by pain: "[S]o long as one is speaking," Scarry remarks, "the self extends out beyond the boundaries of the body, occupies a space much larger than the body" (33). Language has the capability to bridge the gap between self and other and extend the self's identity beyond the body, possibly transgressing the boundaries of pain. Metaphor may serve as a medium of extension and connection between the self in pain and the recipient other.

Referring to the "McGill Pain Questionnaire" by Ronald Melzack and W.S. Torgerson (1971), for example, Scarry concedes that "through the mediating structures of this diagnostic questionnaire, language ... has begun to become capable of providing an external image of interior events" (Scarry 8). This external image is, as we can see in the questionnaire, metaphoric in nature. The pain is flickering and quivering like a flame; it beats and pounds like a hammer; it stabs and cuts like a knife; it bores, it drills, it pinches (cf. Scarry 7-8). In order to translate the intangible presence of pain into comprehensible terms, we must resort to metaphor. Scarry holds that there are only two major groups of metaphors that communicate pain. The first, according to Scarry, "specifies an external agent of the pain, a weapon that is pictured as

---

[3] Mirror neuron theory, although disputed, is fascinating in its suggestion that our bodies seem to be immediately related to the bodies of others through neuronal mirroring processes. In tests with macaque monkeys, researchers noted that the monkeys activated the same neurons in their brains when watching a specific action as when they personally performed that same action. The same mirror neuron system was then also exhibited in the human brain. This has led to a range of speculations regarding human beings' capacity for empathy. For more information regarding mirror neuron theory and communication, cf. Rizzolatti and Arbib or Rizzolatti and Sinigaglia.

producing the pain; and the second specifies bodily damage that is pictured as accompanying the pain" (15). To illustrate the former, Scarry gives the example of comparing pain to a hammer coming down on one's spine (one can also consider some of the examples given in the McGill questionnaire), and, for the second group of metaphors: "'It feels as if my arm is broken at each joint and the jagged ends are sticking through the skin'" (15). Although Scarry criticizes that "[p]hysical pain is not identical with (and often exists without) either agency or damage" (15) and sees a danger in the "conflation of pain with power" caused by "the particular perceptual confusion sponsored by the language of agency" (18), this use of metaphor nevertheless succeeds in bringing the inner pain outward by drawing it toward "the external boundary of the body" (15-16). Scarry acknowledges that "it begins to externalize, objectify, and make sharable what is originally an interior and unsharable experience" (16).

This movement toward an objectification of pain, then, becomes central to Scarry's opposition of pain and the imagination. While pain, unlike other sensations like hunger or desire, is always objectless, the imagination always needs an object. As Scarry explains, pain is "an intentional state without an intentional object, [while] imagining is an intentional object without an experienceable intentional state" (Scarry 164). It is essential, then, that Scarry links pain and the imagination by underlining that an intentional state by definition needs to be directed toward an object, so that, in order to be defined as an intentional state, pain must already be linked to the imagination. Scarry states, "in isolation, pain 'intends' nothing; it is wholly passive; it is 'suffered' rather than willed or directed. . . . [P]ain only becomes an intentional state once it is brought into relation with the objectifying power of the imagination" (Scarry 164).

This relation between pain and the imagination is established through metaphoric expression. Scarry gives several examples in which the imagination steps in to create an object in the attempt to eliminate an objectless state. For example, if a person experiences hunger but does not have any access to food, the imagination may conjure up berries or grain or anything edible, a referential content to a formerly objectless state. I want to argue, then, that the imagination creates metaphors in order to provide referential content for the objectless state of pain. In such cases, the object, as Scarry points out, "comes into existence specifically to *eliminate* the condition" (167). While the imagined bottle of Gatorade won't quench our thirst, and the metaphor of pain will of course not eliminate the pain, the intentional movement toward an object does eliminate the objectless state of these conditions and deliver the self from its emptied, aimless, negative state to a directed and positive movement toward an object and, therefore, into the world.

Metaphors in Illness Narratives

How then do writers of illness narratives employ metaphors in their attempts to communicate pain, to "make sharable what is originally an interior and unsharable experience" (Scarry 16)?[4] Audre Lorde's *The Cancer Journals* (originally published in 1980) offers an excellent illustration of the power of language to carry the individual in pain beyond isolation, into a collective sphere of understanding and agency. Lorde highlights the importance of expression and communication in her introduction to the *Cancer Journals*: "I am a post-mastectomy woman who believes our feelings need voice in order to be recognized, respected, and of use" (7), to strive against "yet another silence" (7) caused by "anger and pain and fear about cancer" (7). Lorde uses strong metaphoric imagery to convey her physical pain and the accompanying emotions of despair. She writes:

> [P]ain fills me like a puspocket and every touch threatens to breach the taut membrane that keeps it from flowing through and poisoning my whole existence. Sometimes despair sweeps across my consciousness like luna winds across a barren moonscape. Ironshod horses rage back and forth over every nerve. (9)

While this vivid metaphoric description may not give the reader an exact impression of the nature of the pain Lorde experiences, the metaphors and similes she uses connect her inner experience to an intersubjective

---

4   In researching metaphoric expressions in illness narratives, I have limited my
    scope to examples of American memoirs. This study has no claims to any
    kind of universality, as the experience of pain and its translation into words
    are, of course, embedded in the self's cultural and linguistic environment.

sphere of commonly perceived symbols and images. Lorde turns her pain into an intentional state by connecting it to concrete objects and entities through her power of imagination. Lorde furthermore makes extensive use of just such metaphors of war that are rejected by Susan Sontag and her followers: The thought of cancer "keeps [Lorde] armed" (12), and she refers to "the war we are all waging with the forces of death" (19) and to herself as "not only a casualty, [but] also a warrior" (19). Lorde engages the war metaphor as a source of agency rather than oppression. Lorde's cancer experience strengthens her links with the community instead of weakening it; she loses her fear of speaking up for black women's rights and feels the responsibility to respond to others' voices and to make herself heard, to break the silence. This emphasis on the need for interaction and community is promoted and assisted by Lorde's use of metaphor as a connecting element between the individual in pain and the community at large.

In *The Camera My Mother Gave Me* (2001), a memoir about her vulvar vestibulitis, Susanna Kaysen also employs metaphors to give a sharable expression to the pain within. Her use of metaphors to describe the searing pain in her vagina has an almost physical effect on the reader: "Some days my vagina felt as if somebody had put a cheese grater in it and scraped. Some days it felt as if someone had poured ammonia inside it. Some days it felt as if a little dentist was drilling a little hole in it" (3). While Kathlyn Conway interprets this passage as an example of the failure of metaphor (80), I think it actually demonstrates that metaphor indeed can help to express the experience of pain. Of course it cannot reproduce it, but the distinct sensations of scraping and drilling evoke a feeling of unease inside the reader that at least echoes Kaysen's sensation. Through the evocation of an external agent of pain, the metaphors Kaysen employs allow the reader to approach her pain. Metaphor creates a link between the internal and the external; it adds tension and directedness to a state that was previously closed off in a wordless space inside.

In her memoir *All in My Head: An Epic Quest to Cure an Unrelenting, Totally Unreasonable, and Only Slightly Enlightening Headache* (2005), Paula Kamen appears to be torn between a rejection of metaphor and a desire to make her readers perceive her otherwise invisible pain through her use of metaphor. She is highly aware of the negative implications of reading illness as metaphor, since a metaphoric interpretation of pain as a message of the body, communicating some hidden psychological fact, can lead to detrimental conclusions about the ill self's personality. Kamen vehemently argues against reading illness as metaphor of any kind. She recounts how members of her fiction-writing group react to the headaches she described in an autobiographical story she shares with them (69) by suggesting various symbolic interpretations—and adds that this is a widespread cultural practice. However, the New Age idea that "[b]asically, the body is one large decoder ring [and that] [g]etting well is a matter of being able to read the body's message about its spiritual and emotional crises" (Kamen 134) bears the danger of placing the blame of illness on a psychological crisis, which would imply that the ill person has the agency to fix herself and just might not be trying hard enough. As Kamen expresses it, "I felt guilty that I had brought this on myself, and when I had pain, I felt that I wasn't working hard enough to change my attitudes" (133).

However, this rejection of a metaphorical exegesis of the body in pain does not imply a dismissal of metaphor as a means of describing her headaches. Kamen envisions her pain by imagining it as being caused by an external agent (cf. Scarry), "a clamp pinching the nerve at various levels of tightness or a dagger piercing through the eye or temple" (7), "a fishhook, pulling backward on the nerves behind the eye, with varying intensities through the day" (7), or "a huge nail [that] had been pounded into my left eye and stuck through the bottom of the bed, pinning me firmly in place" (49). These metaphors give shape to the invisible pain in Kamen's head and make it communicable to others. While most likely none of her readers have had the experience of having their eye pounded by a nail, the intensity of the image is effective because of probable physical memories of pinching, piercing, or pounding and the violent connotations of a nail, a dagger, or a fishhook.

In her memoir *The Body Broken* (2009), Lynne Greenberg, an English professor at Hunter College in New York City, describes the obstacles she encounters in her struggle to give expression to an onset of extreme pain she experiences about twenty years after a car accident during which she had broken her neck. As the doctors soon discover, her neck is in fact still broken. In her description of the aftermath of the original accident, Greenberg writes, "I learned the many faces of pain, his different guises, sensations, and methods, and how clever he is at shape shifting" (xii). This shape-shifting quality of pain, its many incarnations, make it difficult to pin down, to circumscribe, or control through a fixed linguistic representation. Greenberg's first attempts to create an "art of pain"—a term she borrows from contemporary American poet Linda Pastan (Greenberg 37)—fail miserably, as she ends up writing half-finished poems and rather flat if somewhat amusing puns like "[m]y bone had refused to re-fuse. I was unnerved, so please unnerve me, doctor; my nerve pain was too nerve-wracking, too enervating; my nerves had some nerve—frankly they were a pain in the neck" (37). The repeated failure of poetry to express her inner states initially leaves Greenberg in a state of frustration:

> Poetic forms, the very architecture of my professional life, seemed to be crumbling all around me. Pain, I realized, does not fit into the tamed heartbeat of iambic pentameter. It pummels through borders. Unremitting, it refuses closure and explodes rhyme and reason. All-consuming, it does not permit the luxury of metaphoric or chiasmic thinking, tropes or symbols, wit or pun. Its sound is unsound, dysphony, a wail, silence. My "art of pain" was an artless descent into chaos, an all-too-perfect emblem for my life. There were no poetic words for this pain, just my racked body to signify it. (38)

Greenberg, though disillusioned by the insufficiency of a form of linguistic expression that has long been at the center of both her professional and personal life, recognizes the importance of finding the right vocabulary to describe the nature of her pain, to create a narrative to pass on to her doctors. In an example of what she calls "carefully crafted, nearly scientific narratives," she does indeed resort to both metaphor and similes in order to facilitate a correct diagnosis:

> Its sinews unfurling, the pain whips through the middle of my head. It feels like an ice-cream headache—the sharp deep freeze of eating or drinking too much of a cold substance too quickly. It is heavier than an ice-cream headache, though; it feels as if an enormous weight lies along the tendon, crushing this central route, tearing my head in half. When spiking, the pain radiates out from the center and disperses. The ice cream has melted, not just freezing my forehead but dripping down to encompass my entire head symmetrically, pooling finally behind my eyes. (43)

This evocative and sensual portrayal of pain in its various stages—from sinewy, crushing, and tearing monster to a melting, dripping and pooling mass—illustrates the many facets of pain and helps to differentiate and approximate them—it makes visible the subterranean and invisible geography (Scarry) of pain. If, as Greenberg stresses, "pain is by its nature isolating," as "the mind finds itself trapped, incarcerated in the carcass of a once-functional body" (66), the above passage highlights once again that metaphor can help reduce the distance between the person in pain and others; it can at the very least evoke images and sensations that bring others closer to an understanding of the invisible pain of the patient.

What Greenberg attempts in her memoir is both a metaphorical representation of the pain itself and a contextualization of her experience of pain in various mythological literary frames. Each chapter is preceded by an epigraph of poetry, and one of the leading metaphors of her narration is the concept of a fall or descent—her own fall out of the car into a cornfield, which caused her neck fracture; the fall from grace as described by John Milton in *Paradise Lost*; Icarus' fall; Newton's falling apple (6, 21); and later, Persephone's descent to the underworld (40). As Greenberg notes, she had "always turned to literature as a lens through which to understand and interpret my life and to find the words to describe what has seemed ineffable in it. Now I relied on this familiar support, finding a literary analogue that put my situation into a new perspective" (40). Moreover, Greenberg draws a direct comparison between literary criticism and medical diagnosis. She soon revises her initial belief that, "unlike literary criticism, medicine did not have to contend with metaphors with multivalent interpretations and associations" (19), realizing that "medicine, contrary to what I had previously thought, is not a science of black-and-white facts but rather an art, capable of endless possibilities and as open ended as literary interpretation" (23). Her father-in-law even goes as far as advising Greenberg to treat her injury as she would a research paper (28-29).

One of the key concerns of Greenberg's memoir is the connectedness of mind and body. Pain penetrating and infiltrating the body causes, as Greenberg illustrates, her "mind to become a desert" (36). Mind and body, in Greenberg's view, become violently disconnected by intense pain, "as the desires and agency of the mind conflict fundamentally with the inability of the body" (51). In a chapter called "The Loss of

Language," Greenberg thematizes the seemingly inevitable erosion of the mind as a result of her fractured body. The constant pain as well as the regimen of pain medications with their manifold side effects make it at times impossible for her to formulate clear thoughts: "[A]ll logic seemed to have fled and language to have abandoned me" (46). To Greenberg, as to many other authors of illness narratives, "[t]he act of creation competes in a deadly struggle with pain. To create is to dislodge pain from the center, to prioritize and privilege the mind over the body" (Greenberg 194). Greenberg envisions this struggle metaphorically as a quest to tame a wild animal, thinking of herself as "a lion tamer, wielding a whip, trying to wrestle pain into control before it whips me" (198). Throughout her memoir, Greenberg brings to the surface a deep anguish and a desire to visualize the inexplicable sensations within and objectify them rather than being swallowed up by the pain. Even if inevitably imperfect, the use of metaphors to identify the unspeakable moves the subject out of its isolated, speechless state and allows for a degree of participation that reconfirms the pact between self and other.

Conclusion

Pain, to use Friedrich Wilhelm Nietzsche's words, can never be "laid out as if in an illuminated glass case," since nature has locked the door to "the coils of the intestines, the quick current of the blood stream, and the involved tremors of the fibers" and "threw away the key" (44). While in some of the texts presented here, the authors show their frustration with the inadequacy of words and the shortcomings of language in framing pain and illness, they nevertheless all exhibit the urgency of struggling against the odds. As Lara Birk writes in "The Listening Room," a personal account of the extreme pain she experiences due to acute compartment syndrome in her leg, the "sudden onset of unfathomable pain" transported her into "a world no sentences could ever wrap their words around no matter how I cast or stretched them" (35). "Pain," she concludes, "cannot be told. Yet, in isolation, it grows. It longs to be wrapped in words" (38).

In her *Autobiography of a Face* (1994), Lucy Grealy notes the diverging movements of body and mind out of which the need to create linguistic representation emerges: "While our bodies move ever forward on the time line, our minds continuously trace backward, seeking shape and meaning as deftly as any arrow seeking its mark" (27). The longing to arrest the chaotic flow of events, to capture the uncontrollable through a retrospective fastening of the body in text, is a desire shared by many people whose lives have been thrown out of balance by illness and pain. Weaving the incoherent physical experience of pain into a coherent narrative may help the ill self regain a sense of wholeness and identity. Paul Guest, an American poet and memoirist who has been a quadriplegic since a bike accident at age twelve, underlines the urgency of hanging on to the world through words: "I couldn't escape the notion that I was alone, in a broken body, stuck in the places between that body and everyone else, and that maybe each word and every line and all the poems I wrote were a tether, a rope by which I could hang on to the world, and not be left behind entirely, which I feared more than anything" (125-26).

Metaphors of pain may never quite reach the center of the inner state they aim to express, may never perfectly fit the shape of pain, but they carry in them an externalized idea of the inner sensation, thus forming a rope by which the ill person may pull herself out of the clutching, muting grip of a "malevolent aggressor, a ruthless torturer, an imprisoning enemy" (Lascaratou 7), and back into the world. Language, as Merleau-Ponty elucidates, has the power "of bringing the thing expressed into existence, of opening up to thought new ways, new dimensions, and new landscapes" (467). Metaphors, though unable to give direct expression to pain, can thus open up new ways, new dimensions, and new landscapes in which we may never actually come into direct contact with the referent, but may feel its presence with a new force. The effect of metaphor can be both destructive and constructive, but its potential for linking pain to an expressible object makes it a powerful medium of communication.

Works Cited

Birk, Lara. "The Listening Room." *Stories of Illness and Healing: Women Write Their Bodies*. Ed. Sayantani DasGupta and Marsha Hurst. Kent: Kent State UP, 2007. 35-38. Print.

Broyard, Anatole. *Intoxicated by My Illness: And Other Writings on Life and Death*. Comp. and ed. Alexandra Broyard. New York: Fawcett, 1992. Print.

Conway, Kathlyn. *Illness and the Limits of Expression*. Ann Arbor: U of Michigan P, 2007. Print.

Couser, G. Thomas. *Signifying Bodies: Disability in Contemporary Life Writing*. Ann Arbor: U of Michigan P, 2009. Print.

Diedrich, Lisa. *Treatments: Language, Politics, and the Culture of Illness*. Minneapolis: U of Minnesota P, 2007. Print.

Grealy, Lucy. *Autobiography of a Face*. 1994. New York: Harper, 2003. Print.

Greenberg, Lynne. *The Body Broken: A Memoir*. New York: Random, 2009. Print.

Guest, Paul. *One More Theory about Happiness: A Memoir*. New York: Harper, 2010. Print.

Hawkins, Anne Hunsaker. *Reconstructing Illness: Studies in Pathography*. West Lafayette: Purdue UP, 1993. Print.

Holub, Miroslav. "Brief Reflection on the Word 'Pain.'" Trans. Ewald Osers. *Intensive Care: Selected and New Poems*. By Holub. Oberlin: Oberlin College P, 1996. 157. Print.

Kamen, Paula. *All in My Head: An Epic Quest to Cure an Unrelenting, Totally Unreasonable, and Only Slightly Enlightening Headache. A Memoir*. Cambridge: Da Capo, 2005. Print.

Kaysen, Susanna. *The Camera My Mother Gave Me*. New York: Knopf, 2001. Print.

Klein, Joe. "Media Noise: The Year of Living Predictably." *Time Magazine*. Time Magazine, 29 Dec. 2010. Web. 10 Jan. 2011.

Lakoff, George, and Mark Johnson. *Metaphors We Live By*. Chicago: U of Chicago P, 1980. Print.

---. *Philosophy in the Flesh: The Embodied Mind and Its Challenge to Western Thought*. New York: Basic, 1999. Print.

Lascaratou, Chryssoula. *The Language of Pain: Expression or Description?* 9th ed. Amsterdam: John Benjamins, 2007. Print.

Lorde, Audre. *The Cancer Journals: Special Edition.* 1980. San Francisco: Aunt Lute, 1997. Print.

Menaker, Daniel. "Cancer: Fighting Words." Opinion. *New York Times Sunday Review* 27 Aug. 2011. Web. 28 Aug. 2011.

Merleau-Ponty, Maurice. *Phenomenology of Perception.* Trans. Colin Smith. London: Routledge, 2002. Trans. of *Phénoménologie de la perception.* Paris: Gallimard, 1945. Print.

Nietzsche, Friedrich Wilhelm. "On Truth and Lie in an Extra-Moral Sense." *The Portable Nietzsche.* Ed. and trans. Walter Kaufmann. New York: Penguin, 1976. 42-46. Print.

Rizzolatti, Giacomo, and Michael A. Arbib. "Language within Our Grasp." *Trends in Neurosciences* 21.5 (1998): 188-94. Print.

Rizzolatti, Giacomo, and Corrado Sinigaglia. *Mirrors in the Brain: How Our Minds Share Actions and Emotions.* 2006. Trans. Frances Anderson. Oxford: Oxford UP, 2008. Print.

Scarry, Elaine. *The Body in Pain: The Making and Unmaking of the World.* Oxford: Oxford UP, 1985. Print.

Slauter, Lauren. *Lying: A Metaphorical Memoir.* New York: Random House, 2000. Print.

Sontag, Susan. *Illness as Metaphor and AIDS and Its Metaphors.* New York: Picador, 1990. Print.

Anca-Raluca Radu

Coming to Terms: Narrating Loss in John Banville's *The Sea* and Richard B. Wright's *October*

Introduction

John Banville's novel *The Sea* (2005) won the Man Booker Prize in 2005 and was hailed by critics as a harbinger of the return of quality or "high" literature in the Booker canon. The novel against which its brilliance was measured in an article dedicated to Man Booker Prize winners is *Life of Pi*, by Canadian novelist Yann Martel (2002).[1] Its literary counterpart in this particular reading is another Canadian novel, *October* (2007) by Richard B. Wright, whereby the terms of comparison will not be the much debated literary "value" or merits of the novels, for which, in Foucauldian terms,[2] the names of the two novelists stand, but the rhetoric of narrative mediation and its ethics.

Whereas much of the literature concerning the intersection between literary text and medical discourse concentrates on the doctor-patient relationship or the autobiographical patient account, by bringing into the spotlight Banville's and Wright's fictions this essay shifts the focus to the witness of the disease, i.e., the bereaved relative of a patient affected by cancer. *The Sea* and *October* are strikingly similar, both in content and form. Both narratives are told from the perspective of the first-

---

[1] Squires praises the aesthetic qualities of *The Sea* that, in her eyes, earn it the distinction of high literature as opposed to what she sees as the commercial impetus and the broad audience appeal that motivated the Man Booker jury to award its prize to *Life of Pi* in 2002.

[2] Cf. Foucault, "What Is an Author?" (1967).

person narrator-protagonists, Max and James respectively, and follow a time scheme which interpolates present and past events. Both narrators are retired academics confronted with a tragic loss in the present that leads them to reminisce about another traumatic loss in the past. Conflations of present and past induce them to ask themselves questions about their own responsibility in the course of events. At the same time, they struggle with the powerlessness of words to express their woe and their remorse, and with an identity quest that seems to hinge on the resolution of past problems. Their confrontation with a terminal disease functions as a catalyst for their memories, making them conscious of their transience, insecurity, faults, and missed responsibilities and chances to make amends.

In *The Sea*, Max Morden has just lost his wife, Anna, to cancer, which occasions his return to the site of one summer holiday in his childhood. Here, his life was fatefully connected with that of the Graces, a well-to-do family spending their summer on the Irish coast in the village of Ballyless. The glamorous Graces fascinate young Max, who is erotically inspired by the mother, and romantically attracted to their cruel daughter, Chloe. Mistaking the infatuation of the governess, Rose, with the mother for an affair with the father, Max likely drives Chloe and her twin brother Myles to kill themselves by drowning in the sea. Now an art historian in his 60s working on a biography of Bonnard, Max conflates his wife's demise with Chloe's death fifty years earlier, trying to come to terms with his trauma (esp. 237-44).

Similarly, James Hillyer, the Canadian protagonist of *October*, loses both his wife and daughter to breast cancer. On what will turn out to be his last trip to England to visit his daughter, James meets Gabriel Fontaine, whom he knew for a short time of eight weeks during his holidays in Quebec as a teenager. The 16-year-old Gabriel, a rich American tourist with a "genuine gift for cruelty" (33), is confined to a wheelchair as a consequence of polio and fashions himself as an insufferable dandy. Now in his late 70s, Gabriel has pancreatic cancer and is on his way to Switzerland, where he commits assisted suicide, attended by James. The figures from the past haunting James's imagination are Gabriel and Odette Huard, a French Canadian chambermaid, with whom both boys were in love. At the same time, the teenage James suffers from a total estrangement from his parents, due to his father's emotional coldness and his mother's enforced isolation after a nervous breakdown.

Both James and Max seek refuge from the present tragedies in their past, but all promises of comfort are deceptive. Max confesses that he looks to the past "for shelter, for comfort, . . . for cosiness" (*Sea* 60), but ironically cannot find any alleviation in it, as the unearthing of his memories of the summer spent with the Graces only troubles his conscience even more. Both protagonists admit that they do not really like the seaside and both like the month of October despite the tragedies that it entails in their personal histories, i.e., the illness of both Max's wife and James's daughter is connected with that month. The sea is treacherously calm when it swallows Chloe and her twin brother Myles; and it is potentially pregnant with enemy submarines in the summer of 1944 around D-Day off the coast of Quebec, where James uses his binoculars to spot the boats. Basically, by returning to the past, James and Max wish to impose order on the chaos of death and disease, only to discover the futility of their endeavor, as James admits: "What must first strike you in such circumstances is the terrible unfairness of it all. But unfairness in what sense? The concept of fairness or unfairness in life implies order and meaning" (*October* 68).[3]

Both Max and James communicate the events and their feelings to a narratee with whom the narrative audience is invited to identify itself. The most conspicuous feature of this process of communication is its ironic self-referentiality. Basically, Max and James communicate to their audiences the fact that words are inept vehicles for the expression of their feelings. They seem to stand in the way of communication instead of facilitating it or, better said, enacting it.

Most significantly, in both texts, the goal of the protagonists' narrative efforts is one of self-discovery; more specifically, of finding out for themselves where exactly they are located in their own narratives of loss. Max and James are, in the first instance, merely witnesses to the progress and final outcome of the disease featured in the novels and as

---

[3] Rimmon-Kenan debates the need to rethink narrative theory not as a method of imposing order on the story, but as a narratology of chaos, a view championed by critics who hold that illness narratives are frustrated by the inability to express the unspeakable happening in the disintegrating body (esp. 243-44).

such invisible in the text of the illness. Their first-person accounts, on the other hand, place them at the center of a text whose main actors, the patients, retreat into the background.[4] In this way, the issue of visibility that preoccupies literary medical accounts and their critical readings takes a new turn, bringing into focus an affected party whose suffering is not physical, but solely emotional and psychological. As a consequence, Max's and James's participation in the text of illness can be labeled "witness involvement" while their role in the narrative is that of ethically located narrators. An appropriate description of their ethical location in the text could be "responsible narration," which situates them in relation to several audiences of the text, the text itself, and the patient-characters about whom they speak.[5]

The terms "witness involvement" and "responsible narration" are part of an attempt to reconfigure classical narratological terminology by highlighting the ethical dimension and rhetorical constituent of story-telling. Instead of asking so-called "moral" questions of old-fashioned pedagogical pedantry, such as whether it is "fair" or "moral" for the narrators to represent the cancer illnesses of their family members as sparking their self-discovering excursions into the past, it is more

---

[4] The issue of visibility or the lack thereof would generate an interesting reading of the novels that exceeds the scope of the present rhetorical analysis. James's daughter, Susan, comments on the insidious invisibility of the cancer stealthily and steadily at work inside her body: "'This thing,' she whispered, 'can go right into my lungs or bones. Maybe my brain. Isn't that an unpleasant thought?'" (*October* 15). Max's wife, Anna, looks pregnant on account of her tumour. In hospital Anna takes pictures of the other cancer patients but their relatives complain and, against the patients' own will, she is ordered to stop. Even more, Susan's comments on what she calls the "genre" of cancer narratives reveals a cynical frustration with the lack of visibility of incurable patients like her and her mother. Susan reads "'cancer memoirs'": "'It must be a new genre. . . . The bookstores have entire shelves devoted to them. They're in with the self-help and yoga stuff. . . . in every book I've read, the cancer was detected early and cleared up. . . . I don't imagine publishers are all that interested in stories about women whose cancer may be too far gone to respond to treatment'" (*October* 13).

[5] The distinction of several levels of responsibility relies on Phelan's explication of four "ethical locations" in Phelan, *Living* 23, and "Rhetorical" 632-33.

appropriate to regard Max and James as ethically located subjects raising and trying to respond to ethical dilemmas. It is indeed present tragedy that awakens their sensitivity to the existence and needs of the "Other" and gives them succour for overcoming their inner conflicts related to the past. Following Craig A. Irvine's analysis of Levinas's definition of ethics as the recognition of the "Other" by the "same," the suggestion here is that stories that describe a quest of the self necessarily spring from a crisis situation in which the destabilization of the Other, and its recognition by the self, lead to a "'calling into question'" (Levinas qtd. in Irvine 9) of the self.

In her 2007 article "What Can Narrative Theory Learn from Illness Narratives?" Shlomith Rimmon-Kenan takes an explicitly ethical approach to narrative. She looks for the answer to her title question through her analysis of "illness autobiographies" (245), but one can adopt her interrogation for narrative theory in general, which, by relying on formality and structure, largely bypasses the need to address ethical issues emergent from the rhetoric of the text. However, the undecided debate about the implied author as well as the difficulty of defining narrative reliability clearly suggest that there are important aspects of a narrative text that cannot be explored satisfactorily and fully through narratological inquiries. The assessment of authorial traces in the text as well as the relationship between the narrator and the audiences of a text, the integrity of which lies in the manipulative hands of the narrator, hinge principally on the way in which the text assumes ethical responsibility for the contents it transmits to the audience. It is for this reason that the acknowledgement of the communicative nature and thus the rhetorical dimension of literary texts is of high relevance for the analysis of the participation of the different textual agents in the production, transmission, and reception of a text: i.e., author and implied author, narrator, and diverse audiences, including the authorial audience, the narratee, the implied reader, and the flesh-and-bone or "specific" (Rimmon-Kenan 247) reader.

The characters' self-doubts and their struggle to make sense of past events emerge quite compellingly from the way they use and meditate on language, the medium they employ to serve their self-searching goals. Despite their pronounced verbosity, both narrators indicate the difficulties they encounter in coming to terms with, i.e., both coping with and finding the right words for, events that they strive to master retrospectively. Narrative perspective emerges in the two novels as a powerful instrument of linguistic manipulation and persuasive rhetoric in the narrators' communication with their audiences. Max and James construct what could be called a "grammar of loss" out of their linguistic paralysis, enacting poststructuralist anxieties about the ineptness of the signifier. The desire to narrate stands in stark contrast to the impreciseness of language, making the need for communication on an ethical level even more acute. The following analysis will deal primarily with the rhetoric of narration and will focus on the use of language for rhetorical communication and self-reflexivity.

Rhetoric of Loss: The First-Person Narrator and the Narrative Audience

The narratives of the two male protagonists involve the readers in the gradual disclosure of their pasts by appealing to them on several levels. James Phelan subsumes the critical concern with the communicative act addressed towards the reader under the term "rhetorical literary ethics," characterizing it as follows:

> [R]ather than focusing only on textual features and their relationships, I am concerned with the multilayered communications that authors of narrative offer their audiences, communications that invite or even require their audiences to engage with them cognitively, psychically, emotionally, and ethically. (*Living* 5)

Both James and Max are highly unreliable narrators. When Max presents the reader with a cruel, wanton, and overly sexual version of 12-year-old Chloe, he seems very convincing, but as he himself has constant quarrels with "Madam Memory" (*Sea* 163), the audience begins to wonder about the accuracy of his rendering. Max gets mixed up about the chronology of certain events as well as the people involved in them, and frequently confesses to the audience that he has invented or imagined the one or the other fact: "[W]as the cart a misremembrance?" (*Sea* 54); "It is only my fancy, I know, but I see the little waves lapping hungrily at her heels" (243); "The shoes I may have invented" (245). James, too, carefully constructs a villainous image of his antagonist, Gabriel, meant to draw the audience onto his side. In a manner similar to Max's, James's reminiscing abilities are revealed in a new light when the audience realizes that his memories of the summer in Quebec partly differ from Gabriel's. Confusingly and disappointingly for the reader, the two men cannot agree upon the name of the key female character of the summer, Odette, whom Gabriel remembers as Yvette; nor does Gabriel share James's memories of a key episode in James's mnemonic exercise, a romantic beach picnic undertaken by the two boys with Odette and her friend Pauline, also a chambermaid. However, as both James and Gabriel have taken great pains to convince us of the extravagance of the other characters involved and of their own "normality," our initial impetus is to join them in their view of things, until we come to recognize that they provide us with every reason to doubt the narratives.

First-person narration is particularly apt for an analysis not only of narrative reliability, but also of responsible story-telling. As characters involved in the story, first-person narrators are to be held accountable not only for their actions, but also for their rendering of the events. Their narratorial pact is, on the one hand, one with the reader (cf. Rimmon-Kenan 248), but also with the other characters and their own conscience. However, it is difficult to decide the question of reliability in any satisfactory way. Like Rimmon-Kenan, Ansgar Nünning, a structural narratologist, sees unreliability as anchored in the text and recognized by the reader in the conflict between his or her values and those of the narrator (25). Such narratological models leave no room for an implied author, whereas rhetorical readings make narrative unreliability itself contingent on this elusive figure. Such is Susan S. Lanser's definition, according to which reliability is "a reader's (complex) determination that the narrator's values and perceptions are consistent with those of the author."

It seems reasonable to assume that the distance that prevents the reader from identifying with Max and James is the outcome of the reader's awareness of an irony constructed by the implied author. For instance, James is somewhat ready to admit that his interpretation of facts was rather awry: "[A]s usual I misread the whole thing" (*October* 56). Max's misreadings persist, however, even in the present account, which is meant to illuminate the past. Max comes to the realization of his confusion later than the audience itself, a structure which clearly shows that an implied author who communicates with the authorial audience is at work in the novel, even circumventing the first-person narrator. Max announces self-assuredly that he "discovered Rose's secret one Saturday afternoon" (*Sea* 226), i.e., her alleged affair with Carlo. However, even though he secretly witnesses two erotic encounters between Rose and Connie, he completely misinterprets them, still asking himself, fifty years later, why Miss Vavasour, or Rose, has never married (38). While the reader is alerted through these signals to the actual romantic constellation, Max remains a victim of dramatic irony and is surprised when Miss Vavasour confesses her love for Connie (262): "And I thought, too, of the day of the picnic and of her sitting behind me on the grass and looking where I was avidly looking and seeing what was not meant for me at all" (263), i.e., Connie Grace's flesh under her skirt, which she was actually exposing for Rose's, not Max's benefit.

Max's and James's trips down the road of memory are full of self-contradictions and self-corrections. In retrospect, James realizes, for example, that his hated Uncle Chester, best-selling author of adventure fiction for young adults, may have been more benevolently inclined towards his adolescent moods than suspected at the time: "[I]t was yet another example of how badly Uncle Chester misread me. At least in my estimation" (*October* 36); "Looking back now I can see how utterly impossible I must have been" (50); "I was beginning to see that my uncle was not exactly the preposterous figure I had always thought him to be" (200). As James exclaims on his coincidental re-encounter with Gabriel, "How we old survivors tend to edit our memories! Had he forgotten how angry I was with him on that last day?" (74).

Aggrieved by the illness and ensuing deaths of their loved ones, Max and James pursue a search of the self that sets them on a path of self-enquiry through introspection. In order to come to terms with their present losses, they retrieve their past and embed it in their narratives— in which the narrating "I" seeks to justify and explain events in which the experiencing "I" was involved as a witness. Confronted with the helplessness of their present situation, in which it is beyond their power to intervene actively and effectively, Max and James seem to wonder whether they might have influenced the outcome of past events by taking responsible and meaningful action. Indeed, while rendering their roles in human tragedy in their childhood as passive and helpless, the mere depth and amplitude of their efforts to describe them as such, as well as the inclusion of these events at the core of their personal crisis, demonstrate that their conscience is still troubled by guilt. Their story-telling is an ethical act because it stems from their conscience, from the acknowledgement of the Other, and leads to a questioning of the self.

Max is haunted by the memory of the two drowned playmates whom he has possibly driven into suicide. James has to cope with his memory of having been an acquiescent witness and even facilitator of Gabriel's affair with Odette and feels the burden of responsibility for her pregnancy. Likewise, he is plagued by feelings of guilt for the way he used to reject his Uncle Chester's adventure books for boys for which Chester was famous and whose qualities he only begins to appreciate now; and he now understands that he should have paid his mother a share of respect equal to the love he had for her.

Max explains his ethical situation in relation to Chloe with great insight, a perspective which may partly belong to the young Max, but most of which seems to stem from the cultivated mind of the adult protagonist. The older Max realizes in retrospect that his encounter with Chloe marks an essential stage in his development. Through her "difference," Chloe makes Max recognize Otherness and develop his conscience. In terms strongly redolent of Lacanian psychoanalysis, the adult Max describes the emergence of his sense of his own self as different from the big whole: "Before, there had been one thing and I was part of it, now there was me and all that was not me" (*Sea* 168). His ethical self also develops at this stage, acknowledging the Other as different from the same, as Irvine puts forward, citing Levinas, and accepting one's responsibility towards the Other. While Max tries to protect Chloe from herself and from the fact that he is also in love with her mother, the younger Max fails lamentably, with tragic consequences. The twins' suicide is to a great extent the result of his indiscreet bragging and of his total misapprehension of the situation.

Max and James perform what Phelan calls two "'telling functions'": "'narrator functions'" that concern the communication between the narrator and the narratee, both located at the level of the text; and "'disclosure functions'" that concern the relationship between the narrator and the authorial audience, the latter being situated outside the text (*Living* 12). Obviously, both narrators are aware of the facts of the past and their consequences, but they do not confront the reader with them bluntly. Instead, by taking the reader into the past, the narrators make him/her retrace their experience, inducing the audience not to judge them prematurely, but to grasp their reasons first. James consistently and understandably blames his harsh judgement of his environment by connecting it with a teenager's identity crisis. The audience, who is more likely to be mature than adolescent, can identify with him in many ways: Readers will have experienced adolescent insecurity as well as its retrospective adult analysis.

This point is of particular relevance in the case of Max's blunder, for which he obviously blames himself now. Interestingly, the entire dimension of his mistake only becomes clear to him upon revisiting the shores of Ballyless after his wife Anna's death. He clearly intimates that breaking the news of their father's adultery to the twins, coupled with Rose's lack of attention, is responsible for their deaths. But what he consistently fails to apprehend is that Rose, now his landlady Miss Vavasour, was not in love with the father Carlo, but his wife, Connie. The disclosure function is dominant here as the reader is slowly taken towards the revelation of suicide at the novel's end.

The text constructs a cognitive imbalance between implied author, narrator, and audience. At first, the audience is given a hint that a crisis occurred, that "something happened," to use Phelan's words ("Rhetorical" 634), but we are not told what exactly took place. Hence, when Max asks about Miss Vavasour, "Does she blame herself for all that happened and grieve for it still?" (*Sea* 72), the audience is ignorant of the events to which he alludes. As Phelan notes, "just as there is a progression of events, there is a progression of audience response to those events, a progression rooted in the twin activities of observing and judging" (Phelan, "Rhetorical" 634). The drowning of the twins is depicted in very few sentences: "All that followed I see in miniature" (*Sea* 243): "Then calmly they stood up and waded into the sea" (244); "We watched them, Rose and I . . . I do not know what I was thinking, I do not remember thinking anything. . . . After that it was all over very quickly" (244); leaving a lot of questions open for the narrator and the audience: "[T]he old, unasked questions came swarming forward again. I would like to ask her [Rose] if she blames herself for Chloe's death—I believe, I should say, on no evidence, that it was Chloe who went down first, with Myles following after, to try to save her—and if she is convinced their drowning together like that was entirely an accident, or something else" (261).

Unlike the events of the past, the news of cancer is not postponed or gradually revealed. The finality of the disease is also clear from the beginning and the narrative audience is exposed to the same shock as the characters. *October*, in particular, is an exercise in harsh realism in dealing with death, but not with the advance of the disease itself, which is described in short, matter-of-fact sentences. Medical detail is present only in succinct form and medical discourse only enters the narrative briefly, readily dismissed and caricatured for its inadequacy. Science is rendered ineffectual: It cannot make Gabriel walk again; it cannot heal cancer; and it cannot cure James's mother's depression. Despite her doctor's undisputed expertise, James's daughter, Susan, notices that the doctor's medical authority is undermined by her lack of options to act as well as a lack of words to communicate with her patient: She "couldn't say. Or wouldn't" because, Dr Patel says, cancer is "wayward": "I got the distinct impression that cancer's unpredictability infuriated her. . . . under that impassive manner of hers. . . . doctors . . . always like to think they're in charge" (14-15). In *The Sea* as well, the medical consultant, Mr. Todd, is reduced to a caricature. Although patient interviews are his profession, he cannot break the silence preceding the bad news, "playing for time" (16) with Anna's file, instead. It is the patient herself who has to assume the leading role in the disclosure of the diagnosis, and the doctor's subsequent "forceful disquisition" on treatments and drugs is dismissed as "speaking of magic potions, the alchemist's physic" (17).

Self-Reflexivity: Metatextuality and Metaphor

Metaphors and euphemisms abound in the two novels as indirect modes of self-expression. Thus, the depression of James's mother is reported as "[going] to bed for the rest of the year" (*October* 43); James's daughter Susan can only start talking about her cancer directly when she has had too much to drink. James's comment on this lack of explicitness contains the vague reference to a "problem": "circulating around the larger problem. The *only* problem if it came to that" (9); Max borrows medical terminology to designate his regular dose of alcohol his "ready supply of anaesthetic" (*Sea* 59); and James allows himself some optimistic moments of speculation about the advance of Susan's disease:

"A door opens just a crack. A glimmer of light in a dark room" (*October* 107-08).

Rüdiger Imhof remarks that Max has a "fancy, punning prose style" (167) and draws attention to the pun contained in his surname, Morden, to kill, which indicates that he feels responsible for the twins' death. So too with the name of his wife's medical consultant "Todd," which might just as well be "De'Ath," as Max comments (*Sea* 13). Max also often mutters a meaningless refrain of "*Deedle deedle deedle*" (8, 9), "*Doodle deedle dee*" (43), in the absence of better-suited formulations of his feelings. Desperate for words, Max exclaims "how imprecise the language is, how inadequate to its occasions" (66).

Puns, like refrains, merely fill in for language, but they cannot replace it, nor can they express meaning. The character thus communicates to the reader the incommunicability of his loss, which the audience is made to feel. Max and James also seem to live in utter isolation despite occasional contacts with family members; the world at large remains insensitive to their suffering, "getting on with their lives" (*October* 27). In the absence of friends to talk to and in a world of answering machines, signs of sympathy remain the domain of the audience. The narratee is a necessary and distinctive presence in both texts. It is obvious that James and Max address their narratives to an audience to whom they wish to tell their stories, but also to justify the respective parts they played in past occurrences. The audiences of the text tend to identify with the "you" directed at the narratee, as these examples show: "Let me explain" (*Sea* 165); and: "What must first strike you in such circumstances . . . (*October* 68). Even more, the narrators draw the reader onto their side, as when, for example, James suggests the commonsensical proposition that "Our primal instinct is to survive" (*October* 18), including the audience in the first-person plural, "our," and thus precluding any possible disagreement. While the characters' self-disclosure frequently borders on self-pity, the audience is challenged to feel its responsibility towards the characters and fill in the gap of sympathy with its own commiseration.

This is not always made easy by the narrators, who occasionally give the audience sufficient reason to doubt them and desist in their efforts to be sympathetic listeners to their stories. While Max makes sexist remarks about his daughter's unappealing physical appearance (*Sea* 63) and indulges in self-pity, James undermines his own claim to credibility by specifying that "I enjoy listening to the secrets of others, and over the years people have opened their hearts to me. This trait has made me seem more trustworthy than I really am" (*October* 103). He calls this his "furtive side" which would have made him "the perfect Renaissance courtier," "a devious sneak," but which now also fills him "with a vague distaste" (103). This comment follows upon the account of the different versions of their sexual escapades delivered by Gabriel and Odette. James listens passively to the two versions, assuming the role of the courtier who is "intelligent enough, but not particularly ambitious, even a bit lazy, happy enough to be out of the spotlight; someone who can keep his mouth shut, listen to both sides and offer the king wise counsel" (103).

Making arrangements for his return to Canada from Switzerland, James observes Gabriel's nurse writing down the details and muses that "I felt the mild trepidation we sometimes experience when we see another person doing just that—writing down things that will arrange our lives in a slightly different way" (*October* 85). On the one hand, this passage underlines the fact that James is not fully in control of the situation and can no longer withdraw his promise to accompany Gabriel on his final trip. On the other hand, though, with this sentence, James formulates a metatextual comment on his own recording of events in his first-person narrative, as a means of arraying their chaotic course. This order serves as an antidote to, first, the internal chaos of personal crisis and confusing memories, and second, the collapse of cancerous bodies.

James's as well as Max's ordering of events is questionable because of the frequent lapses into self-pity. James paraphrases King Lear's mourning for his beloved Cordelia and quotes "*Never, never, never, never, never*" (*October* 70). The reader feels compelled to commiserate with James when he bemoans the approaching death of his daughter. The intertextual reference lends itself beautifully to an illustration of the complex layering of the addressees of a text. By using this quotation, James clearly appeals to an informed narratee who has read *King Lear* and can thus realize the full implications of James's situation. At the same time, the quotation also appeals to the sensibilities of the audience if that audience is ignorant of the origin of the words, but is also either a parent or someone capable of occupying that position vicariously, in his or her imagination. If parental experience is not given, then the repetition of the hyperbolic "never" renders the experience that James shares here excruciatingly painful and final, helping the audience to understand James's feelings indirectly and cognitively, by undertaking a rhetorical analysis of the words, as exemplified here. In the same way, the (implied) author has similar audiences in mind, excepting the narratee, who is the direct recipient of the narrator's communication and thus instrumental to the comprehension of the narrator's true intentions and strategies.

Harry E. Shaw's designation of the classical narratological definition of the narratee according to its actual presence in the text as "restricting" is part of his criticism of the constrictions of what he calls the "information" mode of reading a text; i.e., as an external observer of the text who completes a structuralist, narratological analysis in which s/he extracts "information" from observation. In contrast, the "rhetoric mode" is one that pays attention to what

> occurs in the mind of the implied author (or sometimes. . . in the mind of the narrator). To be sure, it is crucial that we keep in mind the possibility that a narrative may be addressed to different audiences simultaneously, and particularly the possibility that (guided by the implied author), the narrator may be addressing one kind of audience through another.

In his analysis of an excerpt from William Makepeace Thackeray's *Vanity Fair* (1847-48), Shaw sees the narrator as a "dramatized ethical and rhetorical agent" who "tries to meet the full ethical complexities of coming to grips with Becky's guilt, her society's guilt, and our guilt as readers." Whereas Shaw underlines the divergences between his and Phelan's interpretations of the narrator's role in the passage in question, it is plausible to hypothesize that their analysis of a homodiegetic narrator, unlike that of Thackeray's heterodiegetic omniscient narrator, would be more convergent. The protagonists of the novels discussed here correspond to Shaw's description above, and their ethical concerns are related to their guilt, making the reader react emotionally, cognitively, psychologically, and ethically to their problems while occasionally virtually stepping into the protagonists' shoes.

In both *The Sea* and in *October*, death comes in the month of October; death's cruelty consisting, among other aspects, in its grim arrival during the most colorful and beautiful month of autumn. The sea also functions as a metaphor with multiple significations,[6] but the metaphors that become a frequent topic of metalinguistic reflection are those related to cancer. As Susan remarks in *October*: "God, I'm mixing my metaphors, aren't I. Funny how the only way we can picture cancer is through metaphor. A grass fire. A sneak thief. A little ravaging fiend inside you" (16); or James: "I imagined the creature in the dark corner grinning hideously at us" (10), "a goblin crouching in a darkened corner of the room, waiting to appear as the centre of attention" (9).

In light of such examples, the romantic status of metaphor as an expression of creativity and creative genius has to be reconsidered. In contemporary use, we live by metaphors, meaning that, as George Lakoff and Mark Johnson suggest in their famous study of metaphor, *Metaphors We Live By*, we not only talk of one thing in terms of another, but we also think accordingly (3-6). This may be a sign of linguistic creativity and cognitive imagination, but too many metaphors have become part of our stock, everyday vocabulary for this description to still fit without further specification. Since the audiences of the text are used to thinking in the "metaphors we live by," the use of metaphor to paraphrase illness would not become apparent in the case of a metaphor like the ones quoted above. The metatextual comment, though, draws attention to the metaphor's existence as a signal of the indirectness and ineptness of language.[7]

Thinking and talking of one thing in terms of another is a gesture of indirection that is a way to circumvent direct expression and thereby the problem of its impossibility. As Jennifer Carol Cook suggests, "[i]mplicit in each symbol and metaphor is both the promise of

---

[6] "The sea stands, of course, for a welter of contrary symbols. It has symbolized chaos and the bridge between orderly lands, life and death, time and timelessness, menace and allure, boredom and the sublime . . . .'the primal source of all that lives.' Furthermore, the sea also evokes death. . . . In *The Sea* however, the sea stands for memory itself, more than for anything else" (Imhof 166).

[7] Both narrators meditate intensely on the destructive power of "Words! Glorious words!" (*October* 125) while also admitting that language is an insufficient tool for true expression. This is illustrated through deliberations about the ambiguity of language (e.g., *Sea* 21, *October* 132), as well as in James's lessons on idiomatic English, given to Odette.

communication and the evidence of its failure" (13). Significantly, Cook speaks of a "promise of communication," not of communication itself, which is essential for the use of metaphor in the two novels under discussion here. While linguistic artifice itself does not give comfort to the protagonists, the act of sharing their stories does, it is suggested, have a healing effect.[8]

Conclusion

The two fictions are not narratives of cancer, but rather dramatizations of the disease's effect on the male protagonists. The cancerous *memento mori* puts them on a track back into their past, the aim of which is to provide an explanation for the present. The actual alleviation of pain and loss and the processing of their trauma, however, lie in their narrative verbalization and address to an ethically responsible audience.

The kind of reading suggested here abides by the definition of the fictional text as a communicative medium. Whereas the addressee of the text is represented by a number of audiences (authorial audience, narratee, narrative audience, real or "specific" reader),[9] the rhetorical reading suggested here also acknowledges the (implied) author and the narrator as communicators. The mono-voiced text in particular has the quality of drawing the reader into the thrall of the first-person narrator because the "I" of the speaker and the "you" of the addressee construct a familiar communicative situation that invites several levels of intimacy and identification. The audience may identify with the speaker ("I") or the narratee ("you") or may identify the speaker with the author (based on the homodiegetic "I") of the text. Lanser discusses the potential for

---

[8] Anderson calls stories the "disciplined invention of language" through which a "healing narrative" is constructed with a liberating effect for the traumatized protagonist (361).

[9] As Phelan notes, the various and numerous audiences of a text need not always be separated from one another, as they often overlap ("Narratee" 135).

attachment of what she calls "equivocal"[10] fictional texts with a view to the identification of the first-person narrator with the authorial first person. She argues, and proves convincingly, that "nonnarrative" or "atemporal" segments of the text tend to blur the distinction between the two entities more than plot elements or temporally situated elements of the story. However, it is more than obvious that "nonnarrativity" or "atemporality" is also instrumentalized by the narrator figures in order to conjure reader identification with the narrator's motives. First-person narrators are charismatic and compelling as well as artfully manipulative of their audiences,[11] to whom they wish to justify themselves. Thus, they often resort to expressions of opinion or statements of general knowledge to which the reader cannot but adhere.[12] This is part and parcel of their communication with their audiences and determines the ethical relationship between narrator and audience reader.

Works Cited

Anderson, Charles M. "*Me acuerdo*: Healing Narrative in *Stones for Ibarra*." *Literature and Medicine* 25.2 (2006): 358-75. *Project Muse*. Web. 10 Aug. 2011.

Banville, John. *The Sea*. London: Picador, 2005. Print.

Cook, Jennifer Carol. *Machine and Metaphor: The Ethics of Language in American Realism*. London: Routledge, 2007. Print.

Foucault, Michel. "What Is an Author?" *Modern Criticism and Theory*. Ed. David Lodge and Nigel Wood. Harlow: Longman, 2000. 174-87. Print.

---

[10] Lanser refers to the "equi-vocation of literature," maintaining that "The 'I' that characterizes literary discourse . . . is always potentially severed *and* potentially tethered to the author's 'I.'"

[11] They are unconscious of the existence of the authorial audience and the real reader. Cf. Phelan, "Narratee" 144-45.

[12] As argued elsewhere, first-person narrators display these characteristics especially in narratives in which they wish to justify themselves to an audience (and to themselves) for a wrongdoing committed in the past. These texts can be read as dramatic monologues in prose.

Friberg, Hedda. "Waters and Memories Always Divide: Sites of Memory in John Banville's *The Sea*." *Recovering Memory: Irish Representations of Past and Present*. Ed. Hedda Friberg, Irene Gilsenan Nordin, and Lene Yding Pedersen. Newcastle-upon-Tyne: Cambridge Scholars, 2007. 244-61. Print.

Imhof, Rüdiger. "*The Sea*: 'Was't Well Done?'" *John Banville*. Spec. issue of *Irish University Review* 36.1 (2006): 165-81. Print.

Irvine, Craig A. "The Other Side of Silence: Levinas, Medicine, and Literature." *Literature and Medicine* 24.1 (2005): 8-18. *Project Muse*. Web. 10 Aug. 2011.

Lakoff, George, and Mark Johnson. *Metaphors We Live By*. Chicago: U of Chicago P, 1980. Print.

Lanser, Susan S. "The 'I' of the Beholder: Equivocal Attachments and the Limits of Structuralist Narratology." *A Companion to Narrative Theory*. Ed. James Phelan and Peter J. Rabinowitz. Blackwell, 2005. *Blackwell Reference Online*. Web. 12 Mar. 2007.

Nünning, Ansgar. "*Unreliable Narration* zur Einführung: Grundzüge einer kognitiv-narratologischen Theorie und Analyse unglaubwürdigen Erzählens." Unreliable Narration: *Studien zur Theorie und Praxis unglaubwürdigen Erzählens in der englischsprachigen Erzählliteratur*. Ed. Nünning. Trier: WVT, 1998. 3-39. Print.

Phelan, James. *Living to Tell about It: A Rhetoric and Ethics of Character Narration*. Ithaca: Cornell UP, 2005. Print.

---. "Narratee, Narrative Audience, and Second-Person Narration: How I—and You?—Read Lorrie Moore's 'How.'" *Narrative as Rhetoric: Technique, Audiences, Ethics, Ideology*. Columbus: Ohio State UP, 1996. 135-53. Print.

---. "Rhetorical Literary Ethics and Lyric Narrative: Robert Frost's 'Home Burial.'" *Poetics Today* 25.4 (2004): 627-51. *JSTOR*. Web. 23 June 2010.

Rimmon-Kenan, Shlomith. "What Can Narrative Theory Learn from Illness Narratives?" *Literature and Medicine* 25.2 (2006): 241-54. *Project Muse*. Web. 10 Aug. 2011.

Semino, Elena. *Metaphor in Discourse*. Cambridge: Cambridge UP, 2008. Print.

Shaw, Harry E. "Why Won't Our Terms Stay Put? The Narrative Communication Diagram Scrutinized and Historicized." *A Companion to Narrative Theory*. Ed. James Phelan and Peter J. Rabinowitz. Blackwell, 2005. *Blackwell Reference Online*. Web. 12 Mar. 2007.

Squires, Claire. "Book Marketing and the Booker Prize." *Judging a Book by Its Covers: Fans, Publishers, Designers, and the Marketing of Fiction*. Ed. Nicole Matthews and Nickianne Moody. Aldershot, UK: Ashgate, 2007. 71-82. Print.

Wright, Richard B. *October*. Toronto: Harper, 2007. Print.

PETER SCHNECK

Finding Words for (Not) Losing One's Mind: Alice James, Charlotte Perkins Gilman, and the Sense of Self in Narratives of Mental Illness

Illness Narratives and the Medical Humanities

Since the early 1980s, the interdisciplinary connection between medicine and literature has developed from its initial conception as a "strange marriage" and the "conjunction of seeming incompatibilities" (Rabuzzi ix) into a thriving and highly diversified field of scholarly research and clinical and therapeutic practices. The subsequent formation of the so-called medical humanities as a more encompassing area of both scientific inquiry and professional practice furthermore testifies to the inherent potential of the conjunction of literary and cultural studies and medicine.

One of the most powerful concepts in this alignment of concerns between the disciplines and their various practices has been the notion of narrative and, in particular, the concept of illness narrative. Within the field of medicine, the reception of the "narrative turn," which had already been acknowledged within the humanities and social sciences (cf. Kreiswirth, "Merely"; "Trusting"), helped to inaugurate new perspectives in scholarship and deeply influenced both clinical practice and practical training. The impact of analytical and qualitative approaches based on insights and concepts from narratology, originally developed in the humanities, led to the emergence of a new approach called "narrative medicine," which embraces a broad range of concerns in terms of diagnosis, therapy, and general health care.[1]

All these developments convincingly demonstrate that inter-disciplinary work and the transfer of concepts from the humanities may be of great benefit to the life sciences. In the case of medicine, it has certainly facilitated the reconciliation of empirically based knowledge and professional treatment with the ethical demands of care and healing ideally understood as a process of subjective recovery, based on the specific collaboration between patients and professional caretakers.

It is, however, less easy to estimate the effects the medical humanities have had or might still have on the formation (and reformation) of knowledge in the fields of literary and cultural studies. Following Shlomith Rimmon-Kenan, who has suggested that "just as narrative theory can elucidate illness narratives, so can illness narratives illuminate, and sometimes problematize, central notions in narratology and narrative theory" (241), the subsequent discussion aims to tackle the notion of the "narrative self" within the larger context of illness narratives and the medical humanities.

More specifically, I will be concerned with the question of how narrative is conceived of as a tool to express, communicate, and, at the same time, negotiate and make manageable the experience of mental illness, especially in regard to the sense of self and reality. This understanding of the essential functions of narratives for people who suffer from severe illnesses has become a central staple in approaches to narrative in the medical humanities. Moving beyond established practices of basic "symptomatic" readings of illness accounts, ap-proaches in narrative medicine insist that these narratives have to be closely scrutinized not only in content but also in form:

> Deconstruction of the structure of the illness account—the rhetorical devices and plot outlines used by the patient to assemble particular events into a more or less integrated story line—can reveal hidden concerns that the patient has not verbalized. (Kleinman 233)

---

[1]   Cf. Hurwitz, Greenhalgh, and Skultans; Engel et al.; Meza and Passerman; Angus and McLeod.

The close attention paid by narrative medicine to the specific construction of illness accounts is a way to transcend the more orthodox professional horizon of understanding which aims at the systematic categorization of subjective experience as symptoms of known diseases. More essentially, narrative medicine attempts to recover an "authentic" perspective on the experience of "being ill" (*Kranksein*) as "an experience essential to the understanding of being a human being" (Martinsen and Solbakk 1).

As Hilary Clark has noted, the growing interest in illness narratives over the past decades must be seen as part of "a general trend in scholarship toward accepting the validity of personal narrative, both written and oral, as a source of knowledge" (3). The central argument underlying the emphatic embrace of personal narratives, Clark observes, is that by "attending to them on their own merits, as opposed to using them in order to come to diagnoses and impose regimes of treatments . . . such narratives give voice to the ill, the traumatized and the disabled . . . and help them navigate the bewildering, impersonal context of medical diagnosis and treatment" (3). In a similar vein, Deborah Flynn has argued for a humanities approach to mental disorders or illnesses such as depression, since "in order to understand the experience of depression one must look beyond the changing definitions to the experience and expression of symptoms. Narrative can provide a window into the understanding of an experience that has been historically difficult to define" (36).

One could thus arguably claim that at the heart of the intense interest in illness narratives lies a "secular desire to limit the sometimes dehumanising effects of a medicalised society, and the effects of forms of medical practice that deliver increasing technical sophistication but fail to offer 'comfort and care' for patients as whole human beings" (Bury 282). In the larger social and cultural context of late modernity or post-modernity (depending on one's perspective), the interest in self-narratives thus also represents a larger trend to regain a sense of self through narrative: "Because an essential part of what it is to be human is to know oneself, narratives can provide a way to reaffirm one's sense of self through an exploration of the experiences and relationships one encounters" (Flynn 37).

From my point of view, this fundamental understanding of the relation between narrative and self-assertion in the context of the medical humanities raises two related questions. The first regards the relation between narrative and experience. The suggestion that narrative is the necessary foundation of a sense of self, is often used as a basis for arguments about the essentially *constructive* function of self-nar-ratives—both as positive ("healing" the self) or negative ("disciplining" the self) constructions of selves. Yet to insist that there cannot be a self without a narrative tends to cancel out self-*experience* as something distinct from, or even contrary to self-*narrative*,[2] a consequence which appears especially bothersome in regard to forms of mental illness that obviously impair the ability to maintain a self-narrative or, rather, where the narrative of self registers an impending loss of self.

Starting out from the observation that the disassociation of self-experience and self-narrative presents a crucial aspect of mental illness, the privileging of narrative has become increasingly debated from various related perspectives concerned with forms of mental illness in cognitive science and neuroscience, psychology, psychiatry, and phenomenology. These approaches all share a strong interest in the dynamic relation between self-experience, self-consciousness, and self-narratives in the constitution of the sense of self, and in particular the way in which the experiential self interacts with the narrative self.[3] I will refer to some of these approaches in order to first carve out and

---

[2]   As aptly summarized by Clark: "From the perspective of the ill, disabled, and/or traumatized subject, then, taking up narrative is seen by many to be empowering .... However, there is an obverse side to this linking of narrative and identity: while telling one's story, bearing witness, can be linked with enhanced agency, it is also the case that the stories one tells are not entirely one's own. The poststructuralist view that identity and knowledge are socially constructed by dominant narratives can lead to the more skeptical conclusion that personal narratives ... are always already ideological ..." (3-4). Clark also refers to alternative critical positions on narrative and self, for instance, Galen Strawson's "episodic self." She does not mention the phenomenological approaches I will discuss below (Zahavi; Gallagher), probably because these approaches, much more than Strawson's, insist on the priority of a non-narrative sense of self. Cf. also Hutto.

[3]   Cf., for instance, Gallagher, *Models*; Zahavi, *Exploring*; Zahavi, "Being"; Kircher and David; and Ratcliffe.

discuss some essential problems regarding illness narratives as self-narratives in the medical humanities.

The second question concerns the status of fictional narratives and literature itself. The argument about the humanizing effects of caring for—and caring with the help of—narratives of illness experience has been extended to fictional accounts of mental illness and depression as well. In a recent paper, for instance, Paul Crawford and Charley Baker have argued from the perspective of psychiatry that biographical and fictional accounts of mental illness may present a more powerful, more encompassing, and probably also more effective representation of the experience of mental disturbance and disease and thus could help the practitioner to develop a more adequate grasp of the nature of experience itself: "Through increasing the understandability of illness experience as explicated through fiction, the clinician can develop a deeper empathic understanding of the breadth of human experience" (239).[4]

While certainly respectable and not entirely refutable, this view has a major shortcoming because it tends to undermine the essential difference between biographical memoirs and fictional compositions of illness experience and illness narratives by actual patients. This difference is crucial, I will maintain, even where the author of a fictional composition relies on her own experience of mental illness and medical treatment. Thus, my conclusion will address the *literary* character of biographical illness narratives and discuss the particular challenge of *fictional* illness narratives for interdisciplinary approaches.

---

[4] In this assessment, the difference between autobiographical narratives and fictional illness narratives seems to be more or less negligible. In contrast, my argument is that there is an important difference between patients' narratives in a clinical context, on the one hand, and written forms of illness narratives and fictional accounts of mental illness, on the other hand. And there is also a crucial differentiation to be made between the latter two, as discussed in my conclusion. Nevertheless, all these modes of self-narrative must be related and compared in order to discuss the central function of narratives and the different roles they may play in different contexts.

Narrative and the Sense of Self

It is certainly no simple task to define in any conclusive way what constitutes a "self" or a "sense of self." The "contemporary discussion [about what exactly it means to be a self]," Dan Zahavi has observed, "is bursting with completing and competing notions of the self" ("Phenomenology" 57). The very same could be said for the notion of narrative. For once, there is obvious agreement about the basic functions of narratives for the self and its relation to others and to reality. For Jerome Bruner, for example, narratives basically organize and stabilize our lives because they "impose a structure, a compelling reality on what we experience" (*Making Stories* 89), which is a fundamental require-ment for a sustained sense of self. In a similar vein, but from a rather different perspective, Daniel C. Dennett has famously described the self as the "center of narrative gravity": a fictional entity which gives our lived experience as bodies and minds in the world an "illusion of greater unity" (113). These and other perspectives on narrative and self all support the idea that the capacity for forming and understanding stories is a necessary disposition that allows humans to develop a sense of self in the first place. While the self may be a fiction that has no essence, its more or less palpable and seemingly natural presence relies on the narratives we are able to tell.[5]

Two other points of convergence are significant for the discussion of illness accounts and their particular status in respect to the relation between sense of self and self-narratives. One regards the inherent dynamic of the narrative construction of the self. While narratives may offer structure and stability to lived experience, experience in turn constantly adds new material and thus enforces constant revisions of particular elements of our "storied life." The "narrative self is . . . an open-ended construction, which is under constant revision" (Zahavi, "Phenomenology" 58). Moreover, the sense of self that we develop and maintain with the help of narratives is a composition that relies to a great

---

[5]   For a concise comparative discussion of these perspectives on the narrative self, cf. Schechtman 394-418. For detailed arguments from evolutionary theory, cognitive science as well as developmental psychology, cf. Donald; K. Nelson; Bruner, *Actual Minds*.

extent on impulses from the outside. Self-narratives are not spontaneous, individual constructions; rather they are elicited by the interaction and intervention of parents and peers from early on. With the help of the self-narratives of others, children are enabled to develop a "level of self-understanding [which] integrates action and consciousness into a whole self, and establishes a self-history as unique to the self, differentiated from others' experiential histories" (K. Nelson 7). The narrative self is consequently subjective and inter-subjective, private and public, and shaped both by the desire for individual distinction and the necessity to conform and adjust one's unique experience to the norms and forms of expression already in place. In effect, primary language acquisition and growing linguistic competence are central for what Shaun Gallagher has termed "narrative competency," which helps us to "gain not only a more complex and extended sense of self" but also "a sophisticated understanding of others" ("Pathologies" 211, 216). Finally, the narrative self is always related to some dimension of temporality and, on the cognitive level, a memory system which allows for the connection of present experience with past events.

Given these intrinsic connections between narrative competency and the development and sustenance of the sense of self, it appears obvious that pathologies of the self may also imply or result in pathologies in self-narratives. Likewise, the revisions of self-narratives will also have an impact on the respective sense of self, so that an impaired sense of self may probably be remedied by developing better self-narratives.[6] The most important aspect of these different options is that they both point to the fact that while the sense of self relies on narratives, it is not identical with these narratives. In his discussion of specific pathologies in narrative structure, Gallagher has described four "necessary conditions" for the "non-pathological" development of narrative competency: "the capacity for temporal ordering, the capacity for minimal self-reference, episodic and autobiographical memory, and the capacity for metacognition" ("Pathologies" 205). While deficiencies in any of these aspects may point to a pathological dimension—as the incapacity for temporal order, an incoherent sense of self, and failure of autobiographical memory may characterize schizophrenic self-narratives

---

[6] On both these points, cf., for instance, Polkinghorne.

(cf. "Pathologies" 220)—the self-narrative proper already presents an extension and fortification of a sense of self which precedes its narrative embellishment, a "minimal self" which in phenomenological approaches is referred to as *ipseity*: "Ipseity is the sense that this experience is my experience. It is the 'mineness' of experience—a minimal sense of self that is an immediate and present self-consciousness" (Gallagher, "Pathologies" 208). This is an important observation (or rather hypothesis), especially for the discussion of self-narratives that reflect on the relation or tension between the narrative self and the minimal self. Although inexorably connected, the essential distinction between the two concepts is that the narrative self is always both subjective and inter-subjective, while the minimal self appears to be a disposition geared towards an original distinction between the "me" and the "not-me":

> To begin to form a self-narrative one must be able to refer to oneself by using the first pronoun. Without the basic sense of differentiation between self and non-self I would not be able to refer to myself with any specification, and self-narrative would have no starting point. The minimal sense of self is what gets extended and enhanced in the self-narrative. (Gallagher, "Pathologies" 208)[7]

For Gallagher, the "minimal self becomes an extremely secure anchor for self-narratives," due to two basic aspects. On the one hand, the use of the first-person pronoun in self-narratives offers a "guaranteed self-reference" ("Pathologies" 208). On the other hand, self-reference through the use of personal pronouns is a foundational, and thus most significant (both narrative and cognitive) operation to link experience to agency: "For the construction of self-narrative the sense of agency is the

---

[7]   For similar arguments for the distinction between the narrative self and other, more foundational forms of self, cf., for instance, Antonio Damasio (from a neurophysiological perspective), who distinguishes between a "core self" and an "autobiographical self" (59); and Dan Zahavi (from a phenomenological perspective), who argues that there is a "minimal experiential self" ("Self and Other" 193), which "must be regarded as a pre-linguistic presupposition for any narrative practices" (Gallagher and Zahavi, *The Phenomenological Mind* 205). For an argument that ties these concepts of minimal sense of self to a basic cognitive structure, cf. Hohwy.

basis for the attribution of action to oneself," hence "a lack of a sense of agency will be disruptive to self-narrative" ("Pathologies" 209).

For obvious reasons, the complex dynamics between the narrative and the experiential self presents a major common concern for discussions about the sense of self in mental illness, where the foundational relation between experience and expression of one's self is threatened or even impaired. These discussions also relate to central issues in literary and cultural studies. However, the question remains whether the notions of narrative and of self are sufficiently compatible to allow for an understanding of the social and cultural frameworks in which the relation between self and narrative is developed and shared to begin with. In the next step, I will discuss two examples taken from clinical contexts, which demonstrate the rather different ways in which this relation may manifest itself—which leads to certain interpretive problems and impasses.

Struggling for Narrative: Illness Work and Illness Identity

Mental illness has grave implications for the self's relation to others and to reality: It is both "intensely private" and "profoundly social" (Estroff et al. 331). Social alienation and self-alienation in connection to mental illness may be deepened by the increasing loss of control over one's own narrative self-description and self-definition. On the one hand, the impeded ability to express and communicate one's inner experience and afflictions to others and, on the other hand, the authoritative ascriptions of symptoms and categories of illness that form the inevitable foundation for potential treatments may result in further isolation and self-alienation:

> By definition and in essence, much of madness is invisible and unknowable to the "other." Yet these uncomprehending others identify, name, and treat madness, both revealed and suspected . . . . Within the embrace of authorized naming and treating, the unknown becomes known and its nature exposed (or constructed, depending on one's point of view) at least to those with the authority to know, name, and treat. (Estroff et al. 332)

The authors of the study quoted above specifically researched, over a one-year period, the correlation of illness accounts and self-narratives by a selected group of patients (169 persons from various ethnic backgrounds, half of them women) with persistent mental afflictions.

What they found, above all, was that most patients were continually struggling with the official definitions and descriptions of their state of mental illness, and they were doing so by means of negotiating the official terms and symptoms with their own personal assessments and descriptions. This "illness-identity work," as the study observed, must be seen as an ongoing process of "defining who and what is inside and outside the boundaries [of normalcy]" (Estroff et al. 336, 363).

The struggle to stay inside the boundaries of normalcy, however, is fundamentally and essentially a linguistic struggle or competition of discourses in which the patient's own verbal representation of the experience and effects of mental illness has to be reconciled with or cast in opposition to accounts of others describing the same experience "from the outside," as it were, based on the interpretation of the patient's symptoms. Finding the right words for losing one's mind becomes a matter of psychic sustenance by making a claim for a normal self regardless of the claims of others and the disturbing and desperate experience of mental illness itself. The conclusion of the study makes these points especially salient:

> The enormous amount of normalizing talk we elicited was at times defiant, urgent, plaintive, and even whimsical. Regardless of the tone, this kind of discourse was always meant to persuade us, and no doubt our informants themselves, that whether mentally ill or not, the individual was worthwhile, one of us—normal. Perhaps chronicity and disability begin when normalizing talk ends, or when the individual thinks that no one else is listening. One compelling challenge for anthropologists and clinicians alike is to keep the conversation going. (Estroff et al. 363)

These observations are most significant, since they insist that narratives of self and illness may help patients to maintain a position of self-description and self-definition in the face of "official" narratives of mental illness. These patients did not deny their symptoms nor did they deny that they were being labeled as mentally ill; rather, they struggled to find expression for their troubled sense of self that could escape the rigidness and inflexibility of clinical categories and allow them to occupy—at least for the time being—a flexible space of acceptable, and thus "normal," mental illness. At the same time, these narratives aimed to resist the "cognitive priming" (Corrigan and Watson 40) and stigmatization created by common stereotypes about mental illness. As one of the patients put it: "Everybody's got a little mental illness. It's just some know and some don't" (Estroff et al. 331).

Pre-Symptomatic Experience

My second clinical example shifts the perspective to the other end of the spectrum by looking at the disturbed relation between self-narrative and self-experience in cases where no diagnosis has yet been made. The significance of being able to find words for the impending loss of a sense of self becomes obvious when we look at studies concerned with the so-called prodrome phase in the early development of schizophrenia and other psychotic disorders.[8] These studies, which have gained increasing attention over the past two decades, aim to detect the moment when psychosis "starts" in order to "identify individuals who are presently free of the overt disease but who would, in the future, develop the disease" (Haroun et al. 174). More than any other form of mental illness, schizophrenia has been described as a "disturbance" of the self characterized by the "loss of the usual common-sense orientation to reality, unquestioned sense of obviousness, and unproblematic background quality that normally enables a person to take for granted so many aspects of the social and practical world" (Sass and Parnas 434). In fact, psychotic disorders threaten the very "center of *experiential* gravity" (B. Nelson et al. 386).

---

[8] The terms "prodromal phase" or "prodromal period" are much more current in Anglo-American research of early stages of psychosis, based on the observation of psychological changes that precede the development of psychosis. Other approaches use different terms to describe typical symptoms, e.g., "basic deficits" that would allow for early-stage diagnosis and intervention. Despite the terminological difference, there is some agreement that prediction based on the symptoms is still rather difficult. Cf. B. Nelson et al.; Bürgy.

Yet, while their effects as fully developed disorders manifest themselves with dreadful clarity and can be described and categorized by their distinctive symptoms, psychotic disorders only emerge slowly and over time. The particular challenge for clinical research and therapy is thus to detect signs of mental disturbances before psychosis "breaks"—a rather difficult task, "since there is no quantifiable point at which healthy thoughts become insane" (Aviv 36). The majority of clinical experts acknowledge the problem of predictability involved in early-stage psychotic disorders research. In fact, the main aspect of "prodromal" states regarding these disorders is that their status as *symptomatic* episodes of "self disturbance" becomes obvious only in retrospect:

> The "prodrome" is a retrospective concept: onset of frank psychosis cannot be predicted with certainty from any particular symptom or combination of symptoms; the fact that an individual was "prodromal" can only be asserted once frank psychosis has emerged. (B. Nelson et al. 384)

In current research and models concerned with the particular manifestations of "pre-symptomatic" psychosis, two perspectives dominate. One is based on the correlation of individual risk factors with a systematic record of symptomatic episodes of (quasi-)psychotic experiences. These so-called UHR (ultra-high risk) studies have become increasingly detailed and sophisticated, yet they have also been criticized for their neglect of the subjective dimension of self-experience. Phenomenological approaches in particular have argued that, because of its dependence on operational definitions, the "empiricist-behavioral" perspective prevalent in the risk approach to mental disorder "sacrifices an understanding of how human *experience* (specifically, its pathological varieties) relates to *expression*." For an understanding of mental disorders, this relation is essential since "if we regard psychopathology as being at least in some sense a disorder of *conscious experience*," the neglect of the expression of subjective experience (the patient's narrative) would leave us "with a profoundly deficient understanding of what psychopathology even is" (B. Nelson et al. 382). As a counterpoint, psychologists like Louis A. Sass and Josef Parnas have insisted on taking the subjective narratives about a disturbed sense of self into account, for these can register in a much more direct way the "subtle anomalies in affective, perceptual and cognitive experience" that might signal the emergence of psychotic states (Parnas qtd. in B. Nelson et al. 383).

Working with persons who are already experiencing slightly psychotic states but do not show the critical symptoms that would allow for a categorization of their experience as fully psychotic, one must read the narratives and verbal accounts these individuals create in order to find words for their disturbing experiences as pre-symptomatic representations of mental states that people find disturbing and which they struggle to communicate: "[E]arly symptoms were nearly impossible to describe, and the only way to communicate them was by making up new phrases." One patient wrote about "migrating electrical sensations" and "the sense that 'words were alive'" (Aviv 37). When asked about her experience, another patient replied: "There are no words. It's like trying to explain what a bark sounds like to someone who's never heard of a dog" (qtd. in Aviv 41). The prodromal period of emerging psychoses escapes descriptive formulas and conventional narratives of the self precisely because the intense experience of self-disturbance it entails affects the sense of self at its very core: It disturbs the *ipseity* of a self taken for granted.

In the context of early diagnosis and prevention of psychosis and schizophrenia, it certainly appears both reasonable and desirable to develop diagnostic tools based on phenomenological approaches to psychopathological states that focus on the subjective dimension of the prodromal period.[9] The phenomenological perspective centers on the experience of a sense of self—even a disturbed sense of self—as the necessary requirement for any self-narrative. A better understanding of the experiential conditions of psychopathological states can only emerge through close attention to the narratives of those who experience it. Subjective experience is thus an indispensable dimension of the illness

---

[9] See, for example, the EASE scale (examination of anomalous self-experience) which combines empirical data and clinical experience with phenomenological models and scaled descriptions of psychopathological states of subjective experience to establish a more comprehensive model for the diagnostic assessment of these self-descriptions (Parnas et al., "EASE"). For another example, cf. Weinman et al.

narrative that is being constructed even when this experience appears fragmented, inconclusive, elusive, or simply beyond the grasp of one's own language.

While the close attention to subjective experience—the experiential self and its narrative—may help to move beyond the boundaries of operational definitions of mental illnesses based on evident, quantifiable symptoms, it does so at the cost of turning narratives of subjective experience into symptomatic narratives. Since these narratives become one major source for identifying subjects who are "at risk" of developing full psychoses at a later stage, their experiences turn into templates for clinical interviews and questionnaires. This problem haunted the debates surrounding the potential inclusion of the so-called psychosis risk syndrome in the most recent version of the *Diagnostic and Statistical Manual of Mental Disorders* (DSM), since it would potentially stigmatize subjects with an "officially" diagnosed syndrome, even though "[t]he probability of actually developing schizophrenia in any individual is unknown . . . and it is likely that at least 50% [of the "at risk" group] will not develop schizophrenia" at all (Haroun et al. 174). Thus, studies concerned with the ethical, psychological, and social implications of prodromal research have strongly suggested that researchers and practitioners should restrain their symptomatic readings of individual experience of "self-disturbance" in the face of the potential psychosocial damage inflicted by a diagnosis that often will fail to come true (cf. Corcoran, Malaspina, and Hercher 181).

The Self as Symptom and Experience

The two clinical examples are obviously situated at opposite ends of a broad spectrum. Yet at the center of both processes lies what Arthur W. Frank has described as "the social construction of illness as a rhetorically bounded, discursively formulated phenomenon" (41). To say that a (mental) illness is a social construction does not mean to disavow the concrete experiential reality of the disruption of the sense of self that comes with this illness. It only calls attention to the fact that the translation of experience into narrative, and also the interpretation of experience through narrative, are both essentially informed by the narrative genres and frames that exist at any particular historical moment in a specific social and cultural environment. As Laurence J. Kirmayer states, the failure to acknowledge "the metaphoric and contextual basis of discourse" severely "limits the physician's comprehension of the patient's life world" (339). This limited contextual understanding may eventually work against the patient's own cognitive efforts to find the right words for her or his experience:

> The overzealous interpreter who ascribes meaning to every action may actually obstruct the sufferer's search for his own metaphor. The suffering individual—for whom the inchoate is less an obstacle than the *prima materia* for self-understanding—may experience the clinician's . . . all-encompassing interpretations as oppression. (Kirmayer 340)

Yet it is not only the distance between professional narratives and the subjective metaphors of suffering which may make a mere diagnostic reading of mental illness narratives highly ambivalent. While this distance presents an obstacle that has to be negotiated in the concrete exchange between the patient and the therapist or physician, the interpretation of illness narratives as a social, cultural, and historical phenomenon has to deal with another distancing device. As Jennifer Radden points out, both clinical "narratives" of mental illness and subjective accounts of the experience of self-disturbance are historically contingent. What Frank calls the social construction of mental illness is thus dependent on historically changing frames that inform the perspective on the relation between subjective experience of mental states and their potential symptomatic status as signs of "illness." For Radden, this poses a bundle of interpretive problems in connection with the difficult relation between self and symptom, since individual accounts of mental illness—especially those written in the form of memoirs—cannot be read as "mere phenomenological reports" but, rather, "reflect the 'framing' ideas and explanations accepted and imagined at their given time and place in history" (25). What complicates the socio-cultural and historical interpretation of illness narratives even further is that these "framings" cannot be easily identified, since they might be affected by the illness itself and also by the "reframing" of the initial experience in the act of narrating:

> Because the relation between self and symptoms may itself become disordered as the result of mental illness, any separation between

accurate report and cultural framing is problematic and leaves epistemic indeterminacy at the heart of our interpretive efforts. Further interpretive complexity comes from the element of "reframing": these narratives will likely reflect the temporary standpoint from which they were written rather than the framing within which the symptoms were first experienced. (Radden 25)

By all accounts, the aspect of reframing in particular would set these narratives apart from illness narratives within a clinical context—yet even in the latter case there is always a delay, a temporal distance between the experience and the act of narration, however fragmentary or inconsistent, that introduces a reframing of the original experience. The "epistemic indeterminacy" that Radden describes thus arguably also applies to the interpretation of accounts of mental illness in clinical contexts, only that in these contexts the phenomenological dimension of narrative tends to be objectified in an attempt to match the subjective descriptions to existing descriptions of symptomatic experience associated with specific diseases or psychopathologies.

Within the more general argument about the particular problematic which besets the interpretation of mental illness narratives, one can easily see the connection or even complementarity between the "illness identity" struggle of patients diagnosed with mental illness and their narrative claims for normalcy, the complex negotiation of the (potential) prodromal experiences of pre-symptomatic risk groups, and the hermeneutic complexities that come to bear on the interpretation of autobiographical accounts of mental illness from different historical periods and their various framings and reframings. The common challenge faced by these distinct perspectives on narratives of a disturbed sense of self is that they are both due to and shaped by an inherent and inescapable tension between the phenomenological, the symptomatic, and the narrative dimensions that are all constitutive of the sense of self.

Authorizing Illness Experience

In conclusion, I want to turn to two specific texts, in an attempt to tackle Shlomith Rimmon-Kenan's question about what the study of narrative in general can learn from illness narratives. My interest is a bit different, though. What concerns me here is the particular status and challenge of literary illness in general, and fictional accounts of illness experience in particular.

My aim is not to present exhaustive readings of Alice James's *Diary* and Charlotte Perkins Gilman's "The Yellow Wallpaper"—both texts have obviously received a great share of scholarly interest and interpretation, and space does not permit for any conclusive discussion of the texts within the larger context of the scholarly response they have elicited.[10] Also, my argument so far was not geared toward a specific reading or interpretation, but rather meant to question and complicate a specific form of reading. This mode of reading aims at the reduction and systematization of phenomenological complexity—the density, dynamics, and corporeality of the embodied experience of the sense of self—in order to capture and make this sense of self legible in reference to existing narrative templates or descriptive categories. Reading only "for the symptoms," however, does not simply present an ethical problem, as suggested by the case of prodromal research, for clinical practice alone. Since the problem is essentially connected to the general concept of the "narrative self," which also forms the strongest link or interface between the different disciplines concerned with illness narratives, it poses a challenge for literary and cultural studies as well. Hence, I want to shift the perspective back to the study of literary narratives and literature and point out how the interpretation of illness narratives in literary and cultural studies struggles with its own tendencies to read "for the symptoms."

---

[10] On Alice James, cf., e.g., Maher; Strouse; Yeazell, and the shorter discussions by Boudreau; Bronfen; Cappello; Duquette; Hoffman; Rasmussen. On Gilman, cf., e.g., Allen; Davis; Davis and Knight; Gilman and Dock; Golden; Hill; Horowitz; Rudd and Gough; and the shorter works by Cutter; Shumaker; Treichler.

In their own specific ways, and despite their obvious differences, both "The Yellow Wallpaper" by Charlotte Perkins Gilman and the *Diary of Alice James* can be seen as responses to the disturbing experience of "losing" one's mind and one's sense of self. Even though Gilman obviously chose to translate her experience into a fictional narrative, whereas James used the non-fictional form of a journal, both "narratives" are *literary* in the sense that they aim at a specific form of reception by their readers and contain highly recursive or self-reflexive elements. This observation relies to a great extent on Peter Lamarque's discussion of the difference between literary, non-literary, and fictional narratives. While Lamarque makes a point of distinguishing "literary" from "real-life narratives," the first category includes, but is not restricted to, narrative fictions. Of the various features which Lamarque describes as characteristic for literary narratives, it is especially "the fact that linguistic resources are not merely contingent elements in literary artifices" (122) which applies in the case of both Gilman's story and James's diary, even though one would hesitate to call the latter an "artifice" in Lamarque's sense. In contrast to Lamarque's various principles of literariness, I would contend that what makes these two texts literary in comparable ways is exactly their particular character as illness narratives, highly conscious of the contingency as well as the power of linguistic resources used to describe and interpret illness experience.[11]

That is, they are not merely "about" the illness experience of their authors—which is more obvious for James's *Diary* than for Gilman's story—both texts also offer a meta-level of reflection aimed at the various conflicting (or colluding) interpretations of the illness experience. In reference to Jennifer Radden's observations about the framings and reframings of self-experience in mental illness narratives,

---

[11] The same case, in fact, could be made for most illness narratives in autobiographical form, but especially those that deal with mental illness and disturbances of the self. These disturbances affect precisely the natural self-evidence of the relation between experience, self, and narrative, so that language is foregrounded as the link between the experience and self—a link, however, that has become loose, brittle, or even severed and thus must be restored and regained. In effect, mental illness narratives are as much about the self as they are about the linguistic resources of the self.

the particular rhetorical strategies in James's journal and in Gilman's story aim at highlighting precisely these framing strategies by linking the attempt at interpretation to the attempt at writing and speaking, that is, to expression.

Hence, if one reads the two texts as attempts to find words for the experience of a disturbed sense of self in order to communicate and negotiate this experience, these attempts are constantly foregrounded and commented upon. Gilman's story and James's various journal entries thus emphasize the ongoing struggle for what Susan Sontag has called the "rhetorical ownership of the illness" (181). The act of writing and forming words and sentences thus becomes a matter of regaining a sense of self and, as Gilman put it, "recovering some measure of power" (qtd. in Golden 46). Similarly, Alice James insisted that, by writing her diary, "I shall at least have it all my own way" (*Diary* 25).

There are more similarities. Both texts are written in the first-person account of a diary. The particular format in both cases offers a space of preliminary and precarious self-writing whose narrative structure is still open and has minimal formal restraints. Through their choice of format, both Gilman and James thus insist on their own search for self-expression and a narrative self that has to depend, as Kirmayer put it, on the "inchoate" (340) as the "*prima materia* of self-understanding." As James writes in her very first entry, quoted here in full:

> I think that if I get into the habit of writing a bit about what happens, or rather doesn't happen, I may lose a little of the sense of loneliness and desolation that abides with me. My circumstances allowing of nothing but the ejaculation of one-syllabled reflections, a written monologue by that most interesting being, *myself*, may have its yet to be discovered consolations. I shall at least have it all my own way and it may bring relief as an outlet to that geyser of emotions, sensations, speculations and reflections which ferments perpetually within my poor old carcass for its sins; so here goes, my first Journal. (*Diary* 25)

The entry immediately calls attention to the *purpose* of the diary. It is meant to console, to bring relief, and to overcome the sense of desolation and loneliness that Alice James felt to be constant features of her illness experience. Moreover, the journal is meant as an "outlet" for the abundance of emotional and cognitive engagement which includes the whole gamut of (mental) experience from sensations to reflections.

The sense of an underlying purpose is important, since it gives the act of writing and narrating a frame of motivation as well as a frame of reflection—both perspectives are obviously prominent in this first as in many subsequent entries. What keeps the two perspectives engaged in a productive relation is the declaration of the central "topic" of the journal: the "most interesting being, *myself.*" The self thus occupies the central position in this programmatic statement, and it does so in its most affirmative mode as an emphatic "*my*self." Yet a careful reading of the passage also reveals that this affirmative emphasis on the self is tinged by the conditional which dominates the implicit reflection about the purpose of the writing: "*if* I get into the habit of writing . . . I *may.*" If the self thus appears situated in this passage as the centering (and controlling) instance, its position is rather precarious and preliminary in the face of a more general dynamic that relates the process of writing to the process of experience itself. The self, indeed, *may* constitute itself at the point where writing and experience *may* converge in expression. In fact, on closer inspection, the initial declaration may be seen as something like a template for many similar entries to follow. While they differ widely, of course, in content, the internal development of the entries looks surprisingly similar. At first the language is, almost invariably, declarative and descriptive, in an attempt, as it were, to set the stage for an increasingly performative rhetoric that moves away from the literal toward the literary, often concluding in strong metaphors that aim to contain the tension between experience, self, and narrative. In the first entry, this movement appears obvious in the contrast between the part before and after the appearance of "myself." The second part is dominated by two rather strong metaphors, the "geyser" and the "carcass," which are both hyperbolic in character, yet differ markedly in that the first points at a perpetuation of force while the second clearly expresses a form of decay and lifeless residue. What is most curious (and most telling) is the third metaphorical term that connects these opposites, namely, the verb "ferments." On the face of it, this seems to be a clear case of mixing metaphors—and thus a failure in rhetorical competence and finesse. Yet while the semantic field of fermentation does not easily overlap with the semantics of "geyser," the particular verb James uses does indeed capture a shared meaning that connects the two. That meaning stresses a certain "perverse" resistance to mental and corporeal decline, since fermentation as a process here connects decay with a perpetual process of proliferation—the building up and release of tension.[12] The rather peculiar metaphorical twist must be read as an oblique (or likewise "twisted") reference to James's "illness."

From the age she was nearly twenty onward, Alice James had suffered from repeated psychosomatic and depressive attacks and collapses; "violent turns of hysteria," as her father described it, which put her "on the verge of insanity and suicide" (Edel 6). In the journal which she kept during the last four years of her life, she tried to find a way to balance the recurring phases of psychosomatic seizures and breakdowns that she experienced with a particular style of narration that oscillates between associative expansion, metaphorical integration, and ironic detachment. Moreover, the diary was also written in part in response to James being diagnosed with breast cancer in 1891. Hence, the central rhetorical strategies in her illness identity work must be assessed in reference to her twofold affliction—which presents a certain embarrassment for symptomatic readings of James's *Diary* as a "hysterical narrative."[13] Thus, for instance, the obvious split or separation between her intense mental and emotional engagement (the "geyser") and the experience of physical deterioration (the "carcass"), which informs more than the initial entry of the journal, have been discussed both as proof of the body's resistance to, and its compliance with, dominant male professional (medical) discourses about female hysteria at the end of the nineteenth century. In these readings, the afflicted subjects "enact" or "perform" symptoms; they are actors who

---

[12] Similar metaphors can be found throughout Alice James's writings, for instance, the "emotional volcano" or the "bottled lightning" which actually was a metaphor used earlier by William James in a letter to his sister. Cf. Strouse 238; Yeazell 144; Dinnage 263.

[13] The concrete nature of Alice James's illness is hard to establish in terms of a definite pathology—in her own time it was called "hysteria" (a term that she herself used) or "neurasthenia." Diagnoses were as varied as treatments and there was and still is no consensus about what brought about James's afflictions. There is no doubt about a certain hereditary disposition, since both her father Henry and her two elder brothers, William and Henry, had encountered psychic disturbances of a similar nature though not to a similar degree or length of time.

might eventually become, as in the case of James, "professional invalids."[14]

The following well-known passage is a particular striking case. It describes a scene after one of James's "attacks," which had been triggered, as it were, by her plan to redraft her will and the arrival of the American consul who was to act as a witness. The appearance of the ambassador, James remembers,

> caused me to "go off" and I had to be put to bed—when the most amusing scene followed. I lay in a semi-faint, draped in as many frills as could be found for the occasion, with Nurse at my head with the thickest layer of her anxious-devoted-nurse expression on, as K. told me after, when thro' a mist I vaguely saw five black figures file into my little bower, headed by the most extraordinary little man, all gesticulation and grimace, who planted himself at the foot of the bed and stroking my knees began a long harangue to the effect that he and his wife had both "laid upon a bed of sickness" which seemed to constitute uncontrovertible reason for my immediate recovery. K. with difficulty restrained him from reading the Will aloud there and then—he has doubtless not forgiven this dam thrown across to arrest the flood of his eloquence—It was so curious for me, just like a nightmare effect and I felt as if I were assisting at the reading of my own Will, surrounded by the greedy relatives, as in novels. (*Diary* 89-90)

The passage is a particularly telling example of the way in which the relation between body and mind (or will) forms the central complication in James's illness experience and thus also in her narrative. Consequently, in many interpretations of the journal, there is a strong tendency to focus on the struggle between the two. For Kristin Boudreau, for instance, the gesture of detachment—both through the obvious irony and the reference to fiction—is strategic and aims at a position of self-control through the "staging" of the body as the other:

> [B]y separating self from body in order to assist at the reading of her own will, she removes the body from the realm of knowable selves— implying that, to the woman writing the *Diary*, the woman in bed is a stranger, a fiction, in the same way that all selves are fictions to each other. At the same time, James posits a Cartesian foundation for her own

---

[14]   Cf. Price Herndl's discussion, especially Chapter 4.

selfhood: she, after all, is the author of Will, will, event and narrative. (Boudreau 62)

Readings like these suggest a scenario in which irony as a literary strategy is employed to express and indeed enable the liberation of self from body, a way in which James could find momentary release from the continuous "fight between my body and my will," as James herself described the enormous tension that fundamentally characterized her illness experience (*Diary* 149).[15] In Boudreau's interpretation of this highly self-conscious passage, the *ironic* self appears as a paradoxical sense of self marked simultaneously by alienation and empowerment. Throughout her journal, James thus rather consciously used her considerable linguistic resources and her rhetorical versatility to effect a sense of self that appears undaunted by her bodily affliction. It is also rather clear that she saw the conflict between her will and her body as the defining aspect of her illness. Nevertheless, the question remains whether this is enough evidence to reduce the complex passage in order to turn it into a representative—or symptomatic—passage for the illness narrative as a whole. While the important function of writing, of linguistic expression and rhetorical "wit," certainly played a major role in Alice James's reflections about her illness and her self in general, to conclude that the act of writing itself was enough to cancel out experience—to write illness "out of" experience, as it were—appears a bit bold: "Writing about illness . . . allows the woman writer to separate the experience of it from herself; becoming a writer who creates narratives of illness allows her to control it, to avoid experiencing the sickness herself" (Price Herndl 128).[16] I do not question the distancing effect of irony, and neither do I doubt that writing about one's illness might be an effective way to maintain "control," however elusive that feeling of control may turn out to be. Nevertheless, I would still argue that the use of irony complicates the notion of control considerably and that, moreover, writing *about* illness experience is not (and cannot be) aimed at avoidance but rather at reconciliation. In the case of Alice

---

[15] For similar readings of the performative aspect of illness in James's text, cf. Koch 60-64; for another reading that emphasizes the role of the "hysterical" body, cf. Bronfen; Cappello; Price Herndl; Hoffman.

[16] Cf. also Hoffman.

James's *Diary*, this becomes rather obvious considering the fact that irony certainly is a rather dominant yet by no means exclusive strategy for negotiating a sense of self in the face of her illness. More importantly, detachment by irony can never become an exclusive mode of writing, since then detachment would lose its particular object and become universal. That is to say that if irony addresses a certain moment of illness experience (like a seizure) the target of irony is not the experience itself but its stereotypical reception and thus its "symptomatic" reading. This difference becomes quite clear in the passage about the will, where, above all, it is the reaction of the American official that is being ridiculed by the ironic description: "the most extraordinary little man, all gesticulation and grimace." The main point, however, is that irony cannot unfold its effects *without* simultaneously acknowledging the reality of the experience or object it is meant to target. As a strategy of detachment and control, it is aimed not at avoidance but containment, not absolute control, but coexistence. Irony does not "write out" experience but re-inscribes experience as overstated, dramatized, and fictionalized precisely in its conventional and symptomatic reception. The ironic self thus presents a problem to any fully symptomatic reading of the text, since it is meant to escape the authority of any other mode of narrating the self.

Compared to the use of irony in Alice James's journal, such a conscious strategy is conspicuously absent from Charlotte Perkins Gilman's "The Yellow Wallpaper." When we find irony in the journal of the unnamed heroine in Gilman's story, it appears a rather unconscious reaction than a consciously adopted "voice" or attitude. Reading the narratives side by side, one would thus get the impression that James's illness narrative is characterized by self-assertion, in contrast to Gilman's narrative, which is so full of self-alienation and self-destruction. The absence of forms of ironic distance or detachment add to the strong "symptomatic" effect of Gilman's fiction; i.e., the impression that what is being described comes rather close to the actual experience of the mental disturbance and the loss of self that the author in fact suffered while undergoing a "rest cure" as a treatment for her depression.[17] At first sight, the difference between James's and Gilman's illness narratives may appear simply the result of the genre used in each case. After all, James is writing a biographical account of her illness experience without using fictional elements. Even though one could certainly argue that some of her rhetorical strategies assume the form or features of fictional narratives (especially, of course, in the passage discussed above), there is hardly any confusion about the fact that the author of the narrative and the protagonist in the narrative are one and the same person. In fact, without this general assumption, the ironic detachment which allows for the self watching the self as another (and yet, as I have argued, never denying or denouncing it as "other") would not work at all.

In contrast, one essential assumption about genre that Gilman's strategies build on is that the author and the main character are not the same person. In reading the story, this assumption is somewhat weakened by the use of the first-person narrative: The personal journal format not only invites Gilman's readers to identify with the narrator, but also allows them to invest this affective identification in interpreting the narrator's voice as Gilman's own. Yet this does not revoke the initial assumption; indeed, it remains the essential frame for two complementary modes of identification that are constantly addressed by Gilman's narrative strategies. The major result is that one can read and interpret the story in two rather different ways: as an exemplary story of the destruction of mind and self, and as the opposite, a story of resisting the destruction of mind and self.[18] Of course, most readers and critics would claim that "The Yellow Wallpaper" ultimately represents both options, and that there would be no contradiction in reading the story both ways. I agree, yet my point is that this is only possible because Gilman's choice of genre enforces an essential distinction between

---

[17] For a comprehensive study of the biographical and medical contexts and Gilman's motivation for writing the story, cf. Horowitz. As Julie Bates Dock has pointed out, the reception of Gilman's story has been rather controversial; the feminist readings after Gilman's "re-discovery" in the 1970s, which led to the canonization of the story, have in particular turned on what I call the "symptomatic" performance of loss of self and the descent into "madness" that forms the major strategy of Gilman's illness narrative.

[18] For an example that combines both readings in one discussion, cf. Quawas.

narrator and real author that she then undermines through her narrative strategies. The weakening of the basic fictional framing is intentional, and it increases the effect and the force of the story tremendously. Due to Gilman's particular strategies, these effects are easily accepted as an expression of the intensity of authentic phenomenal experience, to the point where the narrative becomes horrifying and almost unbearable, indeed "too terribly good to be printed," as William Dean Howells declared.[19] Howells's assessment also reminds us that Gilman consciously used devices from established literary traditions and genres, like the gothic tale and the horror story, in order to increase the effect of her illness narrative on her audience. But Gilman also carefully embedded these literary elements in a narrative structure which builds on the increasing tension between the experience of self and the act of narrating. In fact, one could argue that the horror which unfolds in "The Yellow Wallpaper" is less connected to the experience of a loss of self due to illness but rather to what appears as the excessive power of narrative to create, project, and control selves. In a way, this is implied in the very form that Gilman uses for the narrative of the unnamed woman, since the diary is an obvious means of interrogating (i.e., questioning as well as affirming) one's self-experience with the help of language. In Gilman's story, the diary is specifically introduced as an act of resistance against the restrictions of the "rest cure," and thus as the only means of (linguistic) self-assertion. The secret diary is also the medium in which both the narrator and her confidants, the readers, become increasingly trapped. The narrative format is as much a mode of confinement as the room with the yellow wallpaper in which the woman is forced to stay during the cure. The framing is echoed by the story within the story, which emerges after the woman discovers another, unnamed, woman "trapped" behind the hideous arabesque pattern of the wallpaper. This narrative becomes more and more dominant as the identification between the two female figures increases. Moreover, the discovery clearly invigorates the main character by giving her a sense of agency and purpose—even if her motivation is clearly delusional. All

---

[19] Cf. Shumaker, who also quotes the *Atlantic Monthly* editor who declined to publish Gilman's story in 1890: "I could not forgive myself if I made others as miserable as I have made myself" (588).

these devices—the diary, the confinement of the room, the wallpaper, the woman behind the wallpaper, the narrative of entrapment, and the concept of liberation—are carefully chosen to impress a chain of identification which connects the actual reader to the fictional character in the same way as it connects the actual character to the trapped woman, a delusion as real for the patient as the patient is for the reader.[20] Yet even this obvious artificiality of Gilman's illness narrative does not prevent most interpretations from assuming that the particular force and nature of the delusions are solidly based on Gilman's own experience. In this way, "fictional" symptoms can be treated as authentic and representative.

This brings me to my last point, the particular challenge fictional illness narratives pose to the concept of narrative and self in the medical humanities. Autobiographical narratives of illness experience are often referred to in order to point out the fundamental function and form of narratives in connection to disturbances of the sense of self that come with severe illnesses. Even fictional accounts may be able to give helpful insights into the disturbing phenomenological dimensions of mental illness, since, as Paul Crawford and Charley Baker have suggested, literature can give particularly effective expression to a self struggling for a narrative. For both assertions, Gilman's story appears a rather convincing example, since it could be read as a textbook illustration for a psychopathological narrative form that violates the "necessary conditions" for the non-pathological self-narratives described by Gallagher ("Pathologies").[21]

And yet, I would insist, the fictional status of Gilman's narrative is essential. For one thing, to lose sight of the careful construction, the particular narrative strategies, and above all the intention that drives

---

[20] "In non-fictional narrative detail is selected from pre-existing facts, in fictional narrative detail is created" (Lamarque 130). The wallpaper has been a particularly effective device to encourage readings to move beyond the autobiographical context of the illness narrative at the core of Gilman's story; cf. Roth for a discussion and a critique of some of these readings.

[21] For a description of typical psychopathological narrative forms, cf. Dimaggio and Semerari. In this regard, it may also be noticed that Gilman's story was praised as a rather convincing description of a specific psychopathology by one of its contemporary readers.

these strategies would mean to reduce the story's full potential and significance as a work of the imagination. Even though Gilman herself did not want to look at "The Yellow Wallpaper" as a piece of literature,[22] and though most readings have stressed the critical and political motivation that made its author write a story with a purpose beyond mere entertainment, it is obvious that the story was *strategically* written as a fiction, and that it employs the repertoire of literary devices and traditions with great success.

Moreover, the choice of the fictional mode allows Gilman to fully unfold the ambivalence of the narrative self—an ambivalence that challenges both the understanding of narrative as a therapeutic device, and its counterpart, which criticizes the normative, repressive power of narratives. This ambivalence mirrors the latent contradiction between illness identity work in patients' self-narratives and the symptomatic classification of self-experience in prodrome research. In the critical reception of "The Yellow Wallpaper," the ambivalence is demonstrated above all by the conflicting interpretations of the story's conclusion. The image of the "creeping woman" at the end has been read both as a symbol of defeat and as a "triumph" of female self-assertion over male repression—particularly since the woman creeps over the body of her husband/doctor, who fainted when he finally faces his wife's "descent into madness."

In light of my discussion, I would tend to interpret Gilman's ending as being as self-assertive as James's strategy of ironic detachment. However, Gilman's ending must be read as an inversion of the strategy used by James. One of the main techniques Gilman's short story employs is the shift between present and past tense—this, of course, is nothing unusual for the journal form, since it may combine and mix the account of present and immediate sensations and the relation of past actions and events. In Gilman's story, the difference between past and present tense is also maintained as the dividing line or cognitive boundary between the personal illness experience and its official interpretations, since almost throughout, the woman's sufferings and delusions are told in the present tense while her interaction with her

---

[22] Cf. Shumaker 599.

husband and their communication about the illness are related in past tense:

> I don't know why I should write this.
> I don't want to.
> I don't feel able. And I know John would think it absurd. But I must say what I feel and think in some way—it is such a relief! . . .
> It is so hard to talk with John about my case, because he is so wise, and because he loves me so.
> But I tried it last night. . . .
> John was asleep and I hated to waken him, so I kept still and watched the moonlight on that undulating wallpaper till I felt creepy. ("Wallpaper" 651-52)

While the present tense is thus the narrative time of illness experience, the narrative proper follows the convention of "proper" prose narrative—the space of representation and interpretation. At the end of the story, this separation collapses to the point of inversion. First, the action of the present tense (the illness experience) is immediately continued in the past tense (the space of narrative), which has a curious double effect since the illness experience both loses its intimate immediacy (of the secret journal entry) and becomes conventional—yet it also takes over the entire remaining narrative space:

> It is so pleasant to be out in this great room and creep around as I please! . . . Why there's John at the door!
> It is no use, young man, you can't open it!
> How he does call and pound!
> Now he's crying for an axe.
> It would be a shame to break down that beautiful door!
> "John dear!" *said* I in the gentlest voice, "the key is down by the front steps, under a plantain leaf!" (656; my emphasis)

By conventionalizing narrative time at its closure, the story also reinstates the difference between the narrator of the illness experience and the actual author of the text. It thus emphasizes the fictional status of the narrative, and it also revokes any ties to the biographical experience. On the level of the fictional illness narrative, the ending may be read as the ultimate loss of self or as the triumph of narrative; for the author herself, it certainly marked a definite point of closure.

Works Cited

Allen, Judith A. *The Feminism of Charlotte Perkins Gilman: Sexualities, Histories, Progressivism.* Chicago: U of Chicago P, 2009. Print.

Angus, Lynn E., and John McLeod, eds. *The Handbook of Narrative and Psychotherapy.* London: Sage, 2004. Print.

Aviv, Rachel. "Which Way Madness Lies: Can Psychosis Be Prevented?" *Harper's Magazine* Dec. 2010: 35-46. Print.

Boudreau, Kristin. "'A Barnum Monstrosity': Alice James and the Spectacle of Sympathy." *American Literature* 65.1 (1993): 53-67. Print.

Bronfen, Elisabeth. "Perversion, Hysterie und die Schrift: Poes 'Berenice' und die Tagebuchaufzeichnungen von Alice James." *Amerikastudien / American Studies* 37.3 (1992): 451-70. Print.

Bruner, Jerome S. *Making Stories: Law, Literature, Life.* Cambridge: Harvard UP, 2002. Print.

---. *Actual Minds, Possible Worlds.* Cambridge: Harvard UP, 1987. Print.

Bury, Mike. "Illness Narratives: Fact or Fiction?" *Sociology of Health and Illness* 23.3 (2001): 263-85. Print.

Bürgy, Martin. "The Concept of Psychosis: Historical and Phenomenological Aspects." *Schizophrenia Bulletin* 34.6 (2008): 1200-10. Print.

Cappello, Mary. "Alice James: 'Neither Dead nor Recovered.'" *American Imago* 45.2 (1988): 127-62. Print.

Clark, Hilary, ed. *Depression and Narrative: Telling the Dark.* Albany: State U of New York P, 2008. Print.

Corcoran, Cheryl, Dolores Malaspina, and Laura Hercher. "Prodromal Interventions for Schizophrenia Vulnerability: The Risks of Being 'At Risk.'" *Schizophrenia Research* 73.2-3 (2005): 173-84. Print.

Corrigan, Patrick W., and Amy C. Watson. "The Paradox of Self-Stigma and Mental Illness." *Clinical Psychology: Science and Practice* 9.1 (2002): 35-53. Print.

Crawford, Paul, and Charley Baker. "Literature and Madness: Fiction for Students and Professionals." *Journal of Medical Humanities* 30.4 (2009): 237-51. Print.

Cutter, Martha J. "The Writer as Doctor: New Models of Medical Discourse in Charlotte Perkins Gilman's Later Fiction." *Literature and Medicine* 20.2 (2001): 151-82. Print.

Damasio, Antonio. *Descartes' Error*. New York: Harper, 1994. Print.

Davis, Cynthia J. *Charlotte Perkins Gilman: A Biography*. Stanford: Stanford UP, 2010. Print.

Davis, Cynthia J., and Denise D. Knight. *Charlotte Perkins Gilman and Her Contemporaries: Literary and Intellectual Contexts*. Tuscaloosa: U of Alabama P, 2004. Print.

Dennett, Daniel C. "The Self as a Center of Narrative Gravity." *Self and Consciousness: Multiple Perspectives*. Ed. Frank S. Kessel, Pamela M. Cole, and Dale L. Johnson. Hillsdale: Erlbaum, 1992. 103-15. Print.

Dimaggio, Giancarlo, and Antonio Semerari. "Psychopathological Narrative Forms." *Journal of Constructivist Psychology* 14.1 (2001): 1-23. Print.

Dinnage, Rosemary. *Alone! Alone! Lives of Some Outsider Women*. New York: New York Review of Books, 2004. Print.

Dock, Julie Bates. "The Legend of 'The Yellow Wall-paper.'" *Charlotte Perkins Gilman's "The Yellow Wall-Paper" and the History of Its Publication and Reception: A Critical Edition and Documentary Casebook*. Ed. Dock. University Park: Pennsylvania State UP, 1998. 1-26. Print.

Donald, Merlin. *Origins of the Modern Mind: Three Stages in the Evolution of Culture and Cognition*. Cambridge: Harvard UP, 1993. Print.

Duquette, Elizabeth. "'A New Claim for the Family Renown': Alice James and the Picturesque." *ELH* 72.3 (2005): 717-45. Print.

Edel, Leon. "Portrait of Alice James." *The Diary of Alice James*. 1964. Ed. Edel. Boston: Northeastern UP, 1999. 1-21. Print.

Engel, John D., et al., eds. *Narrative in Health Care*. London: Radcliffe, 2008. Print.

Estroff, Sue E., et al. "Everybody's Got a Little Mental Illness: Accounts of Illness and Self Among People with Severe, Persistent Mental Illnesses." *Medical Anthropology Quarterly* ns 5.4 (1991): 331-69. Print.

Flynn, Deborah. "Narratives of Melancholy: A Humanities Approach to Depression." *Medical Humanities* 36.1 (2010): 36-39. Print.

Frank, Arthur W. "The Rhetoric of Self-Change: Illness Experience as Narrative." *Sociological Quarterly* 34.1 (1993): 39-52. Print.

Gallagher, Shaun. *Models of the Self*. Exeter: Imprint, 2000. Print.

---. "Pathologies in Narrative Structures." *Royal Institute of Philosophy Supplement* 60.1 (2007): 203-24. Print.

360   Peter Schneck

---, and Dan Zahavi. *The Phenomenological Mind*. London: Routledge, 2008. Print.

Gilman, Charlotte Perkins. "The Yellow Wall-Paper." *New England Magazine* 11.5 (1892): 647-56. Print.

Gilman, Charlotte Perkins, and Julie Bates Dock. *Charlotte Perkins Gilman's "The Yellow Wall-Paper" and the History of Its Publication and Reception: A Critical Edition and Documentary Casebook*. Ed. Julie Bates Dock. University Park: Pennsylvania State UP, 1998. Print.

Golden, Catherine J. *Charlotte Perkins Gilman's The Yellow Wall-Paper: A Sourcebook*. New York: Routledge, 2004. Print.

Haroun, Nasra, et al. "Risk and Protection in Prodromal Schizophrenia: Ethical Implications for Clinical Practice and Future Research." *Schizophrenia Bulletin* 32.1 (2006): 166-78. Print.

Hill, Mary A. *Charlotte Perkins Gilman: The Making of a Radical Feminist, 1860-1896*. Philadelphia: Temple UP, 1980. Print.

Hoffman, Anne Golomb. "Is Psychoanalysis a Poetics of the Body?" *American Imago* 63.4 (2006): 395-422. Print.

Hohwy, Jakob. "The Sense of Self in the Phenomenology of Agency and Perception." *Psyche* 13.1 (2007): 1-20. Print.

Horowitz, Helen Lefkowitz. *Wild Unrest: Charlotte Perkins Gilman and the Making of "The Yellow Wall-Paper."* New York: Oxford UP, 2010. Print.

Hurwitz, Brian, Trisha Greenhalgh, and Vieda Skultans. *Narrative Research in Health and Illness*. Malden: BMJ/Blackwell, 2004. Print.

Hutto, Daniel D., ed. *Narrative and Understanding Persons*. Cambridge: Cambridge UP, 2007. Print.

James, Alice. *The Diary of Alice James*. 1964. Ed. Leon Edel. Boston: Northeastern UP, 1999.

Kircher, Tilo, and Anthony S. David. *The Self in Neuroscience and Psychiatry*. Cambridge: Cambridge UP, 2003. Print.

Kirmayer, Laurence J. "The Body's Insistence on Meaning: Metaphor as Presentation and Representation in Illness Experience." *Medical Anthropology Quarterly* ns 6.4 (1992): 323-46. Print.

Kleinman, Arthur. *The Illness Narratives: Suffering, Healing, and the Human Condition*. New York: Basic, 1989. Print.

Koch, Lisa M. "Bodies as Stage Props: Enacting Hysteria in the Diaries of Charlotte Forten Grimké and Alice James." *Legacy: A Journal of American Women Writers* 15.1 (1998): 59-64. Print.

Kreiswirth, Martin. "Merely Telling Stories? Narrative and Knowledge in the Human Sciences." *Poetics Today* 21.2 (2000): 293-318. Print.

---. "Trusting the Tale: The Narrativist Turn in the Human Sciences." *New Literary History* 23.3 (1992): 629-57. Print.

Lamarque, Peter. "On the Distance between Literary Narratives and Real-Life Narratives." *Royal Institute of Philosophy Supplement* 60 (2007): 117-32. Print.

Maher, Jane. *Biography of Broken Fortunes: Wilkie and Bob, Brothers of William, Henry, and Alice James*. Hamden: Archon, 1986. Print.

Martinsen, Elin Håkonsen, and Jan Helge Solbakk. "Illness as a Condition of Our Existence in the World: On Illness and Pathic Existence." *Medical Humanities* (2012): 1-6. *JMH Online*. 2 Jan. 2012. Web. 21 May 2012.

Mesa, James P., and Daniel S. Passerman, eds. *Integrating Narrative Medicine and Evidence-Based Medicine*. London: Radcliffe, 2011. Print.

Nelson, Barnaby, et al. "The Phenomenological Critique and Self-Disturbance: Implications for Ultra-High Risk ('Prodrome') Research." *Schizophrenia Bulletin* 34.2 (2008): 381-92. Print.

Nelson, Katherine. "Narrative and Self, Myth and Memory: Emergence of the Cultural Self." *Autobiographical Memory and the Construction of a Narrative Self*. Ed. Robyn Fivush and Catherine A. Haden. Mahwah: Erlbaum, 2003. 3-28. Print.

Parnas, Josef, et al. "EASE: Examination of Anomalous Self-Experience." *Psychopathology* 38.5 (2005): 236-58. Print.

Polkinghorne, Donald E. "Narrative and Self-Concept." *Journal of Narrative and Life History* 1.2 (1991): 135-53. Print.

Price Herndl, Diane. *Invalid Women: Figuring Feminine Illness in American Fiction and Culture, 1840-1940*. Chapel Hill: U of North Carolina P, 1993. Print.

Quawas, Rula. "A New Woman's Journey into Insanity: Descent and Return in *The Yellow Wallpaper*." *Journal of the Australasian Universities Modern Language Association* 105 (2006): 35-53. Print.

Rabuzzi, Kathryn Allen. "Editor's Column." *Literature and Medicine* 1.1 (1982): ix-x. Print.

Radden, Jennifer. "My Symptoms, Myself: Reading Mental Illness Memoirs for Identity Assumptions." *Depression and Narrative: Telling the Dark.* Ed. Hilary Clark. Albany: State U of New York P, 2008. 15-28. Print.

Radley, Alan. "The Aesthetics of Illness: Narrative, Horror and the Sublime." *Sociology of Health and Illness* 21.6 (1999): 778-96. Print.

Rasmussen, Barbara. "Alice James and the Question of Women's Exile." *Renaissance and Modern Studies* 34 (1991): 45-63. Print.

Ratcliffe, Matthew. *Feelings of Being: Phenomenology, Psychiatry and the Sense of Reality.* Oxford: Oxford UP, 2008. Print.

Rimmon-Kenan, Shlomith. "What Can Narrative Theory Learn From Illness Narratives?" *Literature and Medicine* 25.2 (2006): 241-54. Print.

Roth, Marty. "Gilman's Arabesque Wallpaper." *Mosaic* 34.4 (2001): 145-62. Print.

Rudd, Jill, and Val Gough. *Charlotte Perkins Gilman: Optimist Reformer.* Iowa City: U of Iowa P, 1999. Print.

Sass, Louis A., and Josef Parnas. "Schizophrenia, Consciousness, and the Self." *Schizophrenia Bulletin* 29.3 (2003): 427-44. Print.

Schechtman, Maya. "The Narrative Self." *The Oxford Handbook to the Self.* Ed. Shaun Gallagher. Oxford: Oxford UP, 2011. 394-418. Print.

Shumaker, Conrad. "'Too Terribly Good to Be Printed': Charlotte Gilman's 'The Yellow Wallpaper.'" *American Literature* 57.4 (1985): 588-99. Print.

Sontag, Susan. *Illness as Metaphor and AIDS and Its Metaphors.* New York: Anchor, 1989. Print.

Strouse, Jean. *Alice James: A Biography.* Boston: Houghton, 1980. Print.

Treichler, Paula A. "Escaping the Sentence: Diagnosis and Discourse in 'The Yellow Wallpaper.'" *Tulsa Studies in Women's Literature* 3.1-2 (1984): 61-77. Print.

Weinman, John, Keith J. Petrie, Rona Moss-Morris, and Rob Horne. "The Illness Perception Questionnaire: A New Method for Assessing the Cognitive Representation of Illness." *Psychology and Health* 11.3 (2007): 431-45. Print.

Yeazell, Ruth Bernard. *The Death and Letters of Alice James.* Berkeley: U of California P, 1982. Print.

Zahavi, Dan. *Exploring the Self: Philosophical and Psychopathological Perspectives on Self-Experience.* Amsterdam: Benjamins, 2000. Print.

---. "Self and Other: The Limits of Narrative Understanding." *Royal Institute of Philosophy Supplement* 60 (2007): 179-201. Print.

---. "Being Someone." *Psyche* 11.5 (2005): 1-20. Print.

---. "Phenomenology of Self." *The Self in Neuroscience and Psychiatry*. Ed. Tilo Kircher and Anthony S. David. Cambridge: Cambridge UP, 2003. 56-75. Print.

ANNA THIEMANN

Shaking Patterns of Diagnosis:
Siri Hustvedt and Charlotte Perkins Gilman

> It is the strangest yellow, that wall-
> paper! . . . But there is something else
> about that paper—the smell! . . . The
> only thing I can think of that it is like is
> the *color* of the paper! A yellow smell.
> (Gilman, "The Yellow Wallpaper" 265)

> [L]ike envy, resentment, class snobbery,
> or racism, sexual prejudice can be
> smelled like an odor in the room, and if
> the smell gets too strong, it prompts a
> fantasy to escape.
> (Hustvedt, "Being a Man" 96)

In their landmark feminist study, *The Madwoman in the Attic* (1979), Sandra M. Gilbert and Susan Gubar present Charlotte Perkins Gilman's short story "The Yellow Wallpaper" (1892) as a "paradigmatic tale . . . *the* story that all literary women would tell if they could speak their 'speechless woe'" (89). According to Gilbert and Gubar, this woe begins when a woman writer realizes her "parallel confinements in texts, houses, and maternal female bodies" (89), and it ends when she manages to "escape from her textual/architectural" (91) prison. Condemned to stay in the former nursery of an "ancestral" mansion to cure her "temporary nervous depression," Gilman's narrator not only writes a diary against her husband's will but also joins her imaginary double in "shaking" and ultimately destroying the pattern of the room's wallpaper, which seems to symbolize the oppressive structures of patriarchal society ("The Yellow Wallpaper" 255).[1]

While some feminist critics have applauded and confirmed Gilbert and Gubar's reading of "The Yellow Wallpaper," others have found it necessary to caution against their universalizing approach. In her review of *The Madwoman in the Attic*, Mary Jacobus criticizes the authors' "Story of the Woman Writer" (517) as a "reductive" (518) myth that is characterized by an "anxiety of authority" and a "desire for wholeness" (519). Jacobus regards Gilbert and Gubar's repetitive and "repressive" interpretation of women's writing as "evasive at the cost of a freedom which twentieth-century women poets have eagerly sought: the freedom of being read as more than exceptionally articulate victims of a patriarchally engendered plot" (522). Similarly, Janice Haney-Peritz has warned of "the side-effects such a monumental reading may have on feminist literary criticism" (121). She diagnoses that, since the publication of *The Madwoman in the Attic*,

> Gilman's short story has assumed monumental proportions, serving at one and the same time the purposes of a memorial and a boundary marker. As a memorial, "The Yellow Wallpaper" is used to remind contemporary readers of the enduring import of the feminist struggle against patriarchal domination; while as a boundary marker, it is used to demarcate the territory appropriate to a feminist literary criticism. (114)

During the last four decades, feminist critics and women writers have continued to resist Gilbert and Gubar's dubious prescription. In the postfeminist era, theorists and authors have not only rejected female victimhood but also insisted on a redefinition of feminism and

---

[1] The notion that Gilman's narrative constitutes a "feminist document" (124) was first put forth by Elaine Hedges. In her influential afterword to the 1973 Feminist Press edition of "The Yellow Wallpaper," Hedges further argues that "the paper symbolizes [the narrator's] situation as seen by the men who control her" (130), a view that was to be confirmed by later critics. Jean E. Kennard, for instance, points out that "[t]he restrictions on women . . . [are] echoed in the patterns of the room's yellow wallpaper" (75).

femininity.[2] Challenging the division of theory and practice, the American essayist and novelist Siri Hustvedt has recently published what I propose to read as a postfeminist reiteration of Gilman's "mistress-plot" (Jacobus 517). *The Shaking Woman, Or: A History of My Nerves* (2010), a hybrid work that is part essay and part autobiographical memoir, plays with the expectations of a "traditional" feminist audience, turning the anxiety of authority into self-determination, and the "desire for wholeness" into multiplicity. Hustvedt evokes Gilman's short story to emphasize her critical engagement with her literary and academic predecessors. To prove these hypotheses, my essay will first provide a brief—and inevitably simplified—overview of the multifaceted postfeminist movement. Secondly, I will substantiate my claim that Siri Hustvedt can be regarded as a representative of this new paradigm, and, thirdly and finally, I will focus on Hustvedt's reconstruction of the mad woman writer in *The Shaking Woman*.

Similar to postmodernism (cf. Hutcheon), the term postfeminism "has become overloaded with different meanings" (Gill 147), and the relationship between postfeminism and its predecessor, second-wave feminism, has come to be defined in terms of rupture and continuity (cf. Genz and Brabon 2-10). According to Sarah Projansky, "postfeminism is by definition contradictory, simultaneously feminist and antifeminist, liberating and repressive, productive and obstructive of progressive social change" (68). Since the 1980s, postfeminism has been associated with such contradictory paradigms as backlash and new traditionalism, girl power, cyberfeminism, and micropolitics. The first mentioning of the term dates back much further to the heyday of the New Woman movement in the early twentieth century. As Nancy F. Cott notes in *The Grounding of Modern Feminism* (1987):

> [A]lready in 1919 a group of female literary radicals in Greenwich Village—the very grassroots of feminism—had founded a new journal on the thinking, "we're interested in people now—not men and women." They declared that moral, social, economic, and political standards

---

[2]   Stephanie Harzewski and Rosalind Gill and Elena Herdieckerhoff use the term "chick lit" to designate postfeminist novels of the 1990s and 2000s. An overview of sociological, media, literary, and cultural theoretical perspectives on postfeminism will be given in the next section of this essay.

"should not have anything to do with sex," promised to be "pro-woman without being anti-man," and called their stance "post-feminist." (282)

I agree with Stéphanie Genz and Benjamin A. Brabon that the prefix "post" in this quote is to be understood "in evolutionary terms as a progression of feminist ideals" (10). Early postfeminism presumed (or anticipated) gender equality as the eventual outcome of first-wave feminism and envisioned a new era in which feminists would no longer have to fight against men. At the same time, the quote dismantles the postfeminist blindness to race and class and, thus, its underlying elitism. This and the fact that U.S. women's suffrage was only achieved in 1920 and equal pay—if only in theory—in 1963 point to the naivety and potential danger of this early proclamation. But postfeminism nonetheless figures as white women's tentative adjustment to a new social order rather than as a hostile backlash against feminism. This notion of a backlash is precisely what sociologists, as well as media and cultural theorists, tend to associate with the contemporary re-emergence of postfeminism. When the term reappeared in the 1980s, it seemed to have acquired a new meaning (cf. Brooks 2). Its sweeping comeback began in 1982, when *The New York Times* printed Susan Bolotin's article about "Voices from the Post-Feminist Generation." Bolotin's autobiographical and sociological essay deals with women's declining interest in the feminist movement, thus predicting its demise rather than its transformation and continuation. The majority of women who were interviewed for the article expressed the view that feminists were grim, man-hating lesbians or would be regarded and stigmatized as such, which rendered the movement highly unattractive. Bolotin's fatal diagnosis turned out to become the dominant reading of postfeminism as a media and pop culture phenomenon, which engendered texts such as *Bridget Jones's Diary*, *Ally McBeal*, or *Sex and the City* as well as various postfeminist pamphlets in the 1990s.

Representatives of the movement like Naomi Wolf, Katie Roiphe, Natasha Walter, and Rene Denfeld see feminism as an oppressive ideology that insists on female victimhood and limits individual agency. Roiphe, for instance, became weary of what she calls the "rape-crisis movement" (44) or "rape-crisis feminism" (62) of the 1970s and 80s, which caused several U.S. universities to enact laws for dating practices and sexual encounters, thereby recasting women in the role of passive and asexual victims. Other postfeminists like Wolf argue that gender equality is no longer an issue, as the current generation of women does in fact have the power of self-realization and simply needs to exploit it. Like Roiphe, Wolf renounces female victimhood as a unifying political factor and proposes to replace it with "power feminism," which envisions women as "unapologetically sexual," "free-thinking," "plea-sure-loving" and "self-assertive" (148, 180). Detractors of post-feminism condemn this discourse as elitist and apolitical, seeing it as a dangerous threat to the ongoing feminist struggle. They regard postfem-inism as a mere market phenomenon that promises women that they can "have it all" while reconstituting them as mere consumers of fashion, pills, and cosmetic surgery (cf. Coppock, Haydon, and Richter 26). Furthermore, postfeminist practices seem to be reserved for affluent Western women, thus operating at the expense of other, less privileged groups. Or, as Yvonne Tasker and Diane Negra put it, "postfeminism is white and middle class by default, anchored in consumption as a strategy (and leisure as a site) for the production of the self" (2). Yet, not all critics of contemporary postfeminism subscribe to the rupture thesis; some theorists choose to reinvigorate the early twentieth-century meaning and interpretation of the term instead. Scholars like Genz and Brabon read the postfeminist interrogation of second-wave feminism as a "sign that the women's movement is continuously in process, trans-forming and changing itself." For them, postfeminism "signal[s] a generational shift in feminist thinking and in understanding social relations between men and women, beyond traditional feminist politics and its supposed threat to heterosexual relationships" (11). Accordingly, they arrive at a largely positive reading of postfeminist individualism, (consumer) choice and self-rule:

> In its most constructive sense, postfeminism offers a different conceptual model to understand political and critical practice—it is not so much a depoliticisation or trivialisation of feminism as an active reinterpretation of contemporary forms of critique and politics that take into account the diverse agency positions of individuals today. (Genz and Brabon 33)

A key reason for Genz and Brabon's positive conception of postfeminism lies in the fact that their study covers not only the popular "backlash and new traditionalism" but also its academic counterpart comprising "queer (post)feminism," "cyber-postfeminism," and "third wave feminism." Yet, most critics of postfeminism insist on distinguishing between the two. For them, popular postfeminism designates a blind and antifeminist trust in gender equality and girl power that came to dominate public discourse in the 1980s and 1990s. Academic postfeminism, on the other hand, refers to a new generation of feminist critics including theorists like Gayatri Spivak, bell hooks, or Judith Butler, who have internalized the lessons of postmodernism and postcolonialism with their deconstructionist politics of difference (cf. Brooks 4). Depending on which discourse critics deem more relevant, they will regard postfeminism either as hostile to second-wave feminism or as the latter's reformed successor.

In view of this overwhelming complexity, Rosalind Gill has lamented "the difficulty of specifying with any rigour the features of postfeminism," which entails the obvious "problem of applying current notions to any particular cultural or media analysis" (148). To overcome these problems, and in an attempt to preserve "the contradictory nature of postfeminist discourses and the entanglement of both feminist and anti-feminist themes within them," she proposes to abandon period-ization and theorization for the recognition of postfeminism as a distinctive "sensibility" or cultural matrix that comprises various themes:

> These include the notion that femininity is a bodily property; the shift from objectification to subjectification; the emphasis upon self-surveillance, monitoring and discipline: a focus upon individualism, choice and empowerment; the dominance of a makeover paradigm; a resurgence in ideas of natural sexual difference; a marked sexualization of culture; and an emphasis upon consumerism and the commodification of difference. (Gill 149)

Gill's pragmatist interest in the question "What makes a text postfeminist?" (148) is highly important for my study, as the label "postfeminist" has so far not been applied to Siri Hustvedt's writing. At the same time, I see Hustvedt's work as more than a mere pop culture phenomenon to be analyzed and categorized, as it also displays a theorist's critical reflection upon the feminist movement. I argue that this double perspective allows Hustvedt's work to crystalize the multi-faceted aspects of postfeminism.

Siri Hustvedt appears to be the perfect embodiment of the ambiguous postfeminist self. A married writer with a Ph.D. in English and, as some critics feel compelled to note, "an icy blonde with the beauty of a Swedish film star" (Wilson), she seems destined to negotiate popular and academic conceptions of postfeminist identity. Mischa Honeck observes that Hustvedt has reinvigorated the "daring and fearless *young heroine*" (169; my translation) of late nineteenth-century fiction, endowing her with characteristics that fit the postindustrial era of late twentieth- and early twenty-first-century America. The major themes of her writing include issues of postmodern identity, "female eroticism and self-determination, as well as the relationship between life and art" (168; my translation). This observation resonates with the notion that the contemporary rise of postfeminism involves a re-emergence and transformation of the "new woman" of Gilman's generation.[3] Meanwhile, Hustvedt's non-fictional writing about cross-dressing and female sexuality has prompted questions such as: "Is it possible for a woman in the twentieth century to endorse the corset and at the same time approach with authority what it is like to be a man?" (*A Plea for Eros*, jacket notes).

Hustvedt's postfeminist redefinition of femininity approximates and combines both academic and popular notions of gender identity. After all, her work bears traces of such diverse critics as Judith Butler and Katie Roiphe. In her essay "Being a Man" (2003), for instance, Hustvedt reiterates Butler's criticism of sex assignment:

> Despite the optimism of some researchers, where biology ends and culture begins is probably a question beyond science. Even infants, whose borderless existence makes the question of sexual identity seem absurd from the inside, have been born into a world in which the boy/girl question is crucial from the outside, is the first question asked after birth: "Is it a boy or a girl?" In other words, before they know, we know. And what we know is part of a vast symbolic landscape in which the lines are drawn between one thing and another in the linguistic act of naming. (97)

---

[3] Discussing femininity and postmodernism, Janet Lee notes that "the term 'new woman' seems to appear with nearly every generation—from the 'new woman' of the late nineteenth century, who so shocked society with her 'independence,' to that of the present day, who so preoccupies the theorists of 'post-feminism'" (168).

In *Gender Trouble* (1990), Butler asks even more radically: "Are there ever humans who are not, as it were, always already gendered? The mark of gender appears to 'qualify' bodies as human bodies; the moment in which an infant becomes humanized is when the question 'is it a boy or a girl?' is answered" (111). In other instances, as in her essay "Eight Days in a Corset" (1996), Hustvedt follows Butler in stressing the performative aspects of identity, claiming it to be "easy to play at being a man, as easy as playing at being a woman" (92). At the same time, however, Hustvedt does not doubt biological determinism and sexual difference. Musing on how her body changed and controlled her sense of self during pregnancy, she insists that "[s]ex and birth are both culturally constructed and facts of nature" (*The Shaking Woman* 184). Hustvedt is very explicit about her interest in biological explanations of human behavior, to the point where she comes close to breaching her alliance with postfeminist constructionists like Butler:

> The recent fashion for social construction—the study of how ideas are formed in a culture and shape our thought—has spawned innumerable books with titles such as *The Social Construction of X* and *The Invention of Y*. Often these books have a political agenda. By revealing how the idea of womanhood, for example, has been "constructed" and "reconstructed" over time, it may be possible to lift the onus of sexism by showing that femininity is not a static entity but a fluctuating idea subject to the influence of history and society. It would be very hard to argue against this, but sometimes the intense focus on the social turns human beings into floating busts. Although there are hermaphrodites, most of us are born either male or female and there are biological differences between the two sexes, which does not necessarily imply they need to oppress one or the other. (*The Shaking Woman* 183-84)

Evidence of Hustvedt's conflicting views on constructionism and essentialism runs through her fictional and nonfictional oeuvre. In her essay "A Plea for Eros" (1996), which also provided the title for her 2006 essay collection, she reduces sexual attraction to a "combination of biology, personal history, and cultural miasma" (58), which challenges the dogmatic foundation of constructionist feminist thinking (49). At the beginning of the same essay, Hustvedt scrutinizes the feminist insistence on anti-rape campaigns and bedroom politics (45-46), and her response is very similar to what Roiphe has to say about this subject. In an earlier essay called "Yonder" (1995), Hustvedt describes her own experience with campus regulations at Columbia University, where women were asked to wear whistles when entering the badly lit corridors of the library (25). From her examples, it is clear that she distances herself from these practices and their underlying conception of female victimhood. In keeping with Gill's catalog of postfeminist themes, Hustvedt offers an alternative perspective on "femininity as a bodily property," following women's new self-understanding as "active, desiring sexual subjects" (Gill 149, 151). Yet, rather than simply perpetuating these new role models, Hustvedt's appropriation of popular stereotypes reveals her pragmatist and anti-foundationalist approach to feminist ideology and female agency:

> Objectification has a bad name in our culture. Cries of "Women are not sexual objects" have been resounding for years. I first ran into this argument in a volume I bought in the ninth grade called *Sisterhood Is Powerful*. I carried that book around with me until it fell apart. Feminism was good for me, as were any number of causes, but as I developed as a thinking person, the truisms and dogmas of every ideology became as worn out as that book's cover. Of course women are sexual objects; so are men. Even while I was hugging that book of feminist rhetoric to my chest, I groomed myself carefully, zipped myself into tight jeans, and went after the boy I wanted most, mentally picking apart desirable male bodies like a connoisseur. ("A Plea for Eros" 46)

This passage turns the relation between feminist activism and postfeminist consumerism on its head. Not only does Hustvedt present feminism as a commodity that she "bought" and "carried . . . around" because it used to be as hip as "tight jeans," but she also characterizes it as a dogmatic "ideology" that a "thinking person" should meet with skepticism.

All in all, Hustvedt seems to represent the "continuity faction" in postfeminism that argues for a renegotiation of feminist endeavors in a "post-traditional" era. Similar to Roiphe, she points out that "American feminism has always had a puritanical strain, an imposed blindness to erotic truth" ("A Plea for Eros" 47), thus running the risk of turning women into asexual and passive victims of the male gaze. Like the radical New Woman of the early twentieth century, Hustvedt celebrates individual freedom, female desire, and "sexual liberation" (Buhle 260). Yet, Hustvedt's quasi-biological argument does not prevent her from taking a critical perspective on women's social situation. She does not see gender equality as an established fact and concedes that sexual prejudice still "prompts a fantasy of escape" ("Being a Man" 96). She insists that all cultures oppress women "to one degree or another" ("A Plea for Eros" 49) and admits that her occasional "dreams of maleness are at least partly about escaping the cultural expectations that burden femininity . . ." ("Being a Man" 96).

Before turning to *The Shaking Woman*, I would like to ponder the potential limitations and risks of Hustvedt's perspective. Like other postfeminist writers, she can be found guilty of re-centering whiteness and heteronormativity (Gill 165), unless her writing is interpreted as the strictly idiosyncratic response of an educated white woman to social conditions that happen to facilitate her self-empowerment. The fact that strong autobiographical elements such as her academic and Northern European background run through her fictional and nonfictional writings seems to protect Hustvedt against generalizing her own experience. As I will show in the next section of my essay, this holds especially true for her recent nonfictional work.

In a nutshell, *The Shaking Woman* deals with the author's involuntary shaking during public speeches, which first occurred during a ceremony in honor of her deceased father, a former college professor, in May 2006. Terrified by this sudden and recurring loss of control, she "decided to go in search of the shaking woman" (7). This search takes her into the fields of neurology, psychiatry, psychoanalysis, and philosophy, as well as medical and personal history. Hustvedt justifies her interdisciplinary approach, which reflects a genuine interest in science, as follows: "The search for the shaking woman takes me round and round because in the end it is also a search for perspectives that may illuminate who and what she is. My only certainty is that I cannot be satisfied with looking at her through a single window. I have to see her from every angle" (73).

Reviewers—mainly women—have been divided on *The Shaking Woman*. Less enthusiastic readers have described the work and its author as "chilly" (Morrice), narcissist and "painfully self-obsessed" (Bradbury), bemoaning that Hustvedt's aloofness and privileged position preclude ready identification with her experience.[4] Other reviewers praise Hustvedt's "clean intelligence" and "exemplary clarity," celebrating her as an "ambitious, cerebral novelist" (Mantel). There is one review published in the German weekly *Die Zeit* from which I would like to quote a longer passage:

> From the very beginning, Hustvedt's astonishingly clear and discrete objectivity allays fears that the reader will ultimately be confronted with the author's imaginary patricide and her debilitating feelings of guilt and meanwhile be bothered with intimate insights into the Hustvedt family that revolve around the small Siri and her overly powerful dad. This book, which hardly deals with private matters, spares the reader such revelations. (von Thadden, "Siri Hustvedt: Warum zittere ich?"; my translation)[5]

I think that these responses mirror more general expectations that audiences identifying themselves as feminist or postfeminist would bring to such a text. The first group of readers sees the lack of intersubjective insight into Hustvedt's experience as a failure, whereas the second group praises her individualism, which transcends the clichéd dictates of feminist sisterhood and its focus on women's victimization.[6]

---

[4] Wilson ends her review with the conclusion that: "Hustvedt shuts the reader out to the point where you cease to care much why she shakes (a problem, in any case, which seems a pretty minor blot on a charmed East Coast existence). She tells us her roots are in Scandinavia, 'where stoicism is highly valued' and swimming in ice water is 'viewed as admirable.' Hustvedt's shaking seems to be the only loss of control in an otherwise poised persona. But she never makes us feel what it is like to swim with her in the icy waters" (Review of *Shaking Woman*).

[5] "Es ist die erstaunlich klare und diskrete Sachlichkeit von Hustvedts Selbsterkundung, die von Anbeginn der Erzählung die Befürchtung zerstreut, nun werde man auf intimen Schleichwegen zum fantasierten Vatermord inklusive lähmender Schuldgefühle geführt und unterwegs mit allerhand Privatem aus dem Hause Hustvedt behelligt, das einem von der kleinen Siri und einem übermächtigen Papa erzählt. Davon kann in diesem Buch, das Privates kaum preisgibt, die Rede nicht sein" (von Thadden, "Siri Hustvedt: Warum zittere ich?").

[6] Interestingly enough, the battle between feminists and postfeminists continues even among the writers and readers of these reviews. Von

Hustvedt clearly distances herself from the tragic "Story of the Woman Writer" (Jacobus 517), but nevertheless constructs her text in a way that stresses her departure from and indebtedness to her feminist predecessors of the nineteenth and twentieth centuries. This strategy is evident from the very beginning since *The Shaking Woman* uses an epigraph taken from Emily Dickinson's "I Felt a Cleaving in My Mind." This poem features prominently in Gilbert and Gubar's *The Madwoman in the Attic* (627-28, 639), which casts Dickinson as the divided heroine of the study. Sylvia Plath's *The Bell Jar* (1963), the last in Gilbert and Gubar's line of feminist texts whose narrators are haunted by controlling men (508), is also evoked, as when Hustvedt's mother compares her daughter's shaking to an "electrocution" (4).[7] Yet the strongest and most obvious intertextual relation is established between *The Shaking Woman* and "The Yellow Wallpaper." Hustvedt echoes Gilman's short story both in her title and elsewhere in the text, beginning with the narrator's account of her first seizure, which occurs after she has married ("Extracts" 220-21). As in "The Yellow Wallpaper," it is the confrontation with visual art that triggers Hustvedt's first attack, which seems to thrust her into her 'proper' place: "In an art gallery in Paris I suddenly felt my left arm jerk upward and slam me backward into the wall" (*The Shaking Woman* 4). This description is strongly reminiscent of Gilman's shaking woman behind the pattern of the wallpaper. On

---

Thadden's interpretation of *The Shaking Women* prompted the following comment by a reader identified as Clara von Kinzet: "The article is ripe with intellectual hubris so that the author Elizabeth von Thadden does not even notice how she discriminates against another woman by publicly defining her in relation to other men, her father, who is a literature professor, and her husband, a famous writer" ("Der gesamte Artikel ist von einem derartigen intellektuellen Hochmut durchsetzt, daß die Autorin Elisabeth von Thadden nicht einmal merkt, daß sie als Frau eine andere Frau, indem sie sie als Tochter eines Literaturprofessors und Frau eines angesehenen Schriftstellers öffentlich über Männer definiert, diskriminiert"; my translation).

[7]   The narrator of Plath's novel finds herself torn between her desire to become a writer and society's expectation that she will get married and have children. She is eventually "cured" by means of electroshock therapy, which is implicitly compared with the electrocution of Ethel Rosenberg, a Communist, during the McCarthy era.

closer inspection, Hustvedt's narrator even appears to be more passive, for she is "slam[med] into the wall" whereas Gilman's woman of the late nineteenth century is shaking the bars "all over," struggling to get out of her prison. After establishing this analogy, Hustvedt repeatedly returns to Gilman's imagery, yet only to deconstruct and revise its meanings. Much later in Hustvedt's narrative, the narrator of *The Shaking Woman* proposes a simple, "scientific" explanation of her first seizure, thus refuting Gilman's analogy between ornamental patterns and patriarchal oppression: "If I look at too many paintings (and I love paintings), I become dizzy and nauseated. This affliction also has a name: Stendhal syndrome. But in me, at least, it is related to migraine and can develop into a full-blown headache" (119).

Hustvedt's persistent focus on her own experience and identity leads me to the main theme of "The Yellow Wallpaper," namely the narrator's split identity, which runs through *The Shaking Woman* as well. Hustvedt insists that "[t]he shaking woman is not the narrating woman. The narrating, interpreting woman continued on while the other shook. The narrator was a fluent generator of sentences and explanations. It is she who is writing now" (54). Yet, in contrast to Gilman's narrator, she is able to reflect on her divided self, seeing it as "two Siris" (40) as it were, and she does not fall into the trap of generalizing her experience. Critics of Gilman's tale have tended to read the woman behind the pattern of the wallpaper "not only as [the narrator's] literary double but as a symbol of the woman's social condition," that is, of "women in the nineteenth century" (Golden 10). Hustvedt, on the other hand, maintains that women's individual problems are entangled in personal histories and that "narrative is part of the sickness itself" (*The Shaking Woman* 37). The covers of the first American and British editions of *The Shaking Woman* seem to illustrate this postfeminist move from sameness to difference and multiplicity. The Henry Holt edition features a split cover with a monochrome yellow on the left and a quivering mix of iridescent colors on the right, whereas the Sceptre cover looks like a naïve watercolor painting with horizontal waves in yellow, red, and blue. Against this background, the subtitle, *A History of My Nerves*, suggests that the book deals with a strictly private and individual self-investigation.

In another implicit homage to Gilman, Hustvedt links her shaking to the location in which it first occurred. On the St. Olaf College campus, where her father used to teach, Hustvedt may be surrounded by "old building[s]" (3), but she is also standing outside, in front of a memorial pine tree. Hustvedt's description of this setting can be read as a twenty-first-century reform of Gilman's "ancestral halls" (255):

> The first time I shook I was standing on home ground. It wasn't only that my father had taught for many years at the college. As a child, I had lived on that campus because my professor father had a second job as head resident of a men's dormitory. That old building has since been torn down, but I remember its murky hallways, its smells, the elevator with its red door, the soda pop machine glowing on the floor below us, and the button on it for Royal Crown Cola. (98-99)

This is not the paternal house in which the female narrator is reduced to a childlike existence, but a place where Hustvedt "walked . . . again and again, not only as a child but as a girl, and then as a young woman when I was a student" (100). There is another interesting setting in *The Shaking Woman* that invites a comparison to Gilman. At one time, Hustvedt experiences the shaking while being on a hiking tour with her husband and a male friend. Unlike Gilman's narrator, she has moved out into the open country,[8] leaving behind not only the "ancestral halls" but also the garden with its "hedges and walls and gates that lock [her in]" (Gilman, "The Yellow Wallpaper" 256)[9]:

> REPORT: June 23, 2008. I am traveling with my husband and a friend. We are spending three days in the Pyrenees together and plan to take a walk in the mountains. J. has found one identified as "moderate" in his guide book that evaluates activities for tourists of varying degrees of prowess. We drive to the place where the walk begins, and I climb up the rocky mountain path, bounding from one stone to another. I am proud of my strength (showing off, if it must be told, for the two men behind me), and then I retire. Breathless, I sit down on a boulder and feel my body go into full-blown convulsions, which then subside. This is not emotional, I think to myself. This is not about my father's death. This is

---

[8]   The narrator of "The Yellow Wallpaper" sees the other women "creep[ing] faster than I can turn . . . away off in the open country" (266). Gilbert and Gubar associate the "open country" with "health and freedom" (91).

[9]   Kennard similarly argues that "the in-door images of imprisonment [are] echoed in the natural world of the garden" (75).

not conversion disorder. I say nothing to my husband or friend, who were too far away to witness my seizure. When I walk back down the mountain, I go slowly. The event has left me weak and unsteady. (Hustvedt, *The Shaking Woman* 151-52)

Hustvedt's intertextual dialogue with Gilman is highlighted not only by the content but also by the form of this passage, which mimics the journal entries in the "The Yellow Wallpaper." I will return to these generic conversions at the end of my essay. In terms of imagery and content, the above-quoted passage is even more reminiscent of another work by Gilman: the poem "An Obstacle" (1890), which personifies male prejudice as a "colossal" (20) obstacle that prevents the unnamed narrator from "climbing up a mountain-path" (1). Hustvedt's narrator physically exerts herself to dispel the prejudice that she is weak and unfit to compete with her male companions. Yet, in the end, it is her own anxiety about this prejudice that throws her into "full-blown convulsions." The narrator's reluctant insertion—"if it must be told"— attests to her late realization that, sometimes, it is the feminist fear of inequality rather than men's controlling influence ("[they] were too far away to witness [her] seizure") that limits women's agency.

Elsewhere, however, Hustvedt recalls what a feminist reader would classify as "gender-typical" responses to her public shaking, as when stating that her dearest sister, Liv, "said she wanted to go over and put her arms around me and hold me up" (4), whereas her husband "was tempted to rush up onto the stage, grab me, and carry me bodily down the stairs" (29). With this description, she evokes both the concept of feminist sisterhood and masculine anxiety over women on the public stage. Yet, Hustvedt disappoints readers who expect her to use these scattered observations to come up with general conclusions about "women's culture" and patriarchal oppression. Her husband's alerting her "repeatedly" that she "read[s] obsessively" (6) may be reminiscent of John's admonishing Gilman's narrator that "the very worst thing I can do is to think about my condition" (256). But such easy analogies are undermined in Hustvedt's acknowledgments, where she expresses her gratitude to her husband Paul Auster, "who has kindly tolerated my passionate immersion in the brain/mind problem and listened to me think aloud (sometimes for hours) about many issues I address in this book" (213). Hustvedt's situation stands in stark contrast to what the narrator in "The Yellow Wallpaper" has to endure, and the juxtaposition is obviously intended. She turns the power relation in Gilman's tale on its head, as, in Hustvedt's text, it is the writer-husband who resigns himself to the role of the passive listener while the narrator proves her mastery of science.

The Shaking Woman abounds with similar revisionary readings that target the logic of feminist literary criticism after *The Madwoman in the Attic*. When Hustvedt describes the circumstances of her first instance of shaking, she recalls that she "had the strong sensation of hearing my father's voice. . . . I even used the phrase 'Were my father here today, he might have said . . .'" (3). Rather than interpreting this as a woman's loss of authority due to her being "possessed" by a tyrannical father, Hustvedt keeps stressing her good and close relationship to both of her parents and even blames herself for not grieving enough "for someone [she] had loved so much" (24). Moreover, she later explains that other family members, male *and* female, used to be haunted by disembodied voices as well. Hustvedt talks about several further instances of shaking, each time feigning a traditional feminist perspective on the incident. For instance, Hustvedt started to shake when her talk followed that of a male colleague, a "well-known popular novelist" (28), which raises the question whether his presence had "created a subliminal idea that after his victorious narrative my comments would be disappointing" (30). However, not only does this novelist owe his fame to an appearance on *The Oprah Winfrey Show*, but he also turns out to be a feminist battling women's (creative) confinements: "He spoke movingly about his work with female prison inmates. His talk was sad, but it had a happy ending. Despite grotesque manipulations on the part of prison authorities to squelch the writing of the women he had taught, his efforts had triumphed in the end" (28).

Hustvedt uses a similar revisionist strategy to reinterpret her relationship to medical science, practitioners, and institutions. At the beginning of her narrative in *The Shaking Woman*, she describes a prolonged hospital stay after a migraine attack in 1982 as follows:

> [T]hose strange drugged days, punctuated by visits from young men in white coats who held up pencils for me to identify, asked me the day and the year and the name of the president, pricked me with needles—Can you feel this?—and the rare wave through the front door from Dr. C., a man who mostly ignored me and seemed irritated that I didn't cooperate

and get well, have stayed with me as a time of the blackest of all black comedies. (5)

Featuring male authorities ranging from physicians to the American president, phallic symbols, and symbolic penetration, this passage can only be read as an ironic parody of feminist discourse. Hustvedt introduces her hospital experience as a long-past event that has taken the shape of a black comedy, a humorous and exaggerated satire. Feeding on these distorted memories, she insists with a wink that her "imaginary analyst is a man. I choose a man because he would be a paternal creature, an echo of my father, who is the ghost somehow involved in my shaking" (19-20). Predictably, the doctors she meets in real life turn out to be "attentive and sympathetic" (31). "My fantasy story about the shaking woman doubles back on itself as, one by one, living persons replace my imaginary doctors" (153). Amongst them are "confident" women who are "at ease with [their] bod[ies]" (155) and show more interest in their patient's infantile febrile convulsions than in her relationship to her father.

Nevertheless, Hustvedt does not hesitate to stress that "none of us is untouched by bias" (149) and that society is still far from achieving gender equality. Shortly before the "mountain path" passage quoted above, she laments the precarious status of women's writing in the twenty-first century, writing that "prejudice . . . plays an important role in reading. . . . Real men like *objective* texts, not the *subjective* wanderings of mere fiction writers, especially female ones, whose prose, whatever its character, is tainted by their sex before a single word has been read" (149). This observation leads me back to the generic features of *The Shaking Woman*. As mentioned above, Hustvedt incorporates several journal entries, reporting not only her everyday experiences (127, 151) but also her dreams (128). Significantly, these scattered entries occur in the second part of the text, whereas previous passages about Hustvedt's life are mainly written in the style of a mainstream autobiography. The diary, a "day-to-day record of the events in one's life, written for personal use and satisfaction, with little or no thought of publication" ("Biography" 27), has often been classified as a "female text" (Lensink 40). At the same time, it has been noted that "American women publish significantly fewer autobiographies than American men" (Culley 6). This is, of course, due to women's traditional lack of political and social agency and their limited access to the public sphere. According to Linda Peterson, the diary attests to the "(feminine) tradition of private self-revelation," whereas the classic autobiography belongs to the "(masculine) tradition of public self-presentation" (33). Hustvedt makes a clear statement against this essentialist division when she deviates from the homogenously "female" life writing of Gilman's narrator. Unlike the latter, Hustvedt does not let her thoughts and sentences be controlled, interrupted, and dissolved, and she analyzes her life rationally and from a distant perspective. In fact, Hustvedt goes even further than mixing "feminine" and "masculine" modes of self-representation. Similar to the narrator in "The Yellow Wallpaper," she reiterates what male scientists say or might say about her condition, but she assumes the role of an essayist and historian of science to do so, thereby appropriating and adjusting the logics of reason and scientific diagnosis for her own purposes. Her historical perspective undermines the authority of the very discourses she evokes by underlining their inherent contingency. In the end, the narrator of *The Shaking Woman* celebrates and embraces her unscientific subjectivity and the fact that she is "hopelessly tender-minded" (143). Her final diagnosis is that the medical gaze cannot control the "ambiguity" of her split (written) self: "It won't fit into the pigeonhole, the neat box, the window frame, the encyclopedia. It is a formless object of feeling that can't be placed" (199).

The imagery, theme, setting, and hybrid genre of *The Shaking Woman* demonstrate the author's indebtedness to *and* departure from "classic feminist arguments" ("A Plea for Eros" 47). Due to the paradigmatic status of "The Yellow Wallpaper," Hustvedt's borrowing and transformation of this particular text must be interpreted as a deliberate and conscious decision. Her complex revision of Gilman's narrative reveals Hustvedt's suspicion of and resistance to Gilbert and Gubar's "mistress-plot," which reiterates and entrenches the victim status of women (writers) in the nineteenth and twentieth centuries. In her foreword to the 2009 essay collection, *Gilbert and Gubar's* The Madwoman in the Attic *after Thirty Years*, Sandra M. Gilbert mentions "some skeptics and some anti-feminists [who] claim that we're living in a 'post-feminist era' marked by indifference or even contempt for the revisionary excitement that animated so many of us three decades ago" (xiii). With my analysis of Hustvedt's writing, I hope to have shown that

Gilbert's conflation of antifeminism and postfeminism is untenable. Yet, despite, or rather precisely because of this, I concur with the authors of *The Madwoman in the Attic* that, contrary to popular belief, the feminist project is still very much thriving.

Works Cited

"Biography." *A Glossary of Literary Terms*. Ed. M. H. Abrams and Geoffrey Galt Harpham. 10th ed. Boston: Wadsworth/Cengage, 2012. Print.

Bolotin, Susan. "Voices from the Post-Feminist Generation." *The New York Times* 17 Oct. 1982: 29. Print.

Bradbury, Lorna. Rev. of *The Shaking Woman, Or: A History of My Nerves*. By Siri Hustvedt. *The Telegraph* 23 Jan. 2010. Web. 5 Jan. 2011.

Brooks, Ann. *Postfeminisms: Feminism, Cultural Theory and Cultural Forms*. London: Routledge, 2007. Print.

Buhle, Mari Jo. *Women and American Socialism: 1870-1920*. Urbana: U of Illinois P, 1983. Print.

Butler, Judith. *Gender Trouble: Feminism and the Subversion of Identity*. New York: Routledge, 1990. Print.

Coppock, Vicki, Deena Haydon, and Ingrid Richter. *The Illusions of "Post-Feminism": New Women, Old Myths*. London: Taylor and Francis, 1995. Print.

Cott, Nancy F. *The Grounding of Modern Feminism*. New Haven: Yale UP, 1987. Print.

Culley, Margo. "What a Piece of Work is 'Woman'! An Introduction." *American Women's Autobiography: Fea(s)ts of Memory*. Ed. Culley. Madison: U of Wisconsin P, 1992. 3-31. Print.

Denfeld, Rene. *The New Victorians: A Young Woman's Challenge to the Old Feminist Order*. New York: Warner, 1995. Print.

Genz, Stéphanie, and Benjamin A. Brabon. *Postfeminism: Cultural Texts and Theories*. Edinburgh: Edinburgh UP, 2009. Print.

Gilbert, Sandra M. Foreword. *Gilbert and Gubar's* The Madwoman in the Attic *after Thirty Years*. Ed. and introd. Annette R. Federico. Columbia: U of Missouri P, 2009. ix-xiii. Print.

---, and Susan Gubar. *The Madwoman in the Attic: The Woman Writer and the Nineteenth-Century Literary Imagination*. New Haven: Yale UP, 1979. Print.

Gill, Rosalind. "Postfeminist Media Culture: Elements of a Sensibility." *European Journal of Cultural Studies* 10.2 (2007): 147-66. Print.

---, and Elena Herdieckerhoff. "Rewriting the Romance." *Feminist Media Studies* 6.4 (2006): 487-504. Print.

Gilman, Charlotte Perkins. "An Obstacle." 1890. *The Yellow Wall-Paper, Herland, and Selected Writings*. Ed. Denise D. Knight. New York: Penguin, 2009. 321-22. Print.

---. "The Yellow Wallpaper." 1892. *The Portable American Realism Reader*. Ed. James Nagel and Tom Quirk. New York: Penguin, 1997. 254-69. Print.

Golden, Catherine. "One Hundred Years of Reading 'The Yellow Wallpaper.'" *The Captive Imagination: A Casebook on The Yellow Wallpaper*. Ed. Golden. New York: Feminist P, 1992. 1-23. Print.

Haney-Peritz, Janice. "Monumental Feminism and Literature's Ancestral House: Another Look at 'The Yellow Wallpaper.'" *Women's Studies* 12.2 (1986): 113-28. Print.

Harzewski, Stephanie. *Chick Lit and Postfeminism*. Charlottesville: U of Virginia P, 2011. Print.

Hedges, Elaine R. "Afterword to the 'The Yellow Wallpaper,' Feminist Press Edition." 1973. *The Captive Imagination: A Casebook on The Yellow Wallpaper*. Ed. Catherine Golden. New York: Feminist P, 1992. 123-36. Print.

Honeck, Mischa. "Siri Hustvedt, *What I Loved*." *Zweiundzwanzig amerikanische Romane aus dem neuen Jahrhundert: Literaturkritische Essays zur Einführung*. Ed. Dietmar Schloss and Heiko Jakubzik. Trier: WVT, 2009. 167-80. Print.

hooks, bell. *Ain't I a Woman? Black Women and Feminism*. Boston: South End, 1981. Print.

Hustvedt, Siri. *A Plea for Eros: Essays*. New York: Picador, 2006.

---. "Being a Man." 2003. Hustvedt, *A Plea for Eros* 95-103. Print.

---. "Eight Days in a Corset." 1996. Hustvedt, *A Plea for Eros* 85-94. Print.

---. "Extracts from a Story of the Wounded Self." 2004. Hustvedt, *A Plea for Eros* 195-228. Print.

---. "A Plea for Eros." 1996. Hustvedt, *A Plea for Eros* 45-60. Print.

---. *The Shaking Woman, Or: A History of My Nerves*. London: Sceptre, 2010. Print.

---. "Yonder." 1995. Hustvedt, *A Plea for Eros* 1-43. Print.

Hutcheon, Linda. *A Poetics of Postmodernism: History, Theory, Fiction*. London: Routledge, 1988. Print.

Jacobus, Mary. Rev. of *The Madwoman in the Attic*. By Sandra M. Gilbert and Susan Gubar. *Signs* 6.3 (1981): 517-23. Print.

Kennard, Jean E. "Convention Coverage or How to Read Your Own Life." *New Literary History* 13.1 (1981): 69-88. Print.

Lee, Janet. "Care to Join Me in an Upwardly Mobile Tango? Postmodernism and the 'New Woman.'" *The Female Gaze: Women as Viewers of Popular Culture*. Ed. Lorraine Gamman and Margaret Marshment. London: Women's P, 1988. 166-72. Print.

Lensink, Judy Nolte. "Expanding the Boundaries of Criticism: The Diary as Female Autobiography." *Women's Studies* 14.1 (1987): 39-53. Print.

Mantel, Hilary. Rev. of *The Shaking Woman, Or: A History of My Nerves*. By Siri Hustvedt. *The Guardian* 30 Jan. 2010. Web. 5 Jan. 2011.

Morrice, Polly. "Seized." Rev. of *The Shaking Woman, Or: A History of My Nerves*. By Siri Hustvedt. *New York Times* 1 April 2010. Web. 5 Jan. 2011.

Peterson, Linda H. *Traditions of Victorian Women's Autobiography: The Poetics and Politics of Life Writing*. Charlottesville: UP of Virginia, 1999. Print.

Plath, Sylvia. *The Bell Jar*. 1963. London: Faber, 2005.

Projansky, Sarah. "Mass Magazine and Cover Girls: Some Reflections on Postfeminist Girls and Postfeminism's Daughters." *Interrogating Postfeminism: Gender and the Politics of Popular Culture*. Ed. Yvonne Tasker and Diane Negra. Durham: Duke UP, 2007. 40-72. Print.

Roiphe, Katie. *The Morning After: Sex, Fear and Feminism on Campus*. Boston: Little Brown, 1993. Print.

Spivak, Gayatri C. "Can the Subaltern Speak?" *Colonial Discourse and Post-Colonial Theory*. Ed. Laura Chrisman and Patrick Williams. New York: Harvester Wheatsheaf, 1993. 66-111. Print.

Tasker, Yvonne, and Diane Negra. "Feminist Politics and Postfeminist Culture." Introduction. *Interrogating Postfeminism: Gender and the Politics of Popular Culture*. Ed. Tasker and Negra. Durham: Duke UP, 2007. 1-25. Print.

von Kinzet, Clara. "'Die Autorin wird zur Ärztin ihrer selbst.'" *Zeit Online* 1 Feb. 2010. Web. 1 Feb. 2011.

von Thadden, Elisabeth. "Siri Hustvedt: Warum zittere ich?" Rev. of *The Shaking Woman, Or: A History of My Nerves*. By Siri Hustvedt. *Zeit Online* 30 Jan. 2010. Web. 1 Feb. 2011.

Walter, Natasha. *The New Feminism*. 1998. London: Virago, 2000. Print.

Wilson, Bee. Rev. of *The Shaking Woman, Or: A History of My Nerves*. By Siri Hustvedt. *The Sunday Times* 24 Jan. 2010. Web. 5 Jan. 2011.

Wolf, Naomi. *Fire with Fire: The New Female Power and How It Will Change the 21st Century*. New York: Random, 1993. Print.

JOHANNA HEIL

Embedding Richard Powers's
The Echo Maker in Narrative Medicine:
Narrativity, Delusions, and the
(De-)Construction of Unified Minds

> It is, of course, memory that weaves
> one's life into a coherent whole.
> (Kandel 372)

The Echo Maker in Context

Richard Powers's *The Echo Maker* is a novel that addresses a number of issues. It truly is a Pandora's box of cultural, medical, and political themes, and it is this article's concern to concentrate on the neurological impairment of the character Mark Schluter, a 27-year-old man who has survived a serious car accident whose cause cannot be reconstructed due to Mark's retrograde amnesia. He has received traumatic brain injury and, as a consequence, suffers from the rare Capgras syndrome (CS), a condition that severs a patient's emotional recognition from the facial recognition of a loved person. Concretely speaking, Mark recognizes the face of his sister Karin but is utterly convinced that she is an impostor because he does not *feel* her to be herself. In order to make sense of his accident and the disappearance of his sibling, he makes up a story to logically explain everything that has happened.

Being confronted with the effects of CS affects not only Mark, who directly suffers from it, but also those in his social environment, such as

Dr. Gerald Weber, one of his attending neurologists. Weber's personal and professional problems, which are successively unveiled as he spends time with Mark, stem from his successful career as a best-selling author of fictionalized narrative case histories of his former patients. While "Famous Gerald"—as his wife teasingly calls him—has become a popular figure in the public sphere, he is often belittled by colleagues who evaluate his "literary" work as anecdotal at best and unscholarly at worst. After having treated patients for decades, Weber is deeply bothered by the harsh criticism of colleagues and book critics who accuse him of exploiting his patients for commercial effects without caring for their recovery. He excruciatingly questions his faithfulness towards his patients and his wife and finds himself unable to keep a professional and personal distance vis-à-vis Mark's condition although he has heretofore never been notably empathetic towards his patients. Thus, Weber's life, too, unravels, and Weber, too, starts to tell a narrative; but while Mark (re)constructs, Weber seems to deconstruct.

Even though Richard Powers's *The Echo Maker* is itself a purely fictional text, it obviously engages in a cultural and medical debate that is, amongst other things, concerned with the benefits of narrative medicine. As Douwe Draaisma shows in his "Echos [*sic*], Doubles, and Delusions: Capgras Syndrome in Science and Literature," *The Echo Maker* may serve as a playfully arranged medical history of CS that underwent "one of those exemplary Gestalt switches in science" (433) in the 1980s. Thereby, the novel is "able to capture some of the earlier thoughts on Capgras Syndrome" (438) that are echoed by one of the attending doctors, i.e., Weber. Based on the medical history of CS, this article begins by examining the discipline of narrative medicine in order to understand the subject matter of both the individual narratives of patients and of physicians as interpreters. Tracing CS as the subject matter of the narrative of medical and cultural history, and as the subject matter of clinical and reductionist medicine that may present itself as narrative, allows me to examine the discussion of CS in *The Echo Maker* as negotiating narrative versus reductionist knowledge of medicine with regard to the sense of a coherent perception of self that narrative establishes.

Narrative Medicine

For the past thirty years, the literature-and-medicine movement has been prospering as part of the medical education of future physicians, and the approach of narrative medicine[1] has become more popular in the treatment of patients.[2] Rita Charon, for example, reports how, as a young doctor in 1982, she was one of the first to be educated in "a monthlong intensive training program in literary theory, texts, and methods salient to medicine" (*Narrative Medicine* 4). This course also focused on the narratives that the young physicians could tell about their own experiences as attending doctors, and, recapitulating her own experiences, Charon illustrates that the narratives that doctors are confronted with usually begin *in medias res*, include unreliable narrators, and present only one scene of a larger structure. The physician, when piecing together the rest of the story without having properly listened to his or her patient, e.g., because he or she has not been properly trained in narrative medicine or is prejudiced, may run a high risk of misinterpreting the story at large and, thus, of misdiagnosing

---

[1]   Charon comprehensively summarizes narrative medicine as follows: "All these features of what we call medical practice—temporality, singularity, intersubjectivity, causality and contingency, and ethicality—are bedrock narrative features. You find them in the tables of contents of the narratology textbooks of Seymore Chatman (1978), Gérard Genette (1972), Shlomith Rimmon-Kenan (2002), Percy Lubbock (1957), and E.M. Forster (1949). . . . So the phrase *narrative medicine* came to me as a way to designate medicine practiced with the narrative competence to acknowledge the urgency of time, to value the singularity of patients and self, to seek the causality and to tolerate the savage contingency of disease, to dare to forge an intersubjective connection to sick people, and to fulfill the ethical duties incurred by hearing the stories of illness" ("Where Does Narrative Medicine Come From" 25). For a more in-depth discussion of narrative medicine, cf. Chapter 3 of Charon's *Narrative Medicine*, "Narrative Features of Medicine" (39-62).

[2]   Cf., for example, Charon, *Narrative Medicine* (2-6); Anne Hunsaker Hawkins and Marilyn Chandler McEntyre's introduction to *Teaching Literature and Medicine*; or Peter L. Rudnytsky's introduction to *Psychoanalysis and Narrative Medicine*.

his or her patient. This, of course, implies that in narrative medicine, we never find only one story (i.e., the patient's) that needs to be considered: First, there is the patient's story, which may or may not be true; the patient may choose to leave out parts that seem unimportant, that are embarrassing, or that do not seem to matter.[3] Second, the attending physician must be careful to concentrate on the patient alone, and not on him- or herself. Previous knowledge may be helpful when it uncovers common patterns that also apply to the patient but it may just as well lead to jumping to conclusions. Charon thus observes that narrative medicine "has become a way to probe the *narrativity* of disease, of health, of healing, and of the relation between the sick person and the one who tries to help" ("Where" 26).

Despite the stumbling blocks posed by narrative knowledge, Charon highlights "its ability to capture the singular irreplicable, or in-commensurable" that "universal or scientific knowledge" lacks (*Narrative Medicine* 45). In this context, she refers to Roland Barthes's notion of the writerly text, which she rightly interprets as "com[ing] into the hands of the reader incomplete, still alive, requiring active creation from each reader it visits. The reader of the writerly text is coauthor of it, not by virtue of observing what its author did but by virtue of performing what the text compels" (Charon, *Narrative Medicine* 45-46). Barthes himself further characterizes the writerly text as a "perpetual present, upon which no *consequent* language (which would inevitably make it past) can be superimposed" (*S/Z* 5)—the same perpetual present, of course, applies to a narrative of illness that remains as a present/presence after it is told. The narrative of a particular illness offers the raw material with which both physician and patient will work during treatment. Even after the treatment has ended, the narrative may persist. Similarly, Barthes regards writerly texts as productions,[4] not as completed products (cf. 5).

---

[3]   The narrative approach to medicine provides physicians with tools to distinguish the actual state of a patient's body (and) mind, and it may present itself in a patient's narrative (cf., for example, Charon, "Where Does Narrative Medicine Come From?" 31-33).

[4]   In this context, Barthes's production can also be read as performance, which I consider not only to be the act of putting a rehearsed or improvised action on (a literal) stage, but a performance in the way Erving Goffman defines it in

Narrative as a mode of thinking has more generally become a central object of study in many academic disciplines. Discussing the significance of narrative in science, for instance, David R. Olson points out that

> [f]rom both epistemological and educational perspectives, then, scientific thinking has to be seen as merely one mode of thought, a Modernist or paradigmatic mode,[5] which may be contrasted with an alternative Postmodern or narrative mode of thought. The latter puts a new emphasis on the more local, domain-specific *contextualized knowledge, which is interpretive in nature and socially or collaboratively constructed.* (3; my emphasis)

Jerome Bruner emphasizes that, although the two modes of thought are "complementary," they are also "irreducible to one another" (11); Richard Powers further claims that "'narrative' may itself *be* the elemental connection between literature, science, cognition, and consciousness" (interview with Kucharzewski 457),[6] and I seek to discuss this connecting trait in respect to narratives of impaired and unimpaired minds and brains as depicted in *The Echo Maker*. A fruitful collaboration between researchers in the fields of literature and

---

his *The Presentation of Self in Everyday Life*: "A 'performance' may be defined as all activity of a given participant on a given occasion which serves to *influence in any way any of the other participants.* . . . Defining social role as the enactment of rights and duties attached to a given status, we can say that a social role will involve one or more parts and that each of these different parts may be presented by the performer on a series of occasions to the same kinds of audiences or to an audience of the same persons" (15-16).

[5] Bruner further defines the paradigmatic (or "logico-scientific" [12]) mode as "mak[ing] use of procedures to assure verifiable references and to test for empirical truth" (13).

[6] Powers's notion has been a prominent one for a number of philosophers of mind in the past 30 years. For a concise overview, cf., for instance, Fireman, McVay, and Flanagan's *Narrative Consciousness: Literature, Psychology, and the Brain.* I also suggest Rouse's *Engaging Science: How to Understand Its Practices Philosophically*, Polkinghorne's *Narrative Knowing and the Human Sciences*, or Nash's *Narrative in Culture: The Uses of Storytelling in the Sciences, Philosophy, and Literature* for further reading.

neurology is presented in the joint research paper "The Neurology of Narrative" by Kay Young—a literary scholar—and Jeffery L. Saver—a neurologist. They, too, stress the importance of narrative, and they, too, quote Barthes, who writes the following in his "Introduction to the Structural Analysis of Narratives":

> The narratives of the world are numberless. Narrative is first and foremost a prodigious variety of genres, themselves distributed amongst different substances—as though any material were fit to receive man's stories. . . . [N]arrative is present in every age, in every place, in every society; it begins with the history of mankind and there nowhere is nor has been a people without narrative. . . . narrative is international, transhistorical, trans-cultural: it is simply there, like life itself. (Barthes 79; cf. Young and Saver 73)

Young and Saver acknowledge "Barthes's nod toward the question of the relation between the structuring of consciousness in story and the productions [or performances] of those stories as representations of self and culture" (73). Coinciding with what I pursue in this article, they wonder "[w]hy . . . the 'I' tell[s] his or her self as story [and] why . . . the 'I' has a story to tell at all?" (Young and Saver 73). They reason that the stories any "I" tells "are in relation to one another, . . . one offers the other the chance at individual presence and mutual recognition" (72). Thus, narratives establish order, coherence, and re-assurance, be they factual or counterfactual.

Keeping the context of narrative medicine in mind, it is noteworthy that *The Echo Maker* starts with an epigraph from A. R. Luria. In the 1970s, the Russian neurologist classified two modes of scientific and medical methodology that correspond to the distinction between paradigmatic and narrative modes of thought:

> Classical scholars are those who look upon events in terms of their constituent parts. . . . One outcome of this approach is the reduction of living reality with all its richness of detail to abstract schemas. The properties of the living whole are lost, which provoked Goethe to pen, 'Gray is every theory, but ever green is the tree of life.'[7]

---

[7] Cf. Maturana and Verala; and Rouse's *Engaging Science*.

> Romantic scholars . . . do not follow the path of reductionism, which is the leading philosophy of the classical group. Romantics in science want neither to split living reality into its elementary components nor to represent the wealth of life's concrete events in abstract models that lose the properties of the phenomena themselves. It is of the utmost importance to romantics to preserve the wealth of living reality, and they aspire to a science that retains this richness. (*The Making of the Mind* 174)

Theory may be all gray but, as Luria admits, "[r]omantic science typically lacks the logic and does not follow the careful, consecutive, step-by-step reasoning" of classical models but "let[s] artistic preferences and intuitions take over" (175). Yet, he also skeptically notes trends towards reductionist approaches in the natural sciences and medicine in which "[s]imple observation and description . . . [often seduce] observers into pseudoexplanations based on their own phenomenological understanding" (177). Luria's point is that "[w]hen done properly, observation accomplishes the classical aim of explaining facts, while not losing sight of the romantic aim of preserving the manifold richness of the subject" (178). Luria's plea for a combination of romantic and classical scholarship also lies at the heart of Charon's *Narrative Medicine*, in which she argues that a "scientifically competent medicine alone cannot help patients grapple with the loss of health" (3). She strongly promotes incorporating the approach of narrative medicine—which she understands "to mean medicine practiced with these narrative skills of recognizing, absorbing, interpreting, and being moved by the stories of illness" (4)—into non-narrative practice. Thus, Charon's narrative medicine approach reflects Luria's romantic science:

> Unlike scientific knowledge or epidemiological knowledge, which tries to discover things about the natural world that are universally true or at least appear true to any observer, narrative knowledge enables one individual to understand particular events befalling another individual not as an instance of something that is universally true but as a singular and meaningful situation. Nonnarrative knowledge attempts to illuminate the universal by transcending the particular; narrative knowledge, by looking closely at individual human beings grappling with the conditions of life, attempts to illuminate the universals of the human condition by revealing the particular. (*Narrative Medicine* 9)

Charon's agenda—institutionalized in courses combining literature and medicine that can be found in at least some medical schools (cf. Hawkins and McEntyre)—draws on narrative skills developed in literature departments and in psychotherapy, amongst others (cf. Charon, *Narrative Medicine* 10). Neither Luria nor Charon, who are/were trained and practicing physicians, deny that biology or classical research are fundamental in advancing medical treatments, especially in research. Eric R. Kandel, reviewing the history of psychiatry, neuropsychology, and neurology, even laments the "indifference to, if not disdain for, biology" of psychoanalysts in the 1960s that "weakened psychiatry's effectiveness" (366)—a case that Draaisma also argues for Capgras syndrome. Kandel advocates that reductionist and evidence-based research must be employed to expedite psychotherapeutic approaches, but he also acknowledges that "in the early years psychoanalysts made many useful and original observations that contributed to our understanding of mind simply by listening carefully to their patients" (365). CS forms an especially interesting case of neuropsychological impairment since the patient does not perceive his or her health to be impaired. He or she does not feel ill; rather, the outside world ascribes a disease that cannot be communicated as such by the patient.[8] The narrative a CS patient tells will thus not be concerned with illness but with delusional and paranoid stories based on subjective and/or objective observations and interpretations of the outside world.

---

[8]   Health, disease, and illness are contested terms whose definitions do not necessarily depend on whether one is a trained physician or a layperson. The way people define these terms seems to be connected to their attitude towards science in general, evoking Luria's definitions of the romantic and the classical scholar. I myself use the terms in the sense that Ian R. McWhinney, amongst others, understands them in "Health and Disease: Problems of Definition." McWhinney is of the opinion that health and disease are qualities and that "one can *only express their meaning by describing or telling stories* about people or things that have these qualities" (815; my emphasis). He further defines "disease" as "a categorization of the patient's disease that has predictive power and, in some cases, enables causal inferences to be made. There remains the difficult but not insoluble problem of distinguishing disease from social deviance" (815). Illness is defined as the subjective experience of a disease by a patient.

Narratives of CS patients, as *The Echo Maker* shows, become both source and pitfall of knowledge.

Tracing Capgras Syndrome as a Medical Text

Before I can present *The Echo Maker* as a text that illustrates how narrative strategies are used mainly to preserve what the fictional characters consider to be their sanity of mind, it is necessary to illustrate the medical history of CS, with its conflicting understandings of the syndrome. In doing so, I am less concerned with the biological basis of medical research than with the cultural, social, and philosophical backgrounds that have influenced the medical research and treatment of CS in the past. This allows me to understand the medical research of CS as a cultural text, as narrative, that establishes coherence. Thus, given that all of cultural production is text, both the patient and his or her illness and disease become a text that has to be read and interpreted before the patient can be diagnosed and the illness and disease treated. In this light, Anne Hunsaker Hawkins and Marilyn Chandler McEntyre discuss "the tension"

> between constructivist and reductionist notions of illness. Few would argue that illness experience, like medical practice, is not in some way shaped by cultural values and assumptions. But it seems clear that the degree of social constructedness varies widely between a disease that has a definable pathogen, such as tuberculosis, and one that seems to derive from cultural norms and values, such as anorexia. (3)

The boundaries between a clearly "definable pathogen" and an illness that is derived from "cultural norms" does not need to be clear-cut, though, which is a point that *The Echo Maker* addresses both playfully and critically by choosing the rare and spectacular CS as the disorder that triggers the disintegration of the unified selves of its protagonists.

Since its first medical identification and description by Joseph Capgras and J. Reboul-Lachaux in 1923 (cf. Luauté 16), CS has in turn been claimed by the disciplines of psychiatry, psychoanalysis, and neurology. This disciplinary dispute about CS certainly lies in its almost fantastic syndromes. Nicola M. J. Edelstyn and Femi Oyebode characterize CS as "the delusional belief that one or a few highly familiar people have been replaced by impostors who are physically very similar to the original/s. The patient acknowledges that the double and known person look alike, but maintains the belief that the significant person, in psychological terms, is absent" (48). More importantly, however, the etiologies of CS purvey the cultural roots that have incisively affected and influenced the medical history of the syndrome's research and treatment. Draaisma traces these developments in a concise fashion and regrets that the initial article published by Capgras "was followed by a series of articles championing psychoanalytical explanations" with which one could argue that "creating a double is a subconscious way of handling mounting tensions between ambivalent feelings: all hostility is projected on the impostor, whereas the lost dear one tends to be idealized" (432). Moreover, CS lent and still lends itself particularly well to psychoanalytical interpretation since "[t]he idea of doubles was in a sense a natural consequence of recognizing a face but not experiencing the warmth and familiarity that comes naturally with seeing this face" (432). Jean-Pierre Luauté shares Draaisma's sentiment that Joseph Capgras "scotomized" (Luauté 9) the possibility of an organic origin of CS but also understands Joseph Capgras's failure to be a matter of the prevailing *Zeitgeist*. In addition to having medical training in psychiatry (cf. Luauté 10-11), Capgras "was oriented toward an understanding of mental disorders as opposed to mere description" (Luauté 12).

One of the key problems in understanding mental disorders at the beginning of the twentieth century was, of course, the lack of biological knowledge of the brain. In tracing the history of neuropsychiatry and the study of memory, Kandel describes how Freud "had written repeatedly about the relevance of the biology of the brain to psychoanalysis" (45). Kandel quotes both "On Narcissism" (1914)—"We must recollect that all of our provisional ideas in psychology will presumably one day be based on organic substructure" (qtd. in Kandel 45-46)—and *Beyond the Pleasure Principle* (1920):

> The deficiencies in our description would probably vanish if we were already in a position to replace the psychological terms by physiological or chemical ones. (qtd. in Kandel 46)
>
> Biology is truly a land of unlimited possibilities. We may expect it to give us the most surprising information, and we cannot guess what answers it will return in a few dozen years. . . . They may be of a kind

> which will blow away the whole of our artificial structure of hypotheses. (qtd. in Kandel 51)

Kandel thus argues that the biological reality of neuropsychological disorders has always been the basis of psychological and psychoanalytical research, and he honors the Viennese origins of psychoanalysis as decisive for both himself as a young researcher and for the discipline of neuropsychology as a whole. It is not particularly surprising, then, that Joseph Capgras's research papers on CS picked up on contemporary psychoanalytic patterns of explanation that at least offered a path, however convoluted, out of the maze that was constituted by "the immaturity of brain science at the time" (Kandel 366).

Although psychotherapeutic practice may seem to antecede the efforts of narrative medicine (cf. Rudnytsky 2), Peter L. Rudnytsky adds that, to Freud, psychoanalysis was never a "specialized branch of medicine" and that psychoanalysis should "include branches of knowledge which are remote from medicine and which the doctor does not come across in his practice: the history of civilization, mythology, the psychology of religion, and the science of literature"—a formulation reminiscent of narrative medicine—while, at the same time, the psychoanalyst was to maintain an "emotional coldness" towards his patients (Freud qtd. in Rudnytsky 3)—a position challenged by narrative medicine. In his "Recommendations to Physicians Practicing Psycho-analysis," Freud reasons that the analyst's affects, sympathy, and empathy may obscure the results that psychoanalysis would otherwise uncover (cf. "Ratschläge" 380-81). Likewise, Freud advises analysts not to take notes during or after the session but to only remember the analysands' reports, since, in taking notes, the analyst will inevitably select certain information as important and dismiss other information as less significant, which would result in an already edited and annotated narrative of a patient's story (cf. "Ratschläge" 378-79). Thus, Freud, like narrative medicine, intended to protect his protégées from mis-diagnosing an analysand due to the analyst's own prejudices. Emotional coldness would thus fulfill the same function as the covering of patients' bodies in surgery: The doctor sees only that part of the human body that needs treatment; the rest of the patient is concealed so that the surgeon may actually have the courage to cut skin and flesh, expose the diseased organ, and perform the surgery that is needed. These musings present the basic dilemma that a physician encounters in his daily work, i.e., that of finding the right dosage not only of medication but also of empathy and compassion. Rita Charon discusses the difficult relationship of narrative medicine and psychoanalysis that arises because the two approaches are not identical, either in method or in the diseases and illness they attend to or the kind of therapeutic relief they can offer; the body as the site of disease hereby plays a major role, according to Charon.[9] She argues that "[i]f psychoanalysis reminds us of the corporeal dimensions of insight, narrative medicine reminds us of the metaphorical dimensions of illness. The body is *not* transparent, however good the MRI may get. ... That the internist *thinks* it is transparent is the problem. That he or she has not been trained to appreciate its opacity is the *real* problem" ("Where" 30). As my analysis will show, Charon here hits the weak spot of the conflict between Weber and his colleague Dr. Hayes in *The Echo Maker*, who mirror the history of CS research by representing two opposing approaches (cf. Draaisma) to CS and Mark as a patient. The issue that distresses Mark's sister Karin, Weber, and the reader revolves around the question in how far the body may transparently portray CS and to what extent a narrative approach to Mark's condition can illuminate the disease and guide therapy.

Joseph Capgras himself first considered CS as an "agnosia of identification" (Luauté 16) in which "'L'Illusion des sosies' [the illusion of doubles / *doppelgänger*] is recognized as a delusional interpretation based 'first on an emotional state, then on a turn of mind'" that "matches the paranoid personality" (Luauté 17). Soon after, Joseph Capgras

---

[9]   Scheurich, for instance, remarks that literature and psychoanalysis "are very much situated in the marketplace of ideas" and that "psychoanalysis is increasingly marginalized in mainstream psychiatry" (248). He sees the reason for this in the development psychiatry has taken towards "evidence-based practice, managed care, and standardized diagnosis [which] have brought psychiatry closer to general medicine" (248) and strengthening a "biologically oriented" (252) psychiatric practice. The mind-body problem that underlies some of the diverging opinions in psychiatry might in the future be solved by research results showing that "talking does not influence a disembodied 'mind' or 'spirit,' but rather the same organ affected by somatic therapies" (252).

interpreted the illusion of doubles as a "secondary symptom of the 'délire d'interprétation' [delusion of interpretation] similar to confabulation, false recognition, illusions of memory" until he, together with two colleagues, "introduce[d] the idea that the delusion could constitute a sort of defense against greater danger, . . . invok[ing] the well-known psychoanalytic concept of delusion as a restitution" (Luauté 17). Draaisma observes that "there were good reasons to think of Capgras [syndrome] in terms of psychodynamic causes" (433) and argues that the varying interpretations of CS constitute "one of those exemplary Gestalt switches in science" (433). Since the 1980s, CS has usually been considered to be a neurological disorder whereas before it was treated as a psychiatric one (cf. Draaisma 433). As Freud had predicted, this paradigm shift was due to "the articulation of a neurological theory" (Draaisma 434) but the re-interpretation has still not resulted in an unambiguous epidemiology or etiology. In 1999,[10] Edelstyn and Oyebode presented a wide range of "aetiology and explanatory hypotheses" (49) addressing the functional context, psychodynamic proposals, organic context, and neuropsychological proposals. The paper concludes not with definitive answers but with a hopeful perspective: "CS is a discrete neuropsychiatric symptom which has interested clinicians and researchers for the past 75 years. It is hoped that its study will lead to an increased understanding of the neuropsychological basis of psychotic experiences and may provide a paradigm for how we approach the study of the psychoses in general" (53). Despite the greatest efforts and vast biological medical progress, mind and brain remain challenging sites of mystery and provide rabbit holes into phantasmagoric realities for scientists and novelists alike.

---

[10] A research paper dating back 13 years would be considered outdated and could not well be used in a medical context. However, I do not intend to present the latest neurological results on CS but rather seek to portray neuropsychological research in its full complexity, topicality, and transience.

Tracing Capgras Syndrome in Fiction

In the fictional case of *The Echo Maker*'s Mark Schluter, CS has clearly been induced by brain injury[11]—we have a definable pathogen—but CS leads Mark to develop secondary conditions, such as (paranoid) delusions. Although Mark's physical perception of reality does not deviate from that of the other characters—he neither hallucinates nor do details slip his perception—he attributes exaggerated importance to very slight changes, to which he normally would not pay any attention. Dr. Hayes explains that "a quarter or more of CS patients go on to develop other delusional symptoms" (207) in order to restore the missing link in their personal narrative: "A story to link the shifting self back to the senseless facts. Reason was not impaired here; logic still worked on any other topic but this" (164). Weber further elaborates:

> In Capgras, the person believes their loved ones have been swapped with lifelike robots, doubles, or aliens. They properly identify everyone else. The loved one's face elicits memory, but no feeling. Lack of emotional ratification overrides the rational assembly of memory. Or put it this way: reason invents elaborately unreasonable explanations to explain a deficit in emotion. *Logic depends upon feeling.* (Powers 106; my emphasis)

He associates memory, feeling, and logic, which, when (successfully) connected, provide us with the narrative of our selves and our lives. Kandel, too, postulates that "[i]t is, of course, memory that weaves one's life into a coherent whole" (372); a shattered world of memories leads to a shattered sense of identity. The psychologist Daniel L. Schacter affirms that "even though memory can be highly elusive in some situations and dead wrong in others, it still forms the foundation for our most strongly held beliefs about ourselves" (7):

---

[11] Rivka Galchen's *Atmospheric Disturbances* (2008) does not grant its readers this certainty. In her novel, Dr. Leo Liebenstein (notably a psychiatrist), wakes up one morning and finds his wife gone and replaced by a "simulacrum" (5). As I will show elsewhere, such a setting alters not only plot and story of the novel but also the use of narrative and narrative as a critical approach.

> Psychologists have come to recognize that the complex mixtures of
> personal knowledge that we retain about the past are woven together to
> form life stories and personal myths. These are the biographies of self
> that provide narrative continuity between past and future—a set of
> memories that form the core of personality. (93)

Throughout *Searching for Memory*, Schacter emphasizes that personal
histories resemble well-constructed narratives which rarely or never
show characteristics of an objective report. This is not to mean, though,
that "we live in a world of wholly fabricated, self-serving fantasies"
(94). Rather, the connections we draw retrospectively and the way we
remember are always accompanied with a feeling that is as dependent on
the intention with which we retrieve a memory as it is dependent on the
actual event that is retrieved. Recalling Freud's "Screen Memories"
(1899), Schacter suggests that "conscious recollections are inevitably
distorted by a person's wishes, desires, and unconscious conflicts" and
that psychoanalysis served, among other things, to "uncover the 'true'
reality hidden behind the screen memory" (100). Intuitively advocating
psychoanalysis, Weber's wife suggests that Capgras "[s]ounds like
something for Sigmund," but Weber himself points out that CS is "at the
same time, the clear result of injury. That's what makes it so fantastic.
It's the kind of neither-both case that could help arbitrate between two
very different paradigms of mind" (105). Being a neither-both case,
Capgras syndrome creates a space that *Weber* nevertheless fills with
aspects of neurology, psychiatry, psychology, and psychoanalysis. It is
thus *Weber's interpretation, Weber's narrative*, of CS that re-negotiates
conceptions of mind, self, and identity. Although he knows that CS is a
"neither-both case," Weber is so keen to believe in the possibility that
Mark's CS results from "psychodynamic responses to trauma"—which
are "large-scale psychological reactions to the disorientation" (Powers
132)—that Weber does not seem to be willing to explore the physical
causes of CS. Weber's version of CS promises to be the more
fascinating one, lending itself to being rendered as a fictional account,
leaving the door open for Freud to enter the case study. However,
Weber's motives in doing so are questionable, since he has almost come
to resent contemporary neurology for denying him philosophical
answers, and not for being inaccurate or counterfactual:

What would he say the following week, to sum up a discipline drifting
away from him? Long after science delivered a comprehensive theory of
self, no one would be a single step closer to knowing what it meant to be
another. Neurology would never grasp from without a thing that existed
only deep in the impenetrable inside. (365)

As if to remind physicians like Weber that medicine requires both
narrative and science, Oliver Sacks writes:

[W]ith human life, human nature...there is drama,[12] there is
intentionality, at every point. Its exploration demands the seeing and
telling of a story, demands a narrative structure of sensibility and
science. Two modes of thought are always required here . . ., and these,
though so different, must be completely intertwined, to produce a unity
greater than either could alone. This is the unity we sense in Luria and
Freud. ("Luria and 'Romantic Science'" 193)

Nevertheless, I would say that Sacks also alludes here to what Charles
Taylor calls an "inescapable feature of human life" (Taylor 47). Taylor
also argues that "in order to make minimal sense of our lives, in order to
have an identity, . . . we grasp our lives in a *narrative*" (47). Our lives
are situated in space and time, in body and in action, not only in mind
and brain. They "exist in this space of questions, which only a coherent
narrative can answer. In order to have a sense of who we are, we have to
have a notion of how we have become, and what we are going to do"
(Taylor 47). Taylor further specifies that "what is in question is,
generally and characteristically, the shape of my life *as a whole*. . . . We
want our lives to have meaning, or weight, or substance, or to grow
towards some fullness. . . But this means our *whole* lives" (50). In the
same vein, Young and Saver write that "[c]onsciousness needs a
narrative structure to create a sense of self based on the features of
storytelling, like coherence, consequence, consecution" (78-79). *The
Echo Maker* illustrates a major challenge to the mechanism of
fabricating a life story that would encompass the continuous story of
one's (whole) life, since Mark's CS creates a gap in his personal history;
his memories are vulnerable (cf. Schacter 6), as his sister Karin's

---

[12] This "drama" relates to Barthes's writerly text, which I read not only as
continuous production but also as continuous performance.

bewilderment about his symptoms shows.[13] Amnestic patients may bridge the gap that memory loss has created by confabulation or delusion. Young and Saver describe confabulation as the phenomenon of affected persons

> restlessly fabricating narratives that purport to describe recent events in their lives but actually having little or no relationship to genuine occurrences. . . . Unaware of their memory disorder, they also appear unaware they are creating fictitious responses to fill in memory gaps. (76)

Confabulation, they argue, "offer[s] an unrivaled glimpse at the power of the human impulse to narrative" (76), especially since confabulating patients do not fabricate the same story over and over again. Their narratives serve to brush over memory gaps but the narratives are not consistent. In principle, it seems that a narrative does *not need to be* coherent as long as it *establishes* coherence. Mark Schluter, though, does not confabulate. It is true that he suffers from a mild form of retrograde amnesia—he does not remember how the accident happened—but his explanatory narrative is nevertheless consistent:

> Mark was remarkably animated, spinning a story that smoothed out all the breaks. He raced through the answers before Weber even asked the questions. He traced a single, clean line of thought: all his friends were conspiring to hide what had happened that night. Cain and Rupp knew; they'd been talking to him on the walkie-talkie just as he flipped over. But they'd lied to him about it. His sister knew, so she'd been replaced, to keep her from telling. . . . [S]he was probably locked up somewhere. (Powers 300)

Although Mark logically reflects upon what has happened, he cannot reveal the source of and reason for either his accident or the

---

[13] Cf. *The Echo Maker*: "It's strange. He glorifies me now. I mean *her*. In fact, he and I—I mean *this* me—struggle pretty much the same way we always did. We had kind of a rough time, growing up. I've tried to keep him from doing all the stupid things I've done, over the years. He needs me to be the voice of reason; he's never had anyone else for that. Used to resent it like crazy, the straighter I kept him. But now he just resents me, and thinks *she* was some kind of saint" (120).

disappearance of his sister. Of course, he is totally unaware of the non-factual basis of his fabrication. A psychopathological diagnosis might thus characterize Mark's narrative as a delusional disorder. Mark advocates his story and maintains his view with infallible, *a priori* certainty. No one is able to challenge his newly found belief, which he defends both emotionally and in an almost grotesquely logical fashion (cf. Linden 4). He sees himself in the middle of a conspiracy that has to be of highest importance to the ones who allegedly tried to murder him—probably members of some secret government agency.[14] He misinterprets or over-interprets almost everything: an incorrectly parked car, or a poster—showing a topless girl—missing from his apartment, which his sister Karin had actually removed because she thought it offensive (delusional perception, *Wahnwahrnehmung*; cf. Linden 6). Mark's delusion, however, is outrightly systematic (systematic delusion, *systematischer Wahn*; cf. Linden 6): His superordinate narrative forms an airtight system that makes it impossible to 'talk sense into him.' His private narrative is more powerful than the shared reality of all persons around him.

Mark's conviction clearly shatters his own world, but it also triggers the unraveling of Weber's identity, which is caught in-between classic and romantic medical scholarship and treatments. "[T]his dilemma" (175), as the novel puts it, drives Gerald Weber into a serious crisis that concerns not only his work and his success as a physician and author, but also the general narrative of his life and his self. Like Luria, Weber believes in the epistemological power of narrative; he is a romantic scholar who refuses to focus solely on the lesions in Mark's head and who seeks to uncover other complex psychological as well as physiological mechanisms in Mark. Weber's romantic strain, however, seems to prevent him from seeing biological facts at all. A good case in point would be the following passage in which Hayes briefs Weber about Mark's brain trauma, showing him an x-ray of Mark's brain: "The young neurologist saw only structures. Weber still saw the rarest of butterflies, fluttering mind, its paired wings pinned to the film in

---

[14] We have to remember that *The Echo Maker* is (purposefully) set in post-9/11 America and allegorically portrays not only a traumatized but also a paranoid nation. Cf. Birgit Däwes's article in this volume.

obscene detail. Hayes traced over the surreal art. This subsystem still chattered; this one had fallen silent" (131).

Hayes is presented as a classic scholar of the reductionist fashion who "only," i.e., exclusively, perceives what he can measure quantitatively. Weber, in contrast, is "still" fascinated by the aesthetic quality the scan offers, which implies that he has not yet reached the stage of Hayes's professionalism; medically speaking, Weber is not up to date. For him, the x-ray almost has the practical effect of a Rorschach interpretation, a highly controversial psychological method, which, nonetheless, shares some basic axioms with Luria's concept of romantic medical scholarship as it "always proceeds with the objective of developing an understanding of the person as a *unique* individual" (Exner 3). Supporters of Rorschach interpretation argue that "[i]t is the sort of information that goes beyond the identification of symptoms and searches out etiological issues that distinguish one person from another, even though both may present the same symptomatology" (Exner 4-5). While Hayes advocates a purely biological assessment, Weber seeks "a more comprehensive explanation":

> But there's a higher-order component to all this, too. Whatever lesions he has suffered, he's also producing psychodynamic responses to trauma. Capgras may not be caused so much by the lesion per se as by large-scale psychological vectors in his life. He stops recognizing his sister because some part of him has stopped recognizing himself. I have always found it worthwhile to consider a delusion as both the attempt to make sense—as well as the result—of a deeply upsetting development. (132)

Weber knows as well as Hayes that "Mark Schluter's Capgras isn't primarily psychiatric" (133). Yet, he is convinced or wants to be convinced, more for philosophical than for medical reasons, that they "owe him more than a simple, one-way, functionalist, causal model" (133). After all, "he'd championed the idea: facts are only a small part of any case history. What counted was the telling" (109). Yet Weber cannot see the individual tree for the forest, so to speak. Having treated too many impaired minds, Weber seemingly deconstructs the idea that "the self presents itself as whole, unified, embodied, continuous, and aware" (381) by giving numerous examples from the history of neuroscience that provide counterexamples for this assumption (cf. 381-

82). The conclusion of this "deconstruction" is that the self only exists in fictional terms when the brain is in its unimpaired condition. One would have to conclude that telling narratives of illness was an equally illusive endeavor since it only enforces one's faith in a make-believe reality. As soon as a brain suffers damage, not only perception and reception but also the self as such becomes unreliable.[15] One of Weber's illustrative examples is the case of epileptics "who'd had their corpus callosum cut" and "ended up inhabiting two separate brain hemispheres. . . . The left claimed to believe in God; the right reported itself an atheist" (381). The self appears to reside in the body and, thus, will suffer once its shelter is harmed, or, as Rita Charon puts it: "The self depends on the body for its presence, its location. Without the body, the self cannot be uttered. . . . Without the body, the self is an abstraction" ("Where" 30). Weber finally concludes that "of selves as the self describes itself, no one had one. Lying, denying, repressing, confabulating: these weren't pathologies. They were the signature of awareness, trying to stay intact" (Powers 382).[16] Thus, Weber not only defends simple truisms such as that we truly are storytelling animals; he moreover, without even realizing it, proclaims indirectly that storytelling itself is an epistemological "neither-both case." While Mark constructs a coherent yet counterfactual reality, Weber attempts to deconstruct the safety net of coherence and certainty that the shared reality of narrative offers. But both are constructions and both constructions are right in a neither-both

---

[15] "Derealization and depersonalization. Anxiety attacks and religious conversions. Misidentification—the whole continuum of Capgras-like phenomena, phenomena that Weber had witnessed his whole life without quite noticing. Eternal love retracted. Entire life philosophies abandoned in disgust" (Powers 381).

[16] At this point, Weber himself, in an almost neurotic fashion, seems to lose a healthy relation to reality. Freud defined neurosis as *the result of a conflict between the ego and the id*" ("Neurosis and Psychosis" 149) for which "the decisive factor would be the predominance of the influence of reality" ("The Loss of Reality in Neurosis and Psychosis" 183). He further posits that "psychoanalytic research finds no fundamental but only quantitative distinctions between normal and neurotic life" (Freud qtd. in Evans 123). Weber's exposure to extreme neurological and psychiatric diseases has certainly left deep wounds in his own perception of the self.

kind of way—a fact that Weber cannot easily acknowledge. Just like Mark, he substitutes one narrative with another, gaining nothing but an equally structured narrative.

In his "Letter to a Japanese Friend," Jacques Derrida notes that in deconstruction "the dismantling of a structure is not a regression toward a *simple element*, toward an *indissoluble origin*" (3). Weber's conclusion that "Capgras [was] truer than this constant smoothing-out of consciousness" (Powers 448), however, discloses simply the negation of a "whole, unified, embodied, continuous, and aware" (381) self and its regression into its opposite. If deconstruction means "to understand how an 'ensemble' was constituted and to reconstruct it to this end" (Derrida 3), Weber never deconstructs or reconstructs, he only constructs.

Concluding Remarks

Considered from a narrative perspective, CS offers more than a diagnostic history that portrays the state of the medical art—which alone would make it a fascinating disorder for the medical historian. I have shown that the narrative history of neuropsychology as such and CS in particular allows for the recognition of the greater mindset that exposes medical research to political, social, philosophical, and cultural trends. This, of course, is the reason why Richard Powers's portrayal of a CS patient and his immediate social environment in *The Echo Maker* makes such a productive text for literary scholars.

Young and Saver conclude their study on "The Neurology of Narrative" by stating that "[t]o desire narrative reflects a kind of fundamental desire for life and self that finds its source in our neurological make-up" (80). Moreover, "[d]efects in fictive self-narrative construction destabilize and distort the human personality. . . . Individuals who have lost the ability to construct narrative, however, have lost their selves" (77-78). In *The Echo Maker*, narrative has the function of both constructing and deconstructing certainty. Mark needs to reconstruct his accident, which *did* happen, and the disappearance of his sister, which he only thinks happened. Weber constructs his alter ego, "Famous Gerald," his faithfulness towards his patients and his wife, and the psychological reasons for Mark's CS. Although Weber wants to deconstruct the notion of a unified mind, he has long sought shelter in newly constructed structures of his self.

In *The Echo Maker*, Mark's mental health is re-established in a *deus ex machina* fashion when, all of a sudden, surgery and medication cure Mark's CS: "The medication is working, the mild shocks, but so gradually there is almost no threshold. The same spin-doctor subsystem that cut him out without his knowing now blinds him to his own return. She watches him turn back into Mark, old Mark, before her appalled eyes" (444). Order seems to return to the chaos of Mark's brain; still, nothing's well even though it ends well. *The Echo Maker* leaves the reader with reasonable and substantial doubt whether CS is actually cured when Mark again implies that Karin is not his real sister—he says that he only wants to tease her. On the other hand, his last words to Karin leave at least a queasy feeling: "It's not all so bad, huh? Just as good, in fact. In some ways, even better. . . . I mean, us. You. Me. Here. . . . Whatever you call all this. Just as good as the real thing" (447). The novel's final pages, then, do not resolve any of the problems that CS has caused. Even though the symptoms may have disappeared, authentic coherence can no longer be established without being consciously marked as production and performance. With Weber, the case is even more pronounced. When leaving Nebraska, he, asked by a stranger whether he isn't "the brain guy," replies: "Not me, . . . I'm in reclamation" (449). He returns home to reclaim his private, professional, and public self, his wife, and his sense of selfhood in general. Only when he finds himself in reclamation can the reader believe that his constructions have begun to wobble. Even though Weber's intended deconstruction fails, in the novel as such, "[d]econstruction takes place" (Derrida 4). It presents narrative as the most powerful mechanism structuring the consciousness of both unified and disunified minds alike and displays the ruptures that accompany any story. As much as the characters struggle to find answers, the novel's only answer seems to lie in presenting narrative as such as operative. In order to make this point, CS is a fitting disease since it displays the power of narrative in a threefold manner: First, CS leads Mark to fabricate extensive delusional narratives to smooth out consciousness. Second, the real-world research and treatment of CS itself has been guided by ideological (master) narratives that are echoed in Mark's doctors, Weber and Hayes. Third, narrative medicine offers an effective method for anamnesis and treatment in that it helps the physician to understand the patient. Neuropsychological diseases like CS are a case in point of how only narratives may actually lead to a diagnosis, although they may also be the results of the delusion of confabulation. *The Echo Maker* presents narrative as powerfully productive, though not necessarily as fact-based.

Works Cited

Barthes, Roland. *S/Z An Essay*. Transl. Richard Miller. New York: Hill and Wang, 1974. Print.

---. "Introduction to the Structural Analysis of Narratives." *Image Music Text*. Comp. and trans. Stephen Heath. New York: Hill and Wang, 1978. 79-124. Print.

Bruner, Jerome. *Actual Minds, Possible Worlds*. Cambridge: Harvard UP, 1986. Print.

Charon, Rita. *Narrative Medicine*. Oxford: Oxford UP, 2006. Print.

---. "Where Does Narrative Medicine Come From?" *Psychoanalysis and Narrative Medicine*. Ed. Peter L. Rudnytsky and Rita Charon. Albany: State U of New York P, 2008. 23-36. Print.

Derrida, Jacques. "Letter to a Japanese Friend." Trans. David Wood and Andrew Benjamin. *Derrida and Différance*. Ed. David Wood and Robert Bernasconi. Warwick: Parousia, 1985. 1-5. Print.

Draaisma, Douwe. "Echos, Doubles, and Delusions: Capgras Syndrome in Science and Literature." *Style* 43.3 (2009): 429-41. *EBSCOhost*. Web. 21 Jan. 2012.

Edelstyn, N[icola] M. J., and F[emi] Oyebode. "A Review of the Phenomenology and Cognitive Neuropsychological Origins of the Capgras Syndrome." *International Journal of Geriatric Psychiatry* 14.1 (1999): 48-59. *Wiley Online Library*. Web. 21 Jan. 2012.

Evans, Dylan. *An Introductory Dictionary of Lacanian Psychoanalysis*. 1996. London: Routledge, 2007. Print.

Exner, John E. *The Rorschach: A Comprehensive System. Basic Foundations and Principles of Interpretation*. Vol. 1. 4th ed. Hoboken: Wiley, 2003. Print.

Fireman, Gary D., Ted E. McVay, Jr., and Owen J. Flanagan, eds. *Narrative and Consciousness: Literature, Psychology, and the Brain*. Oxford: Oxford UP, 2003. Print.

Freud, Sigmund. "The Loss of Reality in Neurosis and Psychosis." 1924. *The Standard Edition of the Complete Psychological Works of Sigmund Freud*. Vol. 19: *The Ego and the Id and Other Works*. Ed. James Strachey. Trans. James Strachey and Anna Freud. London: Vintage, 2001. 183-87. Print.

---. "Neurosis and Psychosis." 1924. *The Standard Edition of the Complete Psychological Works of Sigmund Freud*. Vol. 19: *The Ego and the Id and Other Works*. Ed. James Strachey. Trans. James Strachey and Anna Freud. London: Vintage, 2001. 149-53. Print.

---. "Ratschläge für den Arzt bei der Psychoanalytischen Behandlung." *Gesammelte Werke*. Vol. 8: *Werke aus den Jahren 1909-1913*. 1945. London: Imago, 1964. 376-87. Print.

Galchen, Rivka. *Atmospheric Disturbances*. London: Harper, 2008. Print.

Gastpar, Markus, Siegfried Kasper, and Michael Linden, eds. *Psychiatrie*. De Gruyter Lehrbuch mit Repetitorium. Berlin: De Gruyter, 1996. Print.

Goffman, Erving. *The Presentation of Self in Everyday Life*. New York: Bantam, 1959. Print.

Hawkins, Anne Hunsaker, and Marilyn Chandler McEntyre. "Teaching Literature and Medicine: A Retrospective and a Rationale." Introduction. *Teaching Literature and Medicine*. Ed. Hawkins and McEntyre. New York: MLA, 2000. 1-25. Print.

Kandel, Eric R. *In Search of Memory: The Emergence of a New Science of Mind*. New York: Norton, 2006. Print.

Kucharzewski, Jan D. "In the Lake House of Language: An Interview with Richard Powers." *Propositions about Life: Reengaging Literature and Science*. Heidelberg: Winter, 2011. 455-61. Print.

Linden, Michael. "Psychopathologie, Deskription und Diagnostik psychischer Erkrankungen." Psychiatrie. Ed. Markus Gastpar, Siegfried Kasper, and Michael Linden. De Gruyter Lehrbuch mit Repetitorium. Berlin: De Gruyter, 1996. 1-17. Print.

Luauté, Jean-Pierre. "Joseph Capgras and His Syndrome." *The Delusional Misidentification Syndromes*. Ed. George N. Christodoulou. Basel: Karger, 1986. 9-21. Print.

Luria, A. R. *The Man with a Shattered World: The History of a Brain Wound*. 1972. Trans. Lynn Solotaroff. Cambridge: Harvard UP, 1987. Print.

---. *The Making of the Mind: A Personal Account of Soviet Psychology.* Ed. Michael Cole and Sheila Cole. Cambridge: Harvard UP, 1979. Print.

Maturana, Humberto R., and Franciso J. Verala. *Tree of Knowledge: The Biological Roots of Human Understanding,* Boston: Shambhala, 1987. Print.

McWhinney, Ian R. "Health and Disease: Problems of Definition." *CMAJ* 136.8 (1987): 815. Web. 21 Jan. 2012.

Nash, Christopher. *Narrative in Culture: The Uses of Storytelling in the Sciences, Philosophy, and Literature.* London: Routledge, 1990. Print.

Olson, David R. Introduction. *Modes of Thought: Explorations in Culture and Cognition.* Ed. David R. Olson and Nancy Torrance. Cambridge: Cambridge UP, 1996. 1-11. Print.

Polkinghorne, Donald E. *Narrative Knowing and the Human Sciences.* Albany: State U of New York P, 1988. Print.

Powers, Richard. *The Echo Maker.* London: Random, 2006. Print.

Rouse, Joseph. *Engaging Science: How to Understand Its Practices Philosophically.* Ithaca: Cornell UP, 1996. Print.

Rudnytsky, Peter L. Introduction. *Psychoanalysis and Narrative Medicine.* Ed. Peter L. Rudnytsky and Rita Charon. Albany: State U of New York P, 2008. 1-19. Print.

Sacks, Oliver. "Luria and 'Romantic Science.'" *Contemporary Neuropsychology and the Legacy of Luria.* Ed. Elkhonon Goldberg. Hillsdale: Lawrence Erlbaum Associates, 1990. 181-94. Print.

Schacter, Daniel L. *Searching for Memory.* New York: Basic, 1996. Print.

Scheurich, Neil. "Reading, Listening, and Other Beleaguered Practices in General Psychiatry." *Psychoanalysis and Narrative Medicine.* Ed. Peter L. Rudnytsky and Rita Charon. Albany: State U of New York P, 2008. 247-60. Print.

Taylor, Charles. *Sources of the Self: The Making of the Modern Identity.* Cambridge: Cambridge UP, 1989. Print.

Young, Kay, and Jeffrey L. Saver. "The Neurology of Narrative." *On the Origin of Fictions: Interdisciplinary Perspectives.* Spec. issue of *SubStance* 30.1-2 (2001): 72-84. *JSTOR.* Web. 24 Aug. 2011.

BIRGIT DÄWES

Traumorama?
The Pathological Landscapes of
Richard Powers's *The Echo Maker*

> [F]acts are only a small part of any case
> history. What counted was the telling.
> (Powers 139)

Introduction

> Turning on the radio to find the world
> blown away. (Powers 344)

During the first decade of the twenty-first century, American literature and literary scholarship have been noticeably overshadowed by the terrorist attacks of September 11. The day that allegedly "changed everything" caused a new vogue for the term "trauma"—both as a literary motif and a critical response. "September 11," Dori Laub writes, "was an encounter with something that makes no sense, an event that fits in nowhere. It was an experience of collective massive psychic trauma" which "shook our world and our assumptions about our lives" (204). This view was shared by a number of mental health professionals and politicians, but also by cultural critics such as E. Ann Kaplan and Judith Greenberg. In the field of fiction, novels such as Jonathan Safran Foer's *Extremely Loud and Incredibly Close* (cf. Uytterschout; Codde; Huehls, Mullins) and Don DeLillo's *Falling Man* (cf. Kauffman; Versluys), for instance, have been extensively analyzed for their traumatized characters. Kristiaan Versluys even speaks of "the first instance of global trauma" ("9/11"), for which we need a new critical vocabulary. It seems that trauma has indeed evolved, as Sabine Sielke suggests, into a "prêt-à-porter trop[e]" ("Why" 387) or even a new master narrative.

While it is true that trauma is a literary motif in many twenty-first century American novels, its viability as a critical concept is less than evident. In this paper, I will specifically call into question the practicality of trauma studies for the context of 9/11 fiction. Following Jeffrey C. Alexander's insight that "trauma is not something naturally existing; it is something constructed by society" (2), I argue that the quest for characters' symptoms actually obscures the inquiry into the cultural dimensions of trauma by distracting from larger historical contexts and repercussions. As Richard Powers's novel *The Echo Maker* exemplarily demonstrates, the forms of medical imagery that have emerged in post-9/11 novels serve a more complex range of functions than merely diagnosing the state of a "wounded" city or nation (cf. E. Kaplan 136 and Greenberg, "Wounded New York" 26). Through a strategy that I will term "neurological metafiction," *The Echo Maker* uses symbolic settings, structural symmetries, and metaphorical nodes in order to map a much wider pathological landscape. It not only liberates 9/11 fiction from the limiting grip of trauma terminology, but it also pinpoints the larger ethical and aesthetic challenges that arise from an era of what Amy Kaplan calls "Homeland Insecurities" (55).

Trauma and 9/11

> Then Pure Terror, Pealing into Air,
> Flipping and Falling. (Powers 12)

In the medical sense of the word—defined as a "psychic injury, esp. one caused by emotional shock the memory of which is repressed and remains unhealed" (*OED*)—the attacks of September 11, 2001, undoubtedly constituted a traumatizing event for those immediately involved. Robert Alan Glick reminds us that "[m]ore than 3,000 children lost parents in the terrorist attacks" (vii, cf. also Cournos 268-72; Elkind 151-60; and Kühner 166); moreover, survivors or witnesses directly exposed to the Twin Towers' collapse in Lower Manhattan (below 14th Street) often showed symptoms of post-traumatic stress disorder (Neria et al. 244). Karen M. Seeley widens the circle of victims by pointing to the "simultaneous trauma" of New York City therapists, who "were in the unusual clinical predicament of treating numerous individuals who were wounded by the same catastrophic events that had also injured them" (4). Furthermore, Barbie Zelizer and Stuart Allan argue that "journalists and news organizations covering the events of September 11 were wounded too" (1). Beyond the immediate victims, however, and beyond the clinical discourse, the question of 9/11's traumatic impact is less than easily settled.[1] As for its functionality for the analysis of fiction, I would like to challenge the term on two accounts.

First of all, the notion of "collective trauma" is a controversial construct (cf. Leys 1-8; Wirth 37). Defined by Kai Erikson as "a blow to the basic tissues of social life that damages the bonds attaching people together and impairs the prevailing sense of communality" (187), "collective trauma" clearly applies to disasters such as the Buffalo Creek flood (Erikson's reference point), or to the forced removal of Native Americans on the Trail of Tears, but the terrorist attacks of September 11 hardly left the city of New York shattered as a community, let alone the American nation or "Western civilization" at large. Jeffrey C. Alexander has convincingly argued that the concept has no ontological

---

[1] In a study conducted by Marnie Brow and Roxane Cohen Silver, the responses "indicated that psychological effects were not limited to those directly affected and the degree of response was not directly proportional to the amount of loss, level of exposure to the attacks, or proximity to the World Trade Center or Pentagon" (Brow and Silver 38). Yet "only 2 percent of respondents reported direct exposure to the events as they were occurring, such as being at, or within view of, the World Trade Center or Pentagon, or on the telephone with someone who was in one of the buildings or airplanes" (38). Interestingly, however, while 40 percent of their respondents reported an increased level of stress two weeks after the attacks (39), these "emotional and psychological responses continued to decline in frequency and intensity" (40) over the next few months. By March 2002, only 6 percent of respondents still showed "high levels of posttraumatic stress symptoms," compared to 17 percent just after the attacks (40). This result is also confirmed by a Mainz University study on "The Emotional Timeline of September 11": According to Mitja Back and his colleagues, who analyzed over 500,000 text messages sent throughout the day, the overwhelming response quickly turned from sadness into anger (cf. Back, Küfner, and Egloff).

foundation: "Traumatic status is attributed to real or imagined phenomena, not because of their actual harmfulness or their objective abruptness, but because these phenomena are believed to have abruptly, and harmfully, affected collective identity" (9-10). In other words, it is the socially attributed "meanings that provide the sense of shock and fear, not the events in themselves" (10).[2] "Cultural trauma," as Alexander terms it (1), thus always relies for its own legitimization on the "meaning work" (12) or narrative framing, by specific interest groups. Applied to the attacks of 2001, this means that each new insistence on the "collective trauma"—in documentary or fictional responses, or in the scholarly analyses thereof—provides the very premise for its own veracity. Radically argued, the discourse of 9/11 as a collective trauma marks a case of circular reasoning.

Second, and especially in light of the recent "literary-critical fascination" (Leys 16) with trauma, one should inquire more deeply into its semiotic economy. Who benefits from the definition of 9/11 as trauma, and its fiction as "trauma literature"? More specifically, which particular discourses are privileged by such a reading, and which are silenced? The concept of trauma emphasizes suddenness and disruption: it is a response "to an unexpected or overwhelming violent event or events that are not fully grasped as they occur" (Caruth 91); or "to events so overwhelmingly intense that they impair normal emotional or cognitive responses" (Vickroy ix). Any approach based on trauma studies thus focuses on the event's effect on the victim—it leaves everyday routines and habits (as well as the causes for their disruption) unquestioned and isolates the experience from its global contexts. "By reaffirming the temporal trajectory of a world before and after September 11, 2001," Sabine Sielke notes, "the claim that 9/11 was a traumatic and transformative cultural experience reproduces in an inverted manner the world view disseminated by the Bush

---

[2]   Cf. Ulrike Tancke, who also doubts the usefulness of applying trauma theory to fiction: "Apart from the oft-voiced criticism that the term may be applied too liberally," she writes, "there is a central dilemma at the heart of trauma studies itself that renders any proposition of trauma as the pivot of subjectivity inherently problematic" (78). This problem is "the central conflict whether trauma erases the subject or, in fact, creates a new, albeit fragmented and precarious subjectivity" (78).

administration—a view that allowed legitimizing changes of policies, violations of international conventions, and the war in Iraq" ("Why" 395). In the case of 9/11, such readings not only underwrite the master narratives of national innocence and exceptionalism, but they also silence critical inquiries into larger political power structures and historical continuities. Rather than scanning 9/11 fiction for traumatized victims, therefore, I am interested in the structural and semantic patterns by which medical imagery translates such complexities into an alternative aesthetics of crisis.

Echoes of Injury: The Neurological Metafiction of Powers's *Echo Maker*

> **A flock of birds, each one burning.**
> Stars swoop down to bullets. Hot red
> specks take flesh, nest there, a body part,
> part body. (Powers 12)

At first glance, Richard Powers's *The Echo Maker* is indeed a "trauma narrative," in which several characters are uprooted by different, yet structurally related, events. The novel's protagonist, Mark Schluter, is torn from his life by a mysterious truck accident. As a consequence of his head injury, he suffers from Capgras syndrome, a form of mental disorder in which the patient is unable to remember his emotional ties to a family member or close friend. In the diagnostic phrase, Capgras is "one of the delusional reduplication syndromes": "a condition characterized by the inability to identify a familiar person, even though one does recognize that person's facial and bodily characteristics. As a result, individuals with Capgras syndrome tend to believe that the person in question has been replaced by a double" (Blom 84). Mark accordingly believes that his sister Karin is an impostor, sent by the government to cover up a major conspiracy, in which his hometown has been replaced by a giant replica. The novel unfolds around the triangular relationship between Mark, Karin, and Dr. Gerald Weber, a cognitive neurologist and TV celebrity from New York, who is both fascinated and unsettled by Mark's case. The characters are connected both through the truck accident and through another disruptive event, which is likewise rendered in psychiatric imagery (as "cinematic insanity" [268] or "shared trauma" [344]): the terrorist attacks of September 11. In 2001, Dr. Weber and Mark both remember the experience of staring in disbelief at the televised images of "the world blown away" (344), and Weber even concludes that "[t]hat one, unthinkable morning was real; everything since had been a narcoleptic lie" (126). A fourth character, Mark's nurse, is most severely affected by the attacks: Barbara Gillespie, it turns out, is a former journalist from New York, who covered 9/11 when it happened, "sticking a video camera in people's faces after the towers" (550) until she broke down, unable to continue her job. Suffering from PTDS, she is sent to Nebraska in order to write a report on migrating cranes—a topic so remote and harmless that it is supposed to heal her wounds. Given this plotline of disruptions and fragmented selves, the methodologies of trauma studies can well be applied to Powers's novel. The "narrative dynamic," to argue from Bert Olivier's point of view, is certainly "impelled by a trauma" (55); and the text also, in Laurie Vickroy's phrase, "reshape[s] cultural memory through personal contexts" (5). However, such a reading limits the process of analysis to mere symptom and does not do justice to the text's aesthetic density. Instead, as I will argue, *The Echo Maker* expands the individual wound into a panorama—or "traumorama"—of global ethics, involving national and transnational, trans-species, and trans-textual connections.

First of all, even if one takes Mark's case of traumatization as a point of departure, the Capgras plot may be read as an allegory of a national misperception, and particularly of American domestic and foreign policies after 2001. Not only is Mark's body explicitly linked to the destroyed Trade Center when he wonders if he should go to New York "and have some airplane slam me" (384), but his conspiracy theories become closely intertwined with the United States' obsession with terrorism, "code-orange" alerts, and the "axis of evil." The notion that Mark's paranoia is, in fact, an accurate perception is increasingly endorsed throughout the novel: When Weber runs a few psychological tests on Mark, he notes that "[h]is emotional maturity tested below average, but . . . [a]ll of America would have tested below average on that, nowadays" (198). Along the same lines, Karin admits that Mark's belief of something being wrong with the surroundings might be accurate: "Kearney, Nebraska: a colossal fake, a life-sized, hollow replica. She'd thought as much herself, all the while growing up" (250).

Whereas, at first glance, Dr. Weber's empirical knowledge (or, Reason) seems to be the solution and cure for the disorder in Mark's brain (or the counter-terrorist paranoia of Homeland Security), the sense of crisis thus turns into a progressively complex and uncontainable problem. In the course of the novel, reality increasingly loses its foothold, and even Barbara cynically agrees with Mark: "The whole place, a substitute. I mean: Is this country anyplace you recognize?" (548). The specific diagnosis of Capgras thus not only serves as a national allegory, but it emphasizes the unreliability of human consciousness at large. Reducing the symptom to a singular traumatic event (such as an accident or a terrorist attack) is, accordingly, merely an attempt at saving what Baudrillard calls "the reality principle" (13): Its logic of cause and effect retains at least the possibility of order and agency. Yet there is no way around "the brain grow[ing] strange to itself" (Powers 294): As Weber repeatedly states, the human mind is completely fallible, because "even a brain that thought it was measuring, orienting, and inhabiting plain-old given space might already, without the slightest notion, have lost as much as half a world" (159). What initially seems to be the effect of a specific trauma is—on the allegorical level—a shared cognitive fallacy.

This fallacy is amplified by Weber's personal and professional unsettlement. As a famous researcher, he is used to speaking with the voice of authority: "When he started to read, prose poured out of him in Old Testament cadences" (234).[3] In the course of the novel, however, this confidence crumbles: Reviewers severely criticize his book; he is humiliated at a public lecture in Australia, and charged with the exploitation of his patients. Weber realizes that his certainties disappear: "He lay awake, thinking of the answers he should have given, seeing the cracks in his ceiling as frozen synapses. Sometime after 3:00 a.m., it occurred to him that he himself might be an extremely detailed case

---

[3] All of the characters undergo severe changes throughout the plot, but Weber's is probably most impressive: Initially, he is distanced and reserved, evaluating Mark's case less as a human tragedy than as an interesting "species he had never seen" (129). It is only when Weber realizes that his success is, in fact, largely based on the dubious methods of a "neurological opportunist" and "[v]iolator of privacy and sideshow exploiter" (346) that he can fully commit to Mark's case and actually help him.

history, a description of personality so minutely realized that it only thought it was autonomous" (294). On a personal level, he then experiences a complete loss of control: He falls in love with Barbara and risks his marriage by sleeping with her. In the passionate moments of "waves of oxytocin and a savage bonding" (544), his theoretical knowledge becomes useless and even unavailable: When he wants to "tell her ten essential things that neuroscience knows for certain" (547), he is unable to do so; "[S]omething has happened to his list. Those that are essential no longer feel certain. And those that are certain can't possibly be essential" (547). The lack of knowledge—or the collective epistemic crisis—that Mark's condition allegorically signifies is universal and all-encompassing: Even the experts, the supposed healers and keepers of academic wisdom, are affected.

The cognitive crisis is aptly translated into the novel's form. *The Echo Maker* is a detective novel, or whodunit, in which Karin tries to find out what happened on the night of her brother's accident. The crucial piece of evidence is a note found on Mark's nightstand:

> I am No One
> but Tonight on North Line Road
> GOD led me to you
> so You could Live
> and bring back someone else. (12)

In their (very different) attempts to restore at least a causal order to the unbearably unclear situation, both Mark and Karin try to solve the mystery of this short text's authorship. Pointing to an unknown witness, the enigmatic note constitutes the structural and symbolic pivot of the interpretational venture: Taken singly, each line provides a title for the novel's five parts, indicating the absent author as the decisive link in the construction of meaning. Furthermore, the signifiers symbolically underline a movement from the loss of individuality ("I am No One") to a relocation of subjective agency in the Other ("bring back someone else"). Through the uncertain signifieds disappearing behind the personal pronouns, the individual neurological crisis is conflated with a collective one, affecting an entire culture's cognitive and epistemic foundations.

This unreliability of signification also emerges in the coordinates of a literal landscape: the novel's setting. While Mark's home of Kearney,

Nebraska, initially looks like a remote, backward, "square state with more cows than people" (191), it is a space deeply invested with cultural, historical, and evolutionary meanings. As the geographical center of the United States, the town of Kearney underlines the representative nature of Mark's individual fate, not only for the nation, but also for the global, trans-species community of living beings that is epitomized by the novel's central symbol, the sandhill cranes. As Richard Powers emphasizes in an interview,

> the town sits right on the crosshairs of two intersecting migratory corridors. On one axis, it lies on or near the great historical American east-to-west routes: Oregon Trail, Mormon Trail, Pony Express, transcontinental railroad, Lincoln Highway, Interstate 80. And on the other, it lies on the choke point of the Central Flyway, that continent-size hourglass used by hundreds of millions of migratory birds, with its narrow waist lying along a sixty-mile stretch of the Platte [River]. (Michod interview with Powers)

Far from remote, Kearney is, in more than one sense, the "American heartland": It turns out to be the crossroads of evolution and history in human and animal migration, representing the principle of (cultural) mobility, from Manifest Destiny to what the novel describes as "the final frontier" (239): contemporary neurological research. Both Mark's injury and the attack of 9/11 are thus elaborately reintegrated into an inclusive historical cartography, which involves patterns much older and more significant than individual human trauma.

The cranes particularly accentuate this universal agenda: Their reliable patterns of migration suggest historical stability as much as transnational border-crossing. With their unfailing memory of travel routes,[4] they not only span the planet in an alternative map of global connections, symbolizing order and continuity, but they also epitomize a particular ethics of difference: Tellingly called "Echo Makers" by the Anishinaabe (229), they share mythical presences in African, Chinese, Greek, Aztec, and Cherokee cultures (cf. 229-30). With the "[a]ncient structures" of their brains, which are still physiologically retained "in

---

[4] "Something in the birds retraces a route laid down centuries before their parents showed it to them. And each crane recalls the route still to come" (4).

ours" (527), the birds are at once the radical Other and the projection
screen of human likeness:

> Those birds danced like our next of kin, looked like our next of kin,
> called and willed and parented and taught and navigated all just like our
> blood relations. Half their parts were still ours. Yet humans waved them
> off: *impostors*. (439)

In terms of the novel's "green politics" (Gibbons 9), our entire race
seems to suffer from Capgras syndrome: Instead of recognizing our
global family members, we destroy their habitat. This rewriting of the
medical leitmotif into a transcultural—and trans-species—ethics of
recognition goes much further, I believe, than the "empathic
unsettlement" that Dominick LaCapra sees as the primary function of
trauma narratives.[5] Charles B. Harris has termed Powers's preoccupation with brain science "neurological realism" (243); a mode of
writing which marks an expansion of Jamesian psychological realism:
"[W]hereas psychological assumptions subtend motives and mental
states in psychological realism, neuroscience, not psychology, subtends
The Echo Maker, the mental states of whose characters reflect the inner
workings of the human brain" (Harris 243).[6] Given the transversal
network of connections in the novel's imagery, however, Harris's
definition seems to fall short of the text's actual effect. The brain's
biochemical processes are not merely reflection screens for the
characters and their states of mind, but their recurrent descriptions serve
as tropes for communicational processes at large; not least for the
novel's own agenda. I would therefore define Powers's text, in contrast
to Harris's reading, as "neurological metafiction": It uses the imagery of
the brain not as an end in itself, but as a metacommunicational device.
The network of synapses, and its translation into a network of poetic

---

[5] "Being responsive to the traumatic experience of others, notably of victims,
     implies not the appropriation of their experience but what I would call
     empathic unsettlement, which should have stylistic effects or, more broadly,
     effects in writing which cannot be reduced to formulas or rules of method"
     (LaCapra 41).

[6] *The Echo Maker*, according to Harris, "is the first fully realized novel of
     neurological realism" (243).

language, thus simultaneously constitutes the imaginary landscape of meaning-making and the map that decodes this landscape.

When Weber, the celebrity researcher, eventually travels home on the plane, he sees an organic microcosm below, brimming with semiotic energy:

> Through the plane's plastic window, the lights of unknown cities blink beneath him, hundreds of millions of glowing cells linked together, swapping signals. Even here, the creature spreads countless species deep. Flying, burrowing, creeping things, every path sculpting all the others. A flashing electrical loom, street-sized synapses forming a brain with miles-wide thoughts too large to read. A web of signals spelling out a theory of living things. (568)

The material American space beneath the plane is rendered as a "creature"; a system of communicating cells which could be located anywhere on the planet. Instead of subscribing to the exclusionary geography of a post-9/11 "Homeland," *The Echo Maker* remaps the nation, through a microscopic lens, as a giant brain within a cosmos of "countless species." Just as the synapses of the American landscape transmit their codes to neighboring cells, observed and interpreted by Dr. Weber, the plot of Mark's cognitive crisis is skillfully interlaced with the semantic fields of the cranes, space, and neuroscience—sending readers a multilayered "web of signals." This communication has been rendered particularly difficult in non-mythical times, as the heterodiegetic narrator reminds us: "When animals and people all spoke the same language, crane calls said exactly what they meant. Now we live in unclear echoes" (231). The only way to approximate these "unclear echoes," the novel ultimately suggests, is through poetic language: only tropes and narrative connections are able to represent the landscape's "thoughts too large to read" (568).

On the novel's diegetic level, the mystery of authorship is solved in the end: It turns out that the accident was caused by Barbara Gillespie, who attempted to commit suicide in the middle of the road. Mark's reaction of swerving his truck off the road saved her life, and it was Mark himself who wrote the text to her, before amnesia erased all traces from his mind. Despite this potemkinesque sense of closure, however, the novel's symbolism (of unresolved traumatic experience, of endless travel and mobility, and of signals being ceaselessly transmitted) persists: The process of making meaning remains open and in flux. Storytelling, *The Echo Maker* insists, is the only viable strategy for not getting lost in the world, and it is also the sole efficacious recipe for recovery:

> That one delusion—*stories came true*—seemed like the germ of healing. We told ourselves backward into diagnosis and forward into treatment. Story was the storm at the cortex's core. And there was no better way to get at that fictional truth than through the haunted neurological parables of Broca or Luria—stories of how even shattered brains might narrate disaster back into livable sense. (524)

Fiction may be illusionary, but it is all the more powerful in its effect. Because of its surplus of signification, fictional narrative resists containment and thus transcends the neurological limits of synapses and biochemical processes. By celebrating, in Mark's tale, precisely such a story "of how even shattered brains might narrate disaster back into livable sense" (524), Powers's neurological metafiction leaves no doubt about its loyalties.

Fiction after the Planes

> The shadows were all wrong: still disorienting, more than eight months on. (Powers 126)

Ten years after the terrorist attacks of September 11, critics widely doubt the literary merits of 9/11 fiction. Adam Kirsch complains about the lack of originality in American novels: "The lesson of most 9/11 books, with their frustrated earnestness," he writes, "may be that American forthrightness is ill-suited to a subject that, like the sun, does not bear looking at directly." The premise for his argument is again the terminology of trauma: "In American fiction, certainly, there's no sign that the trauma has been resolved." In a similar manner, Richard Gray voices his disappointment with the formal and political failure of most novels to react adequately to the 9/11 attacks: "In place of a necessary imaginative encounter with disaster, and the recalibration of feeling and belief that surely requires, most of th[is] fiction . . . betrays a response to crisis that is eerily analogous to the reaction of many politicians and the mainstream American media after 9/11: a desperate retreat into the old sureties" (*After the Fall* 16). The twenty-first century American novel, Gray specifies elsewhere, fails to accommodate the event's historical and political reverberations, and to provide a space for the negotiation of other highly relevant issues, such as immigration, deterritorialization, and "the U.S. as cultural borderlands" ("Open Doors" 135).

Through its focus on victimhood and personal experience, the methodological context of trauma studies smoothly dovetails with the discourse of the domestication of crisis. As Richard Powers's *The Echo Maker* demonstrates, however, fiction also offers powerful counter-narratives to the exceptionalist *grand récit* of 9/11 as an event that "changed everything," and it is a perfect example of how the personal is by nature political. While a reading of Powers's novel as a "trauma narrative" is possible, a focus on symptoms and on the medical discourse's literal level fails to register these counternarratives. The allegorical implications of Mark's accident-induced Capgras syndrome tie individual trauma to national, transnational, and trans-species concerns and involve a politics of difference, both on the levels of plot and form. Through its structure of elaborately interwoven symbols and its metafictional trajectories, *The Echo Maker* thus integrates the repercussions of a disruptive event into a larger pathological landscape of medical, cognitive, ethical, and aesthetic crises. Just like the blinking signals of human life merge into a larger organic unit when seen from the plane, Powers's neurological metafiction turns individual trauma into a catalyst for the negotiation of the global experience of "what it means to be alive," as the author phrases it elsewhere (cf. Williams). "Fiction," according to Powers, "has the potential to be the most complex set of experimental networks ever built, one that can model feedback passed among all other gauges of speculation and inhabitation, fact and concern, idea and feeling. Story alone can refract vast, voiced, complex interactions between local and global that no single discipline can know inclusively or pretend to master" ("Making the Rounds" 309). The scientist's (or reader's) act of attentively heeding these signals is thus precisely the "imaginative exercise in experiencing the impossible" that Gayatri Spivak called for after the 2001 attacks: "stepping into the space of the other" (94). Particularly in the "unclear echoes" (Powers 231) of post-9/11 paranoia and counter-terrorist profiling, *The Echo Maker* thus makes a strong case for an ethics of empathy: It also shows that the fiction of September 11 goes far beyond the mere registration of a "traumatic" event.

Works Cited

Alexander, Jeffrey C. "Toward a Theory of Cultural Trauma." *Cultural Trauma and Collective Identity.* Ed. Jeffrey C. Alexander et al. Berkeley: U of California P, 2004. 1-30. Print.

Andersen, Tore Rye. "Blurry Close-ups: American Literature and 9/11." *Danish Network for Cultural Memory Studies.* Dec. 2008. Web. 3 Jan. 2011.

Back, Mitja D., Albrecht C. P. Küfner, and Boris Egloff. "The Emotional Timeline of September 11, 2001." *Psychological Science* 21.10 (2010): 1417-19. Print.

Baudrillard, Jean. *Simulacra and Simulation.* Trans. Sheila Faria Glaser. Ann Arbor: U of Michigan P, 1994. Print.

Blom, Jan Dirk. *A Dictionary of Hallucinations.* New York: Springer, 2010. Print.

Brow, Marnie, and Roxane Cohen Silver. "Coping with a Collective Trauma: Psychological Reactions to 9/11 across the United States." *The Impact of 9/11 on Psychology and Education: The Day that Changed Everything?* Ed. Matthew J. Morgan. New York: Palgrave, 2009. 37-47. Print.

Burn, Stephen J., and Peter Dempsey, eds. *Intersections: Essays on Richard Powers.* Champaign: Dalkey, 2008. Print.

Butollo, Willi. *Leben nach dem Trauma: Über den therapeutischen Umgang mit dem Entsetzen.* München: Pfeiffer, 1998. Print.

Caruth, Cathy. *Unclaimed Experience: Trauma, Narrative, and History.* Baltimore: Johns Hopkins UP, 1996. Print.

Coates, Susan W., Jane Rosenthal, and Daniel S. Schechter, eds. *September 11: Trauma and Human Bonds.* Hillsdale: Analytic, 2003.

Codde, Philippe. "Philomela Revisited: Traumatic Iconicity in Jonathan Safran Foer's *Extremely Loud & Incredibly Close.*" *Studies in American Fiction* 35.2 (2007): 241-54. Print.

Cournos, Francine. "Lessons for High-Risk Populations from Attachment Research and September 11: Helping Children in Foster Care." *September 11: Trauma and Human Bonds.* Ed. Susan W. Coates, Jane Rosenthal, and Daniel S. Schechter. Hillsdale: Analytic, 2003. 255-72. Print.

Däwes, Birgit. *Ground Zero Fiction: History, Memory, and Representation in the American 9/11 Novel.* Heidelberg: Winter, 2011. Print.

Davis, Walter A. "Trauma and Tragic Transformation: Why We Learned Nothing from 9/11." *The Impact of 9/11 on Psychology and Education: The Day that Changed Everything?* Ed. Matthew J. Morgan. New York: Palgrave, 2009. 139-48. Print.

DeLillo, Don. *Falling Man.* New York: Picador, 2007. Print.

Dewey, Joseph. *Understanding Richard Powers.* Columbia: U of South Carolina P, 2008. Print.

Diao, Keli. "'The Human Race Is Still a Work in Progress': An Interview with Richard Powers." *Foreign Literature Studies/Wai Guo Wen Xue Yan Jiu* 29.4 (Aug. 2007): 1-6. Print.

Elkind, David. "The Effects of Horrific Trauma on Children and Youth." *The Impact of 9/11 on Psychology and Education: The Day that Changed Everything?* Ed. Matthew J. Morgan. New York: Palgrave, 2009. 151-60. Print.

Erikson, Kai. "Notes on Trauma and Community." *Trauma: Explorations in Memory.* Ed. Cathy Caruth. Baltimore: Johns Hopkins UP, 1995. 183-99. Print.

Felman, Shoshana, and Dori Laub. *Testimony: Crises of Witnessing in Literature, Psychoanalysis, and History.* New York: Routledge, 1992. Print.

Gibbons, James. "Beyond Recognition." *BookForum* 13.3 (Sept./Oct./Nov. 2006): 9-10; 35. Print.

Glick, Robert Alan. Preface. *September 11: Trauma and Human Bonds.* Ed. Susan W. Coates, Jane Rosenthal, and Daniel S. Schechter. Hillsdale: Analytic, 2003. vii-ix. Print.

Granofsky, Ronald. *The Trauma Novel: Contemporary Symbolic Depictions of Collective Disaster.* American University Studies 55. New York: Peter Lang, 1995. Print.

Gray, Richard J. *After the Fall: American Literature since 9/11.* Oxford: Wiley Blackwell, 2011. Print.

---. "Open Doors, Closed Minds: American Prose Writing at a Time of Crisis." *American Literary History* 21.1 (2009): 128-51. Print.

Greenberg, Judith, ed. *Trauma at Home: After 9/11.* Lincoln: U of Nebraska P, 2003. Print.

---. "Wounded New York." *Trauma at Home: After 9/11*. Ed. Greenberg. Lincoln: U of Nebraska P, 2003. 21-35. Print.

Harris, Charles B. "The Story of the Self: *The Echo Maker* and Neurological Realism." *Intersections: Essays on Richard Powers*. Ed. Stephen J. Burn and Peter Dempsey. Champaign: Dalkey, 2008. 230-59. Print.

Huehls, Mitchum. "Foer, Spiegelman, and 9/11's Timely Traumas." *Literature after 9/11*. Ed. Ann Keniston and Jeanne Follansbee Quinn. New York: Routledge, 2008. 42-59. Print.

Johnson, Jenell. "To Find the Soul, It Is Necessary to Lose It: Neuroscience, Disability, and the Epigraph to *The Echo Maker*." *Intersections: Essays on Richard Powers*. Ed. Stephen J. Burn and Peter Dempsey. Champaign: Dalkey, 2008. 215-18. Print.

Kaplan, Amy. "Homeland Insecurities: Transformations of Language and Space." *September 11 in History: A Watershed Moment?* Ed. Mary L. Dudziak. Durham: Duke UP, 2003. 55-69. Print.

Kaplan, E. Ann. *Trauma Culture: The Politics of Terror and Loss in Media and Literature*. New Brunswick: Rutgers UP, 2005. Print.

Kauffman, Linda S. "World Trauma Center." *American Literary History* 21.3 (2009): 647-59. Print.

Kirsch, Adam. "In the Shadow of the Twin Towers." *Prospect* 183 (25 May 2011). Web. 23 July 2011.

Kühner, Angela. *Kollektive Traumata: Konzepte, Argumente, Perspektiven*. Gießen: Psychosozial Verlag, 2007. Print.

LaCapra, Dominick. *Writing History, Writing Trauma*. Baltimore: Johns Hopkins UP, 2001. Print.

---. *History in Transit: Experience, Identity, Critical Theory*. Ithaca: Cornell UP, 2004. Print.

Laub, Dori. "September 11, 2001—An Event without a Voice." *Trauma at Home: After 9/11*. Ed. Judith Greenberg. Lincoln: U of Nebraska P, 2003. 204-15. Print.

Leys, Ruth. *Trauma: A Genealogy*. Chicago: U of Chicago P, 2000. Print.

Michod, Alec. "The Brain Is the Ultimate Storytelling Machine, and Consciousness Is the Ultimate Story: An Interview with Richard Powers." *Believer Magazine* 5.1 Feb. 2007. Web. 28 Oct. 2010.

Morgan, Matthew J., ed. *The Impact of 9/11 on Psychology and Education: The Day that Changed Everything?* New York: Palgrave, 2009.

Mullins, Matthew. "Boroughs and Neighbors: Traumatic Solidarity in Jonathan Safran Foer's *Extremely Loud & Incredibly Close.*" *Papers on Language and Literature* 45.3 (2009): 298-324. Print.

Neal, Arthur G. *National Trauma and Collective Memory: Major Events in the American Century.* New York: Sharpe, 1998. Print.

Neria, Yuval, et al. "PTSD in Urban Primary Care Patients Following 9/11." *9/11: Mental Health in the Wake of Terrorist Attacks.* Ed. Yuval Neria, Raz Gross, and Randall D. Marshall. Cambridge: Cambridge UP, 2006. 239-63. Print.

Olivier, Bert. "Trauma and Literature: Derrida, 9/11, and Hart's *The Reconstructionist.*" *Journal of Literary Studies* 24.1 (2008): 32-57. Print.

Peknik, Patricia. "'City of the World!': A New Generation's American Exceptionalism." *The Impact of 9/11 on Psychology and Education: The Day that Changed Everything?* Ed. Matthew J. Morgan. New York: Palgrave, 2009. 265-71. Print.

"Posttraumatic Stress Disorder." *Diagnostic and Statistical Manual of Mental Disorders: DSM-IV-TR.* Ed. American Psychiatric Association. 4th ed. 2000. Arlington: American Psychiatric Association, 2004. 463-68. Print.

Powers, Richard. *The Echo Maker.* New York: Vintage, 2006. Print.

---. "Making the Rounds." *Intersections: Essays on Richard Powers.* Ed. Stephen J. Burn and Peter Dempsey. Champaign: Dalkey, 2008. 305-10. Print.

Rees, Ellen. "Some Clinical Observations after September 11: Awakening the Past?" *September 11: Trauma and Human Bonds.* Ed. Susan W. Coates, Jane Rosenthal, and Daniel S. Schechter. Hillsdale: Analytic, 2003. 165-90. Print.

Rothberg, Michael. "A Failure of the Imagination: Diagnosing the Post-9/11 Novel. A Response to Richard Gray." *American Literary History* 21.1 (2009): 152-58. Print.

---. "'There Is No Poetry in This': Writing, Trauma, and Home." Greenberg 147-57. Print.

Seeley, Karen M. *Therapy after Terror: 9/11, Psychotherapists, and Mental Health.* Cambridge: Cambridge UP, 2008. Print.

Sielke, Sabine. "'The Subject of Literature,' or: (Re-)Cognition in Richard Powers' (Science) Fiction." Ideas of Order: Narrative Patterns in the Novels of Richard Powers. Conference. University of Erlangen-Nuremberg. 26-28 Nov. 2010. Conference paper.

---. "Why '9/11 Is [not] Unique,' or: Troping Trauma." *Trauma's Continuum: September 11th Reconsidered.* Ed. Andrew S. Gross and MaryAnn Snyder-Koerber. Spec. issue of *Amerikastudien/American Studies* 55.3 (2010): 385-408. Print.

Spivak, Gayatri. "Terror: A Speech after 9-11." *Boundary 2* 31.2 (2004): 81-111. Print.

Tancke, Ulrike. "Uses and Abuses of Trauma in Post-9/11 Fiction and Contemporary Culture." *From Solidarity to Schisms: 9/11 and after in Fiction and Film from Outside the US.* Ed. Cara Cilano. Amsterdam: Rodopi, 2009. 75-92. Print.

Uytterschout, Sien. "Visualized Incomprehensibility of Trauma in Jonathan Safran Foer's Extremely Loud and Incredibly Close." *Zeitschrift für Anglistik und Amerikanistik: A Quarterly of Language, Literature and Culture* 56.1 (2008): 61-74. Print.

Versluys, Kristiaan. *Out of the Blue: September 11 and the Novel.* New York: Columbia UP, 2009. Print.

---. "9/11: The Discursive Responses." 9/11 Ten Years After: History, Narrative, Memory. International Conference. Bavarian American Academy, Munich. 14-15 July 2011. Conference paper.

Vickroy, Laurie. *Trauma and Survival in Contemporary Fiction.* Charlottesville: U of Virginia P, 2002. Print.

Williams, Jeffrey. "The Last Generalist: An Interview with Richard Powers." *Cultural Logic* 2.2 (1999). Web. 1 Nov. 2011.

Wirth, Hans-Jürgen. *9/11 as a Collective Trauma and Other Essays on Psychoanalysis and Society.* Hillsdale: Analytic, 2004. Print.

Zelizer, Barbie, and Stuart Allan. Introduction. *Journalism after September 11.* Ed. Zelizer and Allan. New York: Routledge, 2002. 1-24. Print.

DIETRICH VON ENGELHARDT

The World of Medicine
in the Medium of Literature:
Structures, Dimensions, Perspectives

The relationship between literature and medicine is complex and reciprocal, consisting of many dimensions with a long tradition stretching from antiquity up to the present.[1] On the one hand, literature and medicine are connected by similarities and influences in both directions. Medicine in itself combines "art" (ars) and "science" (scientia), consisting as it does of the natural sciences and humanities. One simple example of this crossover can be seen in the mutual influence of medicine on literary descriptions of disease and of literature on the medical imagination, as S. J. London noted in a 1968 article, "The Whimsy Syndromes." Published in the journal *Archives of Internal Medicine*, the article notes that many names of diseases are taken from literature: the "Oedipus complex," "Electra complex," "Rapunzel syndrome," "Münchhausen syndrome," or recently the "Oblomov syndrome" from the novel *Oblomov* (1859) by Ivan Aleksandrovich Goncharov (1812-1891). Oblomov syndrome describes a specific incapacity to cope with the normal challenges of life. As the eponymous protagonist in Goncharov's novel experiences the syndrome: "Brain and voli-

---

[1] Numerous literary examples and many scientific studies on this topic exist. Cf., for example, Binet and Vallery-Radot, *Médecine et littérature* (1965); Carmichael, *Medicine* (1991); Ceccio, *Medicine in Literature* (1982); v. Engelhardt, *Medizin in der Literatur der Neuzeit* (1991/2000); v. Jagow and Steger, *Literatur und Medizin* (2005); Rhodes Peschel, *Medicine and Literature* (1980); Trautmann and Pollard, *Literature and Medicine* (1975; rev. 1982).

tion alike had become paralyzed, and, to all appearances, irrevocably—the events of his life had become whittled down to microscopical proportions. Yet even with them he was powerless to cope—he was powerless to pass from one of them to another" (71). The arts have played a role in both treating and diagnosing illness since antiquity. According to Aristotle (384-322 B.C.E.), tragic theater has a cathartic effect—very similar to physiological concepts of medicine—which works through a "purgation" of the emotions of "pity" (éleos) and "fear" (phóbos) provoked by the action on the stage (cf. Aristotle 1449b). However, literature always exceeds the ordinary therapeutic aims of medicine and psychotherapy. From this perspective, Franz Kafka ascribes to literature the function of being an "Axt für das gefrorene Meer in uns" (Letter to Oskar Pollak 28).

On the other hand, the relationship between literature and medicine is also marked by differences in regard to the relationship to reality, tradition and progress or historical change, conceptual structure, phenomena, and external causes and immanent dynamics. Physicians and especially psychiatrists often revered literary representations and interpretations. Karl Jaspers was deeply convinced of the value of literature: "It is not mere chance . . . that poets have used symbols and figures of madness for the essence of human life in its highest and most horrible possibilities, in its greatness and decline. Thus Cervantes in *Don Quixote* and Ibsen in *Peer Gynt*, Dostoevski in *The Idiot*, Shakespeare in *Lear* and *Hamlet*" (786). Given the ontological difference between literature, medicine, and reality, the philosopher Georg Wilhelm Friedrich Hegel (1770-1831) observes that art nevertheless has a specific advantage: "Die harte Rinde der Natur und gewöhnlichen Welt machen es dem Geiste saurer zur Idee durchzudringen als die Werke der Kunst" (Hegel 30). The Russian writer Fyodor Mikhailovich Dostoyevsky (1881-1821) underscores the higher reality of literary figures in comparison to figures of reality: "Authors for the most part attempt in their tales and novels to select and vividly and artistically represent, in their entirety, types rarely met with in actual life, though they are nevertheless almost more real than real life itself" (423). For his part, Thomas Mann (1875-1955) is convinced of a major difference between literature and reality: "der Wesensunterschied nämlich, welcher die Welt der Realität von derjenigen der Kunst auf immer scheidet" ("Bilse und ich" 16). Aldous Huxley (1894-1963) defines science as "nomothetic" or generalizing in the sense of establishing explanatory laws whereas literature is "idiographic" or individualizing and not concerned with laws and regulations (cf. Huxley, *Literature and Science* 8).

Intuition, spontaneity, and imagination are important for medical practice. Surgery, for instance, requires artistic skills; overcoming disease and producing health is a creative act; communication with patients transcends the logic of "evidence based medicine" and needs empathy, fantasy, nonverbal, and nonvocal capacities; and lectures and scientific publications can reach artistic or literary levels. Literature on the other hand can be helpful in diagnosis and treatment as well as all the other arts.[2] The effects of reading and writing literature have to be empirically evaluated, in order to differentiate specific dimensions of diagnosis, treatment, prevention, rehabilitation, patient consultation, and the therapeutic and personal atmosphere of a hospital.

To sum up, the following aspects could be singled out as central elements of the intersecting fields of literature and medicine: the relationship between medicine, literature, and reality; the literary function of medicine; the medical function of literature; and the genuine function of fictionalized medicine. This essay will not explore literature and literary representations from the point of view of a literary critic, but from the perspective of the medical humanities to bring into focus the mutually overlapping and reciprocally influential interests of literature and medicine.

Medical Dimensions: Literary Representations

An entire world of medicine has been represented in literary texts—with different emphases being given in different historical epochs, specific genres, and individual œuvres. Essential dimensions of these literary representations are: 1) pathophenomenology or the description

---

[2] For example, cf. Downie, *The Healing Arts* (1994); v. Engelhardt, *Bibliotherapie* (1987); Petzold and Orth, *Poesie und Therapie* (1985); Rubin, *Using Bibliotherapy* (1978); Zifreund, *Therapien im Zusammenspiel der Künste* (1996).

of disease, 2) etiology or causality of disease, 3) subjectivity and patient behavior, 4) the image of the physician, 5) diagnosis and treatment, 6) the medical institution, 7) social reactions, and 8) symbolism.

Pathophenomenology

Pathophenomenology means the objective or real description of disease. Authors differ from doctors in medical knowledge. François Rabelais (1493-1553), Tobias George Smollett (1721-1771), Oliver Goldsmith (1730-1774), John Keats (1795-1821), Anton Pavlovich Chekhov (1860-1904), Arthur Schnitzler (1862-1931), Georges Duhamel (1884-1966), Alfred Döblin (1878-1957), Gottfried Benn (1886-1966), Hans Carossa (1878-1956), and Walter Vogt (1927-1988) were physicians and poets with specific consequences for their work. According to Chekhov, the representation of medical phenomena is ultimately a task for physicians who are at the same time poets: "In order to settle such problems as degeneration, psychosis, etc., one must have scientific knowledge of them" (Chekhov, Letter to E. M. Shavrova, 28 Feb. 1895, 256).

Honoré de Balzac (1799-1850) compares his *Comédie Humaine* with nature, discussing the contributions to literature made by the famous French naturalists Georges-Louis Leclerc de Buffon (1707-1788), Georges Cuvier (1769-1832), and Étienne Geoffroy Saint-Hilaire (1772-1844). Balzac underlines the differences between culture and nature beyond their similarities: "L'État Social a des hasards que ne se permet pas la Nature, car il est la Nature plus la Société. La description des Espèces Sociales était donc au moins double de celle des Espèces Animales . . ." (Balzac, "Avant-Propos" 9).

Thomas Mann's physician, Dr. Behrens, in *Der Zauberberg* (1921) underlines the value of medical knowledge for the poet; for example, in physiology, anatomy, or dermatology:

> Es ist eben gut und kann gar nicht schaden, wenn man auch unter der Epidermis ein bißchen Bescheid weiß und mitmalen kann, was nicht zu sehen ist,—mit anderen Worten: wenn man zur Natur noch in einem andern Verhältnis steht als bloß dem lyrischen, wollen wir mal sagen; wenn man zum Beispiel im Nebenamt Arzt ist, Physiolog, Anatom und von den Dessous auch noch so seine stillen Kenntnisse hat. (361)

The whole spectrum of physical and psychical diseases is described in the nineteenth-century novels of Balzac, Adalbert Stifter (1805-1868), Charles Dickens (1812-1870), Dostoyevsky, L. N. Tolstoy (1828-1910), and Émile Zola (1840-1902). In the Romantic era, metaphysical descriptions and interpretations of medical phenomena dominate the texts of Novalis (1772-1801), E.T.A. Hoffmann (1776-1822), Achim von Arnim (1781-1831), Clemens Brentano (1778-1842), George Byron (1788-1822), and Percy Bysshe Shelley (1792-1822). Cancer, tuberculosis, and madness are central topics in the literature of the twentieth century: Mann's *Der Zauberberg* (1924), Carson McCullers's (1917-1967) *Clock without Hands* (1961), A. I. Solzhenitsyn's (1918-2008) *Cancer Ward* (1967), Simone de Beauvoir's (1908-1986) *Une mort douce* (1964), Robert Musil's (1880-1942) *Der Mann ohne Eigenschaften* (1930/43), Virginia Woolf's (1882-1941) *Mrs. Dalloway* (1925), Elsa Morante's (1912-1985) *La Storia* (1974), and Thomas Bernard's (1931-1989) *Wittgensteins Neffe* (1982) are only a few important examples.

A concrete portrayal of plague is given in Giovanni Boccaccio's (1313-1375) *La Decamerone* (1349/53) and Albert Camus's (1878-1956) *La Peste* (1947) and of cholera in Mann's *Der Tod in Venedig* (1924), complete with statistical figures, a depiction of the normal development, and mortal end. Alfred de Musset's (1810-1857) novella *Pierre et Camille* (1844) features a child who is born deaf and dumb: "À mesure qu'elle grandissait, on fut surpris de lui voir garder une immobilité étrange. Aucun bruit ne semblait la frapper; elle était insensible à ces mille discours que les mères adressent à leurs nourrissons" (Musset 574).

The eleven-year-old Jeanne in Zola's novel *Une Page d'amour* (1878) suffers from pathological jealousy of her mother, Hélène Grandjean, due to Jeanne's extreme sensibility, and dies at the end of the novel from an acute and mortal tuberculosis: "Jeanne regardait Paris de ses grands yeux vides. Sa figure de chèvre s'était encore allongée, avec des traits sévères, une ombre grise descendue des sourcils qu'elle fronçait; et elle avait ainsi dans la mort son visage blême de femme jalouse" (Zola, *Une Page d'amour* 1071).

At the age of 15, the hemophiliac Charles—a member of Zola's Rougon-Macquart family—physically resembles a child of twelve and psychically a child of five, and at the same time—with his indistinct features—his great-great grandmother Adélaïde Fouque and her desiccated face.

> L'enfant avait levé le regard sur la folle, et tous deux se contemplèrent. À ce moment, leur extraordinaire ressemblance éclata. Leurs yeux surtout, leurs yeux vides et limpides, semblaient se perdre les uns dans les autres, identiques. Puis, c'était la physionomie, les traits usés de la centenaire qui, par-dessus trois générations, sautaient à cette délicate figure d'enfant, comme effacée déjà elle aussi, très vieille et finie par l'usure de la race. (Zola, *Docteur Pascal* 1101)

Detailed descriptions of the external symptoms of disease can be found in literary texts, including patients' gestures, miming, and language, as depicted for instance by Robert Musil in his novel *Der Mann ohne Eigenschaften* (1930/43) in regard to madness and Janet Frame (1924-2004) in the novel *Owls Do Cry* (1957) in regard to epilepsy. The epileptic Toby, in the latter novel, has problems not only in writing, but also in speaking, especially long words: "He might stumble in speech sometimes and be slow, with his tongue lolling at the corner of his mouth" (Frame 56).

Pain is described in all its central different aspects: perception, expression, valuation, behavior, treatment, social reactions, and cultural context. In the novella *Cancer* (1830) by the English physician and writer Samuel Warren (1807-1877), the ill female protagonist gains support and strength during the very painful amputation of her breast without any anesthetics by reading the love letters of her absent husband. "Her eyes continued riveted, in one long burning gaze of fondness, on the beloved handwriting of her husband; and she moved not a limb, nor uttered than an occasional sigh, during the whole of the protracted and painful operation" (Warren 20). The limitations of literary representations are repeatedly stressed. The poet Rainer Maria Rilke is convinced of the anonymous and inhumane world of pain: "ce plan insituable et si peu humain" (Letter to Jules Supervieille 536).

Literature is not medicine; literary nosology differs from medical nosology, and literary classification is not the same as the modern "International Classification of Diseases" (ICD-10), which is accepted worldwide. Health and disease are physical, social, psychological, and spiritual phenomena that can be represented in concepts that are both descriptive and normative, although these two types or dimensions of concepts and perspectives have not always been clearly distinguished in medicine and literature.

Diseases must not always and only be negative. The poet and naturalist Novalis was convinced that chronic diseases afford the opportunity to practice the art of living and to gain in personal development: "Lehrjahre der Lebenskunst und der Gemütsbildung" (*Fragmente und Studien* 686). According to Jean Paul (1763-1825), diseases can force "Ash Wednesdays" on people which provide a perspective on and guide their entire lives: "Aschermittwoche, die zuweilen das ganze Leben sichten und lenken" (895). Men and women not only determine what will be regarded as health and disease, they also interpret these experiences and decide how to respond to them. No universally valid definition of health has been found until now nor a universally valid definition of disease. From this perspective, literature is rich with substantial suggestions and stimulations for medicine (here, the medical function of literature).

Etiology

Etiology or causality of disease is a decisive element in diagnosis and treatment, not only for medicine and the physician, but also for the patient, his or her family, and society. Aristotle differentiates four types of causes of disease: efficient cause (*causa efficiens*), final cause (*causa finalis*), material cause (*causa materialis*), and formal cause (*causa formalis*), whereas medicine during modern times concentrates upon the first type, i.e., efficient cause (*causa efficiens*), with, due to this orientation, important progress in treatment.

Literature, on the other hand,—and this is a further important contribution to medicine—keeps the three other types continuously in mind, especially the final cause (*causa finalis*), the sense or function of disease. The epileptic child Useppe in Elsa Morante's *La Storia* (1974) demands in his childish language to know—not only from his mother, but more from a metaphysical destiny—the reason of his being ill: "E con lo stupore di una bestiola, disse in una voce disperata: 'A'mà ... pecché?' In realtà, questa sua domanda non pareva rivolgersi proprio a Ida là presente: piuttosto a una qualche volontà assente, immane, e inspiegabile" (499-500; ellipsis in orig.).

In the Aristotelian tradition, which is also taken up by the philosopher Arthur Schopenhauer (1788-1860), the value of the *causa formalis* and *causa materialis* is explicitly acknowledged by the physician Dr. Behrens in Thomas Mann's *Der Zauberberg,* when he defines life as a specific union of the flux of matter and the continuity of form: "Leben ist, daß im Wechsel der Materie die Form erhalten bleibt" (372). In a holistic integration of nature and culture, body and soul—one can speak, if this is allowed, of "cultural-socio-psycho-somatics"— Mann conceives the cause of disease from the perspective of these four dimensions: culture influences society, society the individual, the individual mind the individual body. Disease is then the consequence of culture.

Human beings are not machines or mere organisms. Only philosophy, theology, art, and literature can provide an answer as to why disease and pain and death exist. According to Michel de Montaigne (1533-1592), life and death immanently belong together: "Mais tu ne meurs pas de ce que tu es malade: tu meurs de ce que tu es vivant" (1140). The evolution of modern forms of virtual medicine, virtual diagnosis, and virtual surgery lies in the Cartesian tradition. Against these objective and reductionist tendencies, philosophy, theology, and the arts remind medicine and society again and again of the subjective, mental, and cultural nature of disease.

But literature is not sacrosanct and cannot be absolutized; it has its limits and risks. An appropriate example are novels written from the perspective of the anti-psychiatric movement. The possibilities of literature in describing madness or psychotic disease and providing causal explanation has been often and controversially discussed; the German psychiatrist Kurt Schneider (1887-1967) marks a specific and fundamental limit or incapacity of literature in this field: "Das Wesen der Psychose ist das Abreißen der Verständlichkeit; das Dichterwerk aber verlangt durchgehende Motivzusammenhänge wenigstens in seinem hauptsächlichsten Geschehen" (10). Substitute another concept of literature and another concept of madness and this judgment will also change.

Patient Subjectivity and Behavior

The word "illness" in the English language refers to the subjective or personal side of disease, whereas "disease" has the connotation of a medical conception of pathological abnormality. The term "sickness" transcends both of these concepts by focusing on social coherences. A person can feel ill without having a disease, and, conversely, can have a disease without feeling ill. The way in which societies vary in their interpretations of physical and mental disorders and in their treatment of and symbolic reactions to them reflects the cultural dimension of disease.

Whereas in medicine the "history of the disease" (objectivity) has more and more replaced the "history of the patient" (subjectivity), literature since antiquity not only mentions disease, but always refers to the ill person as well (cf. F. Hartmann). The Middle Ages gave the name "scribendo solari" to the practice of writing as an aide in coping with disease and pain. In 1916, the term "bibliotherapy" was coined by Samuel McChord Crothers (1857-1927). Today, arts and literature are acknowledged as helpful in coping with disease, pain, and death. Contemporary biblio-counselling, bibliotherapy, or poetry therapy depends on several dimensions including the production and reception of literature in health and disease; the influence of different diseases; the influence of specific types of treatment; the influence of the patient's personality, interests, and culture; the literary work's mediation; the professional education of the bibliotherapist; and the integration of literature and the different arts.

Processes of naturalization, secularization, and individualization deeply influence the image of the patient in modern times. Idealism and romanticism in the 1800s, with metaphysical concepts of nature and spirit, determined the perception of illness and death and the physician-patient relationship. The positivist nineteenth century separated the natural sciences and medicine from the humanities and laid the foundations of scientific medicine; the concept of disease becomes objective. Undoubtedly the length and the quality of life are increased by means of anaesthesia, antisepsis, and bacteriology; at the same time, however, medicine is experiencing anthropological losses and scientific reductions.

In the twentieth century, the patient's subjectivity and ethics in medicine come to the fore once again. The "introduction of the subject" refers, according to the anthropological physician Viktor von Weizsäcker (1886-1957), to the patient, the doctor, and medicine.[3] The psychiatrist and philosopher Karl Jaspers (1883-1969) emphasizes the fundamental importance of the methodological dualism of "explaining" (science) and "understanding" (humanities) for medicine and especially psychiatry (cf. Jaspers). From the sociological perspective, the patient has a role with four different aspects: 1) an exemption from being responsible for incapacity, 2) an exemption from normal role and task obligations, 3) the obligation to try to "get well," and 4) the obligation to seek competent help (Parsons, "Definition" 117).[3]

Literature reflects these developments and positions without losing sight of the cultural, social, and individual dimension of disease and pain. All the aspects of individual patients, their conscience, feelings, thoughts, wishes, language, and behavior are repeatedly illustrated and judged in literary texts: the fears, hopes, thoughts, and actions of the tubercular Raphaël in Balzac's *La Peau de chagrin* (1831); the sensations and inner experiences of the epileptic Myshkin before and after the attacks and seizures in Dostoyevsky's *The Idiot* (1868/69); the detailed account and analysis of physical and psychic feelings in Marcel Proust's (1871-1922) *À la Recherche du temps perdu* (1913/27); the emotions and actions of the insane Moosbrugger before he commits a sex murder in Musil's *Der Mann ohne Eigenschaften*; the individual conscience of the ill and dying apothecary Malone in Carson McCullers's *Clock without Hands*; and the thoughts, behavior, and social contacts of the schizo-phrenic Paul Wittgenstein in Thomas Bernhard's (1931-1989) autobio-graphical novel *Wittgensteins Neffe* (1982).

Immediately before an epileptic attack (aura), Myshkin experiences profound sensations of "the highest synthesis of life," notwithstanding the severe and destructive character of his disease:

> He remembered among other things that he always had one minute just before the epileptic fit (if it came on while he was awake), when suddenly in the midst of sadness, spiritual darkness and oppression, there seemed at moments a flash of light in his brain, and with extraordinary impetus all his vital forces suddenly began working at their highest tension. The sense of life, the consciousness of self, were multiplied ten times at these moments which passed like a flash of lightning. His mind

---

[3] Cf. Weizsäcker, "Der Arzt und der Kranke" (1926).

and his heart were flooded with extraordinary light; all his uneasiness, all his doubts, all his anxieties were relieved at once, they were all merged in a lofty calm, full of serene, harmonious joy and hope. (Dostoyevsky, *The Idiot* 208)

In *The Sound and the Fury* (1929), William Faulkner (1897-1962) illustrates the language of the feeble-minded, deaf and dumb Benjy Compson using inner monologue as a narrative parallel: "I was trying to say, and I caught her, trying to say, and she screamed and I was trying to say and trying and the bright shapes began to stop and I tried to get out. I tried to get it off of my face, but the bright shapes were going again" (53).

Objectivity and subjectivity are connected. Disease changes the perception of time and space, especially in the case of psychiatric and neurological diseases. "Alzheimerland is a foreign country. Time doesn't move the same way here, calendars are fuzzy, the days and months shuffled like cards in a deck. And space is different too—the land seems to wobble, the signposts shift. You stumble through mud or sand, through mines and traps" (Moore 51).

All these examples—of literature as well as the other arts—manifest and demonstrate that subjectivity has a meaning that is both individual (the conscience of a single person) and general (culture) while objectivity also has individual meaning (the body of a single person) and general meaning (nature).

The Image of the Physician

In literary texts, all types of physicians, practitioners, and medical researchers are taken up: positive and negative, empathic and indifferent, general and specialized—often corresponding to philosophi-cal or scientific concepts, but sometimes also in an independent fiction-al sphere.

Plato's and Aristotle's typology of three physicians who model three different patient-doctor relationships (cf. Plato, *The Laws* 107) can be encountered in literature as well as in reality. The "slave doctor" commands, and the patient has to obey; the "doctor to free men" explains the treatment to the patient as well as to the patient's family and does not start unless the informed patient has given his or her consent; the doctor

understood as a "medically educated lay person" represents the individual who takes responsibility for his or her own health, sickness, and
death.

Karl Jaspers develops different types of explaining and
understanding: causal explaining, static understanding, genetic understanding, rational understanding, spiritual understanding, existential
understanding, and metaphysical understanding (cf. *General Psychopathology*). Viktor von Weizsäcker pleads for medicine as the double
union of disease and treatment and patient and physician. In addition to
explanation and comprehension, it is important for a doctor to have a
transjective understanding, which von Weizsäcker describes as
understanding how the patient understands himself (20). From the
sociological perspective, according to Talcott Parsons, the physician has
a role with specific aspects: 1) affective neutrality, 2) collective
orientation, 3) universal attitude, 4) medical competence, and 5)
functional speciality ("Social Structure" 428-79).

There are many impressive and stimulating examples of literary
physicians from the perspective of these concepts.[4] For example, in
Proust's *À la Recherche du temps perdu*, Dr. Boulbon stresses the
inherent relationship between disease and culture, consoling the author's
ill grandmother by saying:

> Vous appartenez à cette famille magnifique et lamentable qui est le sel
> de la terre. Tout ce que nous connaissons de grand nous vient des

---

[4]   There are the different physicians representing specific medical positions in
      Balzac's *La Peau de chagrin* (1831); the physicians who become ill in Robert
      Louis Stevenson's (1850-1894) *The Strange Case of Dr. Jekyll and Mr. Hyde*
      (1886), as well as in Charles Dickens's *A Tale of Two Cities* (1859), in
      Chekhov's *Ward No. 6* (1892), and in Walker Percy's (1916-1990) *The
      Thanatos Syndrome* (1987); the opposed physicians Dr. Boulbon and Dr.
      Cottard in Marcel Proust's *À la Recherche du temps perdu* (1913/27), Dr.
      Behrens and Dr. Krokowski in Thomas Mann's *Der Zauberberg*, and Dr.
      Hymes and Dr. Bradshaw in Virginia Woolf's *Mrs. Dalloway* (1926); the
      physician as scientist in Jean Paul's *Dr. Katzenbergers Badereise* (1809), in
      Zola's *Le Docteur Pascal* (1893), in Herbert George Wells's (1866-1946)
      The Island of Doctor Moreau (1896), in Sinclair Lewis's (1885-1951)
      Arrowsmith (1925), and, more recently, in Richard Powers's (*1957) *The
      Echo Maker* (2006).

nerveux. Ce sont eux et non pas d'autres qui ont fondé les religions et composé les chefs-d'œuvre. Jamais le monde ne saura tout ce qu'il leur doit et surtout ce qu'eux ont souffert pour le lui donner. Nous goûtons les fines musiques, les beaux tableaux, mille délicatesses, mais nous ne savons pas ce qu'elles ont coûté à ceux qui les inventèrent, d'insomnies, de pleurs, de rires spasmodiques, d'urticaires, d'asthmes, d'épilepsies, d'une angoisse de mourir qui est pire que tout cela, et que vous connaissez peut-être. (Proust 601)

The empathic physician Sir Lake Strett in *The Wings of the Dove* (1902) by Henry James (1843-1916) offers his patients in his limited time a "great empty cup of attention" (150). The patient Esther in *The Bell Jar* (1963) by Sylvia Plath (1932-1963) gives her doctor Nolan her "trust on a platter and told her everything, and she had promised, faithfully, to warn me ahead of time if ever I had to have another shock treatment" (223). Dr. Ravic in Erich Maria Remarque's (1898-1970) *Arc de Triomphe* (1946) conceals the inoperable cancer out of pity for his patient Kate Hegström, who is totally aware of her situation. The apothecary Malone (a name which could be interpreted as *I am alone*) in McCullers's novel *Clock without Hands* asks the physician for information, but expects reassurance and not the diagnostic truth. The ill physician Ljudmila Afanasjewna Doncova in Solzhenitsyn's *Cancer Ward* (1968) also rejects information and wishes simply to confide in her colleagues.

Mario Tobino (1910-1991), a psychiatrist in a mental hospital (Manicomio) near Lucca in Tuscany, applies the established modern treatment methods of psychiatry in his autobiographical novel *Le libere donne de Magliano* (1963) alongside psychopathology. Tobino thereby stresses the metaphysical dimensions of the hallucinations and delusions of his mad patients ("sue frasi avevano qualche cosa al 'di sopra dell'uman'" [129]), which cannot be found in the ICD-10, the standard diagnostic reference work for scientific classification of diseases.

The difference between patient and physician is not absolute—in the words of Proust's Dr. Boulbon: "Dans la pathologie nerveuse, un médecin qui ne dit pas trop de bêtises, c'est un malade à demi guéri, comme un critique est un poète qui ne fait plus de vers, un policier un voleur qui n'exerce plus" (602). The psychiatrist Manette in Dickens's *A Tale of Two Cities* (1859) becomes ill and through his illness indicates to his friend—a unique example in literature—the right means of being healed. Both Dr. Behrens and Dr. Krokowski in *Der Zauberberg* suffer from the diseases they try to cure, whereas the patients Castorp and Settembrini are active in art therapy (literature and music) and attending dying persons. The physician in Franz Kafka's novella "Ein Landarzt" (1918) is rejected by a young wounded boy on account of the doctor's incapacity to treat him insofar as the physician himself is ill: "Du bist ja auch nur irgendwo abgeschüttelt, kommst nicht auf eigenen Füßen" (127-28).

Diagnosis and Treatment

Concepts of disease, concepts of treatment, and concepts of the physician-patient relationship are interrelated. Thus, a mechanical or technologically structured understanding of disease (viewing the human as a defective machine) requires a corresponding mechanical or techno-logically structured treatment (in the sense of repair) and a mechanical or technologically structured healer-patient therapeutic relationship (a relationship of technician to defective machine). More personal or holistic concepts compel the respective types of treatment and healer-patient relationships.

In literary texts, certain forms of diagnostics can be problematized or rejected. The literary reception of the anti-psychiatry movement, for example, is depicted in the novels of Ernst Augustin (*1927) (*Raumlicht* [1976]), Heinar Kipphardt (1922-1982) (*März* [1976]), Walter Vogt (*Schizogorsk* [1977]), and criticized in Tobino's novel *Le libere donne di Magliano* (1963). In Thomas Mann's *Der Zauberberg*, for instance, medical radiology is judged as immoral; x-ray photographs are images of death: "Und Hans Castorp sah, was zu sehen er hatte erwarten müssen, was aber eigentlich dem Menschen zu sehen nicht bestimmt ist und wovon er auch niemals gedacht hatte, daß ihm bestimmt sein könne, es zu sehen: er sah in sein eigenes Grab" (306). Moosbrugger in Musil's *Der Mann ohne Eigenschaften* detests all psychiatrists who try to classify his complex nature using the scientific categories of medicine: "[er] haßte niemand so inbrünstig wie die Psychiater, die glaubten sein ganzes schwieriges Wesen mit ein paar Fremdworten abtun zu können, als wäre es für sie eine alltägliche Sache" (72). Whereas melancholia is no longer a medical category in modern medical classification, it continues to be examined in literature. The epileptic child Useppe in Morante's *La Storia* reacts to diagnostic examination with a fit of rage, but subsequently endures the process almost indifferently, as if witnessing some "abstruse ceremony" ("astrusa cerimonia") (Morante 398).

Medical treatment consists principally of dietetics, medication, and surgery. The system of dietetics involved much more than regulation of food and drink in antiquity; it embraced six areas of life that, although natural, did not regulate themselves as did such physiological functions as respiration and digestion and were therefore called "non-natural" (*sex res non naturales*): (1) air and light, (2) food and drink, (3) waking and sleep, (4) motion and rest, (5) secretions, and (6) emotions. Professor Schneider, a psychiatrist and Myshkin's teacher, suffering from epilepsy, cures his mentally ill patients following the logic of classical dietetics, "with cold water and gymnastics, training them also, and superintending their mental development generally" (Dostoyevsky, *The Idiot* 26). Medicine in modern times reduces dietetics more and more to diet (*cibus et potus*), or in the words of Dr. Grabow in Mann's novel *Buddenbrooks* (1901), to "ein wenig Franzbrot, ein wenig Taube" (37).

All types of surgery are exemplified in literature, even organ transplantation and specifically xeno transplantation. The living heart transplantation in Hartmann von Aue's medieval Middle High German verse poem *Der arme Heinrich* (circa 1195) depends on the informed and free consent of the young child, as the physician explains to her: "'Mein Kind, hast du diesen Entschluß selbst gefaßt oder bist du dazu durch Bitten oder Drohungen deines Herrn gebracht worden?' ... 'Wenn du stirbst, dich aber nicht aus freiem Willen geopfert hast, dann bist du junges Wesen tot, und es nützt uns leider überhaupt nichts! Deshalb offenbare mir, wie es zu deinem Entschluß kam. Ich sage dir, was mit dir geschehen wird'" (59, 61).

Treatment and research can come into conflict. In Dostoyevsky's *The Brothers Karamasov* (1879/80), Smerdjakov's extremely life-threatening epileptic attacks provoke less human condolence than scientific interest in the district medical officer: "'Such violent and protracted epileptic fits, recurring continually for twenty-four hours, are rarely to be met with, and are of interest to science,' he declared enthusiastically to his companions, and as they left they laughingly congratulated him on his find" (541).

Medical Institutions

The medical institution comprises hospitals, practice, and various corresponding initiatives of medicine and the health system of prevention, treatment, and rehabilitation. Thomas Mann's *Zauberberg*— a sanatorium in the Swiss Alps for patients suffering from tuberculosis—represents a classic example of the literary sanitorium based on the old medical adage *natura sanat, medicus curat*; the physician treats, nature cures. Mann's "großes Kolloquium über Gesundheit und Krankheit" (Mann, *Zauberberg* 621) debates the fundamental questions of health and disease, burial, corporal punishment, torture, religion, and enlightenment. The cause of disease, according to the author, transcends the physical and individual sphere and unifies nature and culture in what might be called a "cultural-socio-psycho-somatics."

The tubercular Settembrini develops a collection of literary texts helpful for different diseases and sufferings that could be compared with the collection of works of music which the physician Behrens supplies his patients in *Der Zauberberg*. In McCullers's *Clock without Hands*, the ill and dying apothecary Malone, suffering from cancer, is offered some books in the hospital. The murder mystery bores him; then his eyes are drawn to a book called *Sickness unto Death* (1849) by the Danish philosopher Soren Kierkegaard (1813-1855): "From the wilderness of print some lines struck his mind so that he was instantly awake. He read the lines again and then again: 'The greatest danger, that of losing one's own self, may pass off quietly as if it were nothing; every other loss, that of an arm, a leg, five dollars, a wife, etc., is sure to be noticed.' If Malone had not had an incurable disease those words would have been only words and he wouldn't have reached for the book in the first place" (McCullers 130).

In Aleksandr Solzhenitsyn's *Cancer Ward* (1967), the medical institution appears as a form of social order, with internal structures and external relations. The rooms in Station 13 are badly ordered, and not even the smallest space exists for the doctors in the radiation treatment department. The hospital isolates them from the world, which in turn further isolates the tumor; the melanoblastoma is considered the queen of all malignant tumors. *Cancer Ward* is not merely the account of a singular hospital, and stands not only for the post-Stalinist Soviet Union, but for the whole world. After his release from hospital, the patient Kostoglotow visits a zoo and discovers a similarity between the animals in their cages and human beings. He then realizes the difficulty of freedom: "[D]eprived of their home surroundings, they had lost the idea of rational freedom. It would only make things harder for them, suddenly to set them free" (Solzhenitsyn 508).

Hospitals can be places of aid and protection, but also of suppression and isolation. In "The System of Doctor Tarr and Professor Fether" (1845) by Edgar Allan Poe, the insane patients become physicians and nurses who themselves are locked up as patients: "The keepers, ten in number, having been suddenly overpowered, were first well tarred, then carefully feathered, and then shut up in underground cells" (628). In a similar reversal, the psychiatrist Ragin in Chekhov's *Ward No. 6* is confronted during his own mental illness with the inhumane conditions of the hospital, for which he was formerly responsible. In Dino Buzzati's "Sette piani" (1937), the ill are distributed on the seven floors of the institution according to the gravity of their illness—on the highest floors are the mildest cases, on the lowest floors, those who are dying. With the descent, the distance to society and nature increases and on the last floor no physicians are still active, only priests. Giuseppe Corte experiences this downward trajectory in the development of his disease and then finally total darkness, which signifies his death: "Con uno sforzo supremo Giuseppe Corte, che si sentiva paralizzato da uno strano torpore, guardò l'orologio, sul comodino, di fianco al letto. Erano le tre e mezzo. Voltò il capo dall'altra parte, e vide che le persiane scorrevoli, obbedienti a un misterioso comando, scendevano lentamente, chiudendo il passo alla luce" (Buzzati 42).

There are also, in contrast, positive examples in literature. The central aim of the Italian psychiatrist Mario Tobino is to transform his hospital for the insane near Lucca into a place of quiet and ordered communication: "Ed il mio desiderio è di fare di ogni grano di questo territorio un tranquillo, ordinato, universale parlare" (76).

Social Reactions to Disease

Social reactions include the reactions of the healthy to the ill, of the ill to the healthy, of one ill person to another ill person, and of a healthy person to another healthy person in regard to illness or those who are ill. The spectrum of these reactions is also great in works of literature, comprising refusal and help, misunderstanding and empathy, compassion and solidarity. The novella *La Chambre* (1939) by Jean Paul Sartre (1905-1980), for example, represents active euthanasia as the promise or readiness of Eve to kill her mad fiancé if he should reach a certain future stage of his madness: "Un jour, ces traits se brouilleraient, il laisserait pendre sa mâchoire, il ouvrirait à demi des yeux larmoyants. Eve se pencha sur la main de Pierre et y posa ses lèvres: 'Je te tuerai avant'" (75). And Paul in Jean Edern Hallier's (1936-1997) novel *Le Premier qui dort réveille l'autre* (1977) continues the life of his dead brother Aubert.

Agathe in Musil's *Der Mann ohne Eigenschaften* gains the capacity of withdrawing from daily demands during her illness, which makes her at the same time open to the deep and metaphysical dimensions of the world:

> Es ist nicht unmöglich, daß dieser Vorteil, den sie unter so eindrucksvollen Verhältnissen kennenlernte, später den Kern ihrer seelischen Bereitschaft bildete, sich dem Leben, dessen Erregungen aus irgendeinem Grund nicht ihren Erwartungen entsprachen, auf eine ähnliche Weise zu entziehen; es ist aber wahrscheinlicher, daß es sich umgekehrt verhielt und daß jene Krankheit, durch die sie sich den Forderungen der Schule und des Vaterhauses entzog, die erste Äußerung ihres transparenten, gleichsam für einen ihr unbekannten Gefühlsstrahl durchlässigen Verhältnisses zur Welt gebildet hatte. (Musil 856)

The birth of the deaf and dumb child Camilla destroys the marriage of her parents, Monsieur and Madame des Arcis:

> Ce qui causa cette séparation soudaine et tacite, plus affreuse qu'un divorce, et plus cruelle qu'une mort lente, c'est que la mère, en dépit du malheur, aimait son enfant avec passion, tandis que le chevalier, quoi qu'il voulût faire, malgré sa patience et sa bonté, ne pouvait vaincre l'horreur que lui inspirait cette malédiction de Dieu tombée sur lui. (Musset 575-76)

Similarly, in Joseph Conrad's novella *The Idiots*, it is suggested that it is the children's mental disability which is responsible for the breakdown of the parents' marriage: Susan stabs her husband Jean-Pierre to death and drowns herself afterwards in the ocean. "The mother of idiots—that was my nickname! And my children never would know me, never speak to me. They would know nothing; neither men—nor God" (Conrad 66).

Balzac's Lady Brandon in *La Grenadière* (1832) recommends that her son conceal his suffering from other persons in order to achieve fortuitous social and family arrangements:

> Mon fils, répondit-elle, nous devons ensevelir nos peines aux yeux des étrangers, leur montrer un visage riant, ne jamais leur parler de nous, nous occuper d'eux: ces maximes pratiquées en famille y sont une des causes du bonheur. Tu auras à souffrir beaucoup un jour! Eh! bien, souviens-toi de ta pauvre mère qui se mourait devant toi en te souriant toujours, et te cachait ses douleurs; tu te trouveras alors du courage pour supporter les maux de la vie. (434)

In *La Storia* by Elsa Morante, the epileptic mother Mancuso assists her epileptic child, Useppe, and experiences in his epileptic seizures what she herself could not see and observe when in this state of non-consciousness: "Stavolta Ida assistè coi propri occhi all'intera vicenda dell'insulto, fino al momento che il *Grande Male* gettò il suo grido, calando come un predatore omicida sul piccolo Useppe" (497). The death of her beloved son causes her madness and refusal to belong to mankind: "Ida prese a lagnarsi con una voce bassissima, bestiale: non voleva più appartenere alla specie umana" (647).

Symbolism, Ideas, Metaphors

Medicine in literature is never simply objective description but always contains metaphorical, symbolic, and ideal interpretations—this refers to disease, patients, physicians, diagnosis, treatment, the medical institution, and social reactions.

The statement by the romantic poet and scientist Novalis that the nature of disease is as dark as the nature of life ("[d]as Wesen der Krankheit ist so dunkel als das Wesen des Lebens"), is adopted by

Thomas Bernhard in his novel *Amras* (1964) as motto (cf. Novalis 595). In the novel *Ulysses* (1922) by James Joyce (1882-1941), the different organs each play specific symbolic roles which may correspond to the real way in which people interpret organ transplantation (kidney, liver, heart, brain, etc.) differently. Many novels of madness manifest the old topos of "wisdom in madness."[5] But only philosophers, according to Balzac, can understand the abyss between deepest stupidity and highest wisdom in the madness of Louis Lambert: "Les philosophes en regretteront les frondaisons atteintes par la gelée dans leurs bourgeons; mais sans doute ils en verront les fleurs écloses dans des régions plus élevées que ne le sont les plus hauts lieux de la terre" (*Louis Lambert* 646).

Leprosy as history of disease and patient in Hartmann von Aue's medieval epic poem *Der arme Heinrich* stands for a tainted soul. The knight's renouncement of the young girl's readiness to sacrifice her life and heart for him liberates the former from his disease and restores his moral integrity. The flickering lights of advertising in London streets are, according to Aldous Huxley, "the epileptic symbol of all that's most bestial and idiotic in contemporary life" (*Antic Hay* 230-31). In Albert Camus's *La Peste* (1947), it is said at the end of the novel that the rats will come back into a happy city: "la peste reveillerait ses rats et les enverrait mourir dans une cité heureuse" (1474). The epileptic Toby and his schizophrenic sister in Janet Frame's *Owls Do Cry* suffer from the "crevice" of the world: "We all carry some kind of mark like that because we are all branded in our lives, as I was. That is true" (Frame 170, 67). Beyond the empirical and scientific perspective brought to bear on Moosbrugger's sexual offense and his insanity in *Der Mann ohne Eigenschaften,* these phenomena are given a deep and symbolic meaning: "Wenn die Menschheit als Ganzes träumen könnte, müsste Moosbrugger entstehen" (Musil 76).

---

[5] See the literary work of, for example, Erasmus von Rotterdam (c. 1467-1536), Miguel de Cervantes (1547-1616), E.T.A. Hoffmann (1776-1822), Balzac, Gérard de Nerval (1808-1855), Poe, Dostoyevsky, Dickens, and Thomas Bernhard.

Perspectives

Medicine in literature or more broadly the conjunction of medicine and literature signifies many dimensions and stimulates debates on the nature of medicine, literature, and reality. In regard to these contributions by art and literature, three types of relationship between medicine and literature seem fundamental: Medicine and medical history contribute to literary interpretations (=the literary function of medicine); the representations of literature stimulate medicine and medical education (=the medical function of literature); literature influences general and individual attitudes towards health and disease, birth and death, and medical institutions and treatment (=the general function of literary medicine).

Health and disease are not merely medical terms; they are also vital themes in literature and art, philosophy, theology, sociology, and psychology. In fact, these very disciplines remind medicine again and again of its "anthropological" character, in the sense that medicine deals with the nature and destiny of humans. Neither medicine nor the concepts of health and disease with which it deals can be properly understood by using the contrasting categories of natural sciences and human sciences as a framework. Just as medicine cannot be reduced to either of the two, it is necessary to connect nature and culture in order to reach an understanding of health and disease. Medical humanities is the modern term for medicine as a unity of sciences and humanities. Both representations and interpretations of literature are fundamental contributions; medicine itself is a science and an art; and living with disease is also an art.

Culture is the cause of disease but culture is equally the product of disease. Culture shapes disease, diagnosis, and treatment, the situation of the patient, the activity of the physician, and social reactions. Subjectivity has an individual meaning (i.e., conscience of a single person) and a general meaning (i.e., culture), and objectivity also has an individual meaning (connoting the body of a single person) and a general meaning (nature). Besides the transcendent transcendence of religion, an immanent transcendence of culture exists, which can be experienced by listening to music, reading books, or looking at paintings. Culture—meaning literature and all the arts—enables an acceptance of the limits of individual life, pain, disease, and death.

Works Cited

Aristotle. *Poetics.* c. 335 B.C.E. *The Complete Works.* Vol. 6. Princeton: Princeton UP, 1984.

Balzac, Honoré de. "Avant-Propos." 1842. *La Comédie Humaine.* Vol. 1. Paris: Gallimard, 1976. 7-20. Print.

---. *La Grenadière.* 1832. *La Comédie Humaine.* Vol. 2. *Études de moeurs: Scènes de la vie privée.* Paris: Gallimard, 1951. 422-43.

---. *Louis Lambert.* 1832. *La Comédie Humaine.* Vol 11. *Études philosophiques.* Paris: Gallimard, 1980. 589-692. Print.

---. *La Peau de chagrin.* 1831. *La Comédie Humaine.* Vol. 10. *Études philosophiques.* Paris: Gallimard, 1979. 47-294. Print.

Bernhard, Thomas. *Amras.* Frankfurt am Main: Suhrkamp, 1987. Print.

---. *Wittgensteins Neffe: Eine Freundschaft.* Frankfurt am Main: Suhrkamp, 1987. Print.

Binet, Léon, and Pierre Vallery-Radot. *Médecine et Littérature.* Paris: Expansion Scientifique Française, 1965. Print.

Buzzati, Dino. "Sette piani." 1937. *La Boutique del Mistero.* Milano: Mondadori, 2006. 25-42. Print.

Camus, Albert. *La Peste.* 1947. Paris: Gallimard, 1967. Print.

Carmichael, Ann G., and Richard M. Ratzan, eds. *Medicine: A Treasury of Art and Literature.* New York: Lauter Levin, 1991. Trans. as *Medizin: In Literatur und Kunst.* Köln: Könemann, 1994. Print.

Ceccio, Joseph, ed. *Medicine in Literature.* New York: Longman, 1978. Print.

Chekhov, Anton Pavlovich. "Ward No. 6." *Ward No. 6 and Other Stories.* New York: Barnes & Noble Classics, 2003. 177-232. Print.

---. *Letters.* Ed. and sel. Avvalim Yarmolinsky. New York: Viking, 1973. Print.

Conrad, Joseph. "The Idiots." 1896. *Tales of Unrest.* Ed. Allan H. Simmons and J. H. Stape. Cambridge: Cambridge UP, 2012. 51-74. Print.

Crothers, Samuel McChord. "A Literary Clinic." 1917. *The Atlantic Monthly* 118.3 (1916): 291-301. Print.

Dickens, Charles. *A Tale of Two Cities.* 1859. London: Penguin Classics, 2011. Print.

Dostoyevsky, Fyodor Mikhailovich. *The Brothers Karamazov.* 1880-81. University Park: Pennsylvania State UP, 2007. Print.

---. *The Idiot*. 1868. New York: Barnes & Noble Classics, 2005. Print.

Downie, Robin S., ed. *The Healing Arts*. Oxford: Oxford UP, 1994. Print.

Engelhardt, Dietrich von. *Medizin in der Literatur der Neuzeit*. Vols.1-2. Hürtgenwald: Pressler, 1991-2000.

---. *Krankheit, Schmerz und Lebenskunst: Eine Kulturgeschichte der Körpererfahrung*. München: C. H. Beck, 1999. Print.

---, ed. *Bibliotherapie*. Gerlingen: Bleicher, 1987. Print.

Faulkner, William. *The Sound and the Fury*. 1929. New York: Vintage, 1990. Print.

Frame, Janet. *Owls Do Cry*. 1957. London: Women's Press, 2002. Print.

Goncharov, Ivan Aleksandrovich. *Oblomov*. 1859. London: George Allen & Unwin, 1915. Print.

Hallier, Jean-Edern. *Le Premier qui dort réveille l'autre*. Paris: Sagittaire, 1977. Print.

Hartmann von Aue. *Der arme Heinrich*. c. 1195. Frankfurt am Main: Fischer, 1997. Print.

Hartmann, Fritz. "Krankheitsgeschichte und Krankengeschichte (naturhistorische und personale Krankheitsauffassung)." *Sitzungsberichte der Gesellschaft zur Beförderung der gesamten Naturwissenschaften zu Marburg* 87.2 (1966): 17-32. Print.

Hegel, Georg Wilhelm Friedrich. *Vorlesungen über die Aesthetik*. Stuttgart-Bad Cannstatt: Fromman, [4]1964. Print.

Huxley, Aldous. *Antic Hay*. 1923. London: Chatto & Windus, 1949. Print.

---. *Literature and Science*. London: Chatto & Windus, 1963. Print.

Jagow, Bettina von, and Florian Steger, eds. *Literatur und Medizin: Ein Lexikon*. Göttingen: Vandenhoeck & Ruprecht, 2005. Print.

James, Henry. *The Wings of the Dove*. 1902. Harmondsworth: Penguin, 1971. Print.

Jaspers, Karl. *General Psychopathology*. Vol. 2. Baltimore: Johns Hopkins UP, 1997. Print.

Kafka, Franz. *Briefe 1902-1924*. Frankfurt am Main: Fischer, 1958. Print.

---. "Ein Landarzt." 1918. *Sämtliche Erzählungen*. Frankfurt am Main: Fischer, 1988. 123-28. Print.

London S. J. "The Whimsy Syndromes: The Fine Art of Literary Nosology." *Archives of Internal Medicine* 122 (1968): 448-52. Print.

Mann, Thomas. "Bilse und ich." 1906. *Gesammelte Werke*. Vol. 10. Frankfurt am Main: Fischer, 1974. 9-22. Print.

---. *Buddenbrooks*. 1901. *Gesammelte Werke*. Vol. 1. Frankfurt am Main: Fischer, 1974. Print.

---. *Der Zauberberg*. 1924. *Gesammelte Werke*. Vol. 3. Frankfurt am Main: Fischer, 1974. Print.

McCullers, Carson. *Clock without Hands*. 1961. London: Penguin, 1965. Print.

Montaigne, Michel de. *Les Essais*. 1580/95. Paris: Gallimard, 2007. Print.

Moore, Jeffrey. *The Memory Artists*. 2004. New York: Phoenix, 2005. Print.

Morante, Elsa. *La Storia*. 1974. Torino: Einaudi, 1995. Print.

Musil, Robert. *Der Mann ohne Eigenschaften*. Hamburg: Rowohlt, 1952. Print.

Musset, Alfred de. *Pierre et Camille*. 1844. *Contes: Œuvres complètes en prose*. Paris: Gallimard, 1960. 571-611.

Novalis. *Fragmente und Studien, 1799/1800. Schriften*. Vol. 3. 3rd rev. ed. Ed. Richard H. Samuel and Paul Kluckhohn. Darmstadt: WBG, 1983. 525-694. Print.

Parsons, Talcott. "Definition of Health and Illness in the Light of American Values and Social Structure." *Patients, Physicians and Illness*. Ed. E. Gartly Jaco. 1958. New York: Free Press, [3]1979. 107-27. Print.

---. "Social Structure and Dynamic Process: The Case of Modern Medical Practice." *The Social System*. Glencoe: Free Press, 1951. 428-79. Print.

Paul, Jean. *Titan*. 1800-03. *Sämtliche Werke*. Ed. Norbert Miller. Part 1, Vol. 3. München: Hanser, 1961. Print.

Peschel, Enid Rhodes, ed. *Medicine and Literature*. New York: Neale Watson Academic Publications, 1980. Print.

Petzold, Hilarion, and Ilse Orth, eds. *Poesie und Therapie: Über die Heilkraft der Sprache. Poesietherapie, Bibliotherapie, Literarische Werkstätten*. Paderborn: Junfermann, 1985. Print.

Plath, Sylvia. *The Bell Jar*. 1963. London: Faber, 1999. Print.

Plato. *The Laws*. c. 347 B.C.E. Chicago: U of Chicago P, 1988. Print.

Poe, Edgar Allan. "The System of Doctor Tarr and Professor Fether." 1845. *The Complete Tales and Poems*. New York: Barnes & Noble, 2007. 613-28. Print.

Proust, Marcel. "Le Côté de Guermantes." I. 1920-21. *À la Recherche du temps perdu*. Vol. II. Paris: Gallimard, 1988. 307-608. Print.

Rilke, Rainer Maria. *Briefe*. Vol. 2. Wiesbaden: Insel, 1950. Print.

Rubin, Rhea Joyce, ed. *Using Bibliotherapy*. Phoenix: Oryx Press, 1978. Print.

Sartre, Jean Paul. "La Chambre." 1939. *Le Mur*. Paris: Gallimard, 1939. 37-75.

Schneider, Kurt. *Der Dichter und der Psychopathologe*. Köln: Rheinland-Verlag, 1922. Print.

Solzhenitsyn, Aleksandre. *Cancer Ward*. 1967. New York: Farrar, Straus and Giroux, 1991.

Tobino, Mario. *Le Libere Donne di Magliano*. 1963. Milan: Arnoldo Mondadori, 1990. Print.

Trautmann, Joanne, and Carol Pollard. *Literature and Medicine: Topics, Titles and Notes*. Philadelphia: Society for Health and Human Values, 1975. Rev. ed. *Literature and Medicine: An Annotated Bibliography*. Pittsburgh: U of Pittsburgh P, 1982. Print.

Warren, Samuel. "Cancer." 1830. *Passages from the Diary of a Late Physician*. Edinburgh: Blackwood, 1868. 18-20. Print.

Weizsäcker, Viktor von. "Der Arzt und der Kranke." 1926. *Gesammelte Schriften*. Vol. 5. Frankfurt am Main: Suhrkamp, 1987. 9-26.

Zifreund, Walther, ed. *Therapien im Zusammenspiel der Künste*. Tübingen: Attempto, 1996. Print.

Zola, Émile: *Le Docteur Pascal*. 1893. *Œuvres Complètes*. Vol. 5. Les Rougon-Macquart. Paris: Gallimard, 1967. 313-1220.

---. *Une Page d'amour*. 1878. *Œuvres Complètes*. Vol. 2. Les Rougon-Macquart. Paris: Gallimard, 1961. 801-1092. Print.

Contributors

CARMEN BIRKLE is Professor of American Studies at the University of Marburg, Germany. She taught at the University of Mainz and was Visiting Professor at the University of Vienna and at Columbia University, New York City. She currently serves as Vice President of the German Association for American Studies and was assistant editor of the journal *Amerikastudien/American Studies* from 1992 to 2002. She holds a Ph.D. in American Studies from the University of Mainz (1994) where she also received her postdoctoral degree (2002). Her publications, research, and teaching focus on ethnic and gender studies, inter- and transculturality, literature and medicine, and popular culture. She is the author of *Women's Stories of the Looking Glass* (1996) and *Migration—Miscegenation—Transculturation* (2004), editor of *Literature and Medicine: Women in the Medical Profession (Parts I and II)* [special issues of the online journal *gender forum* (Sept. and Dec. 2009)], and co-editor of *(Trans)Formations of Cultural Identity in the English-Speaking World* (1998), *Frauen auf der Spur: Kriminalautorinnen aus Deutschland, Großbritannien und den USA* (2001), *Sites of Ethnicity: Europe and the Americas* (2004), *Asian American Studies in Europe* (2006), *"The Sea Is History": Exploring the Atlantic* (2009), *Living American Studies* (2010), and *Emanzipation und feministische Politiken* (2012). Her current book project focuses on the intersections of literature, gender, and medicine in nineteenth-century America.

CARLA BITTEL is Associate Professor of History at Loyola Marymount University in Los Angeles. She received her Ph.D. in American history at Cornell University in 2003. Her research focuses on gender issues in the history of medicine; she has examined the history of women's health, women physicians, and the role of science in medicine. Bittel is the author of *Mary Putnam Jacobi and the Politics of Medicine in Nineteenth-Century America* (U of North Carolina P, 2009). She has also published in the *Bulletin of the History of Medicine* and contributed to the edited volume *Women Physicians and the Cultures of Medicine* (Johns Hopkins UP, 2009). Her research has been supported by several grants, including a Scholars Award from the National Science Foundation. Her new work examines the politics of gender and phrenology in antebellum America.

STEPHANIE BROWNER is Dean of Eugene Lang College at The New School for Liberal Arts in New York City. Formerly she was the Academic Vice President and Dean of Faculty at Berea College in Kentucky, known nationwide for providing a tuition-free liberal arts education to low-income students. Browner is the author of *Profound Science and Elegant Literature: Imagining Doctors in Nineteenth-Century America* (U of Pennsylvania P, 2005), which was named an outstanding academic title of the year by *Choice* magazine, and her articles on literature and medicine have appeared in *American Quarterly*, *PMLA*, and *Texas Studies in Literature and Language*. In addition, she is a co-author of *Literature and the Internet: A Guide for Students, Teachers, and Scholars* (Routledge, 2000) and recently published an essay on "Digital Humanities and the Study of Race and Ethnicity" in *The American Literature Scholar in the Digital Age*. She is the founder and editor of the Charles Chesnutt Digital Archive and serves on the Board of NINES (Networked Interface for Nineteenth-Century Electronic Scholarship). Lecturing widely both in the U.S. and abroad, Dr. Browner has given keynote addresses to graduating medical students and to the medical school faculty at the University of Kentucky. She holds a Ph.D. and an M.A. in American Literature and American Studies from Indiana University and a B.A. from the University of Chicago.

BIRGIT DÄWES is Professor (Juniorprofessorin) of American Studies at Johannes Gutenberg University, Mainz. She received her Ph.D. and postdoctoral degree (habilitation) from the University of Würzburg, Germany, and she has been fortunate to spend some of her academic time at University College, Galway, Ireland, at Amherst College, Massachusetts, at Stanford University, California, as well as the National Sun Yat-sen University in Kaohsiung, Taiwan; partly with research grants from the German Academic Exchange Service (DAAD) and the German-American Fulbright Commission. Her publications include the two award-winning monographs *Native North American Theater in a Global Age: Sites of Identity Construction and Trans-difference* (Winter, 2007) and *Ground Zero Fiction: History, Memory, and Representation in the American 9/11 Novel* (Winter, 2011). Most recently, an edited collection on *Indigenous North American Drama: A Multivocal History* was published by the State U of New York P (2013).

ANTJE DALLMANN received her Ph.D. in American Studies and her M.A. in American and British Studies, Cultural Studies, and French from Humboldt University Berlin with a dissertation on *ConspiraCity New York: Großstadtbetrachtung zwischen Paranoia und Selbster-mächtigung*, published in 2009. At present, she teaches American literature and culture at Humboldt University Berlin. Her research interests focus on the representation and symbolization of medicine and the "medical romance," urban literature and culture, visual cultures, and Minority Studies.

DIETRICH VON ENGELHARDT studied Philosophy, History, and Slavic Languages and received his Ph.D. in 1969 and his medical habilitation in 1976. From 1983 to 2007, he was Director of the Institute for the History of Medicine and Natural Sciences at the University of Lübeck. He has been a member of the *Deutsche Akademie der Naturforscher Leopoldina* since 1995 and has taught at the Internationale Hochschule für Kunsttherapie und Kreativpädagogik Hamburg since 1998 and at the Asklepios Medical School in Budapest/Hamburg since 2009. His research interests are the philosophy of medicine, the history of medical ethics, medicine in literature, science and medicine in the epoch of Idealism and Romanticism, historical consciousness in the natural sciences, coping processes of patients, and art therapy.

SONJA FIELITZ is Professor of English Literature at the University of Marburg, Germany. She studied English, Latin, and German at the University of Munich and received her Ph.D. in 1992 with a study of Shakespeare's *Timon of Athens*. Her postdoctoral thesis, published in 2000, examines the status of Ovid's *Metamorphoses* within the various theoretical and critical discourses in eighteenth-century England. She is the editor of two (German) book series and has furthermore edited five collections of essays in English on various topics. Her further publications include two textbooks on how to analyze dramas, respectively novels, a study of Shakespeare's *Othello*, and numerous articles on the early modern period, the long eighteenth century, children's literature, high school and university novels, and postmodern drama with particular reference to performance criticism.

INGRID GESSNER is Assistant Professor of American Studies at the University of Regensburg. She also taught at the University of Mainz and the University of Michigan, Ann Arbor, and is the recipient of research grants from the German Academic Exchange Service (DAAD), the German-American Fulbright Commission, and the German Research Foundation (DFG). She is the author of *Kollektive Erinnerung als Katharsis? Das Vietnam Veterans Memorial in der öffentlichen Kontroverse* (2000) and of the award-winning *From Sites of Memory to Cybersights: (Re)Framing Japanese American Experiences* (2007). Further publications include articles on cultural memory, visual culture, the digital and transnational turns in American Studies, and on teaching American Studies. She is currently finishing a book on the cultural dimension and representation of yellow fever in nineteenth-century U.S.-American literature and visual culture.

ASTRID HAAS is a researcher and instructor of American literature and culture at Bielefeld University, Germany. She studied English and American Studies, History, and Art History at the University of Münster, Germany, where she received her Ph.D. in 2007, and the College of William and Mary, Williamsburg, Virginia. Her research interests include travel writing of the Americas, U.S.-American drama and autobiography, ethnic and gender studies, literature and medicine, sports culture, and the visual arts and media. Besides various contributions to journals and edited volumes, her publications include the monograph *Stages of Agency: The Contributions of American Drama to the AIDS Discourse* (2011). Together with María Herrera-Sobek she co-edited *Transfrontera: Transnational Perspectives on the U.S.-Mexico Borderlands*, a special issue of the *American Studies Journal* (2012). Her current research project, financed by the German Research Foundation, is a comparative analysis of U.S.-American, Mexican, and German travel writing on Texas, 1821-1861.

MARCEL HARTWIG is research and teaching assistant at the University of Siegen, Germany. He studied English and American Studies at Chemnitz University of Technology and the University of Glasgow. He was both a junior lecturer in English and American Studies and Ph.D. student at TU Chemnitz. Hartwig is author of *Die traumatisierte Nation?: "Pearl Harbor" und "9/11" als kulturelle Erinnerungen* (transcript, 2011). He has published articles in academic readers as well as European journals in the fields of literary criticism, gender studies, and popular culture. These include essays on Andy Warhol, F. Scott Fitzgerald, Sinclair Lewis, Bret Easton Ellis, and Michael Chabon. Hartwig is co-editor of *Media Economies* (due to be published in 2013) and is currently working on his postdoctoral project in the field of transatlantic studies entitled *Transit Cultures: Early Medical Discourses in England and the New World*.

JOHANNA HEIL studied at the University of Marburg, Germany, and at Trinity College Dublin and received her M.A. in 2008. Since then she has worked as instructor in American Studies at the University of Marburg, teaching classes in American literature and culture and working on her doctoral thesis (working title: "An Inquiry into Knowing: Narrative, Sciences, and Works of Art in Richard Powers's Fiction"). She was a visiting scholar at the University of Illinois at Urbana-Champaign in 2010 and 2012 with grants from the German Academic Exchange Service (DAAD). Her research interests include contemporary literature, critical and cultural theory, literature and medicine, psychoanalysis, the neuroscientific turn, and dance and performance studies.

IMKE KIMPEL studied at Boston University and the University of Marburg, Germany, and majored in English Literature with an M.A. thesis on "William Shakespeare's *Troilus and Cressida*: Texts and Contexts" at the University of Marburg in 2008. She is currently pursuing a Ph.D. in early modern English literature (working title: "Shakespeare's Histories") and teaches classes on early modern and modern English literature as an instructor in the Department of English and American Studies at the University of Marburg.

MARTIN KUESTER teaches English and Canadian Literature at the University of Marburg, Germany, and is Director of the Marburg Centre for Canadian Studies. A graduate of German and Canadian universities (M.A. Trier, Ph.D. Manitoba, Dr. phil. habil. Augsburg), he has written and/or edited several books and numerous essays on Canadian and English literature. His monographs include *Framing Truths: Parodic Structures in Contemporary English-Canadian Historical Novels* (U of Toronto P, 1992) and *Milton's Prudent Ambiguities: Words and Signs in His Poetry and Prose* (2009). He co-wrote *Basislexikon anglistische Literaturwissenschaft* (2007) and co-edited, amongst other works, *Writing Canadians: The Literary Construction of Ethnic Identities* (2002), *Reading(s) from a Distance: European Critics on Canadian Women's Writing* (2008), and *Narratives of Crisis / Crisis of Narrative* (2012). From 2011 to 2013, he was President of the Gesellschaft für Kanada-Studien (Association for Canadian Studies in German-Speaking Countries).

RÜDIGER KUNOW is Chair of the American Studies program at Potsdam University. He is also Director of the Ph.D. School "Cultures of Mobility." His major research interests are cultural constructions of aging and illness, transnational American Studies, and the sub-continental diaspora in the U.S. From 2005 to 2008 he served as President of the German Association for American Studies.

CHRISTINE MARKS is Assistant Professor in the English Department at LaGuardia Community College (City University of New York). She received her Ph.D. from Johannes Gutenberg University in Mainz, Germany with a dissertation on intersubjective identity constellations in the works of the contemporary American novelist and essayist Siri Hustvedt. Her academic interests also include literature and medicine, food and culture, gender studies, hybrid identities, and theories of the gaze. She has taught courses in composition, cultural studies, American literature, and world literature.

MARC PRIEWE is Professor of American Studies and New English Literature at the University of Stuttgart. From 2007 to 2008 he worked as a Visiting Assistant Professor of Early American Literature at St. Lawrence University. From 2008 until 2010 he was a part-time online instructor at the New School in New York City. In 2009 he was awarded a Fulbright Fellowship to work in the History of American Civilization Program, Harvard University. His books include *Writing Transit: Refiguring National Imaginaries in Chicana/o Narratives* (Winter, 2007) and *Imagined Transnationalism: U.S-Latino/a Literature, Culture, and Identity* (co-edited, Palgrave, 2009). His second monograph deals with literary and cultural representations of illness, healing, and medicine in colonial New England and is funded by the German Research Foundation.

ANCA-RALUCA RADU teaches English Literature and Culture at the University of Göttingen. She holds a Ph.D. from the University of Marburg, Germany, for her dissertation "Intertextuality in English-Canadian Artist Novels" (2009). Her publications are in the field of Canadian Studies, and her research interests are contemporary British and Canadian fiction, the contemporary first-person novel, and the rhetoric and ethics of narration.

KATJA SCHMIEDER earned her Ph.D. (2008) at the University of Leipzig. Her field of interests stretches from literature of every shade via art and art history to the natural sciences along with their history and philosophy. In her doctoral thesis she explored the relevance of C. P. Snow's statement about the allegedly unbridgeable gap between the "two cultures"—literature and science—and argued for their reconciliation in American crime novels of the late twentieth century. Thus, it comes as no surprise that—along with her regular participation in meetings and symposia in the field of American Studies—she engages in seemingly unrelated areas of research. In this context she has presented at conventions of forensic psychiatrists and at conferences of the Society for Literature, Science, and the Arts, published on the German perception of American crime fiction, and participated in a postmortem as part of an interdisciplinary research project. She is currently engaged in a project on fictions about age difference.

PETER SCHNECK is Professor and Chair of American Literature and Culture at Osnabrück University. He studied American Studies and Media and Communication Studies at the Free University Berlin and at Yale University and received his Ph.D. from the FU Berlin in 1996.

Between 1997 and 2006 he taught as an assistant and associate professor at the Amerika-Institut in Munich. He was a fellow at the National Museum of American Art, Smithsonian Institution in Washington D.C. and a visiting scholar at the University of California at Irvine, Nottingham University, and the University of Torino, Italy. His publications include *Rhetoric and Evidence: Legal Conflict and Literary Representation in American Culture* (DeGruyter, 2011); *Bilder der Erfahrung: Kulturelle Wahrnehmung im amerikanischen Realismus* (Campus, 1998); *Iconographies of Power: The Politics and Poetics of Visual Representation* (co-ed., 2003); *Making America: The Cultural Work of Literature* (co-ed., 2000); *Hyperkultur: Zur Fiktion des Computerzeitalters* (co-ed., 1996); as well as articles on literature and visual art, media history, cultural studies, and law and literature. Since 1997 he is also co-editor of *PhiN.Philologie im Netz*, an online journal for literary and cultural studies and linguistics. From 2008 to 2011, he was president of the German Association for American Studies (GAAS). He participated in the joint committee of the GAAS and the German Association for English Studies for the development of national standards in teachers' education in 2008/09.

ANNA THIEMANN obtained her M.Ed. (*Erstes Staatsexamen*) and M.A. (*Magistra Artium*) in English, German, Philosophy, and Communication Studies from Westfälische Wilhelms-University Münster, Germany. Since 2007, she has been a research and teaching assistant to the chair of American Studies at WWU Münster. Her teaching and research interests include contemporary and nineteenth-century American literature, literature and science, visual culture, ethnic studies, and gender studies. She is currently finishing her Ph.D. project about trauma, neuroscience, and the contemporary literary imagination, which she developed at WWU Münster and Duke University, North Carolina. Her publications include "Metaphor and (Dis)Embodiment: Inside the Autistic Mind" (2008), co-authored with Annette Kern-Stähler, *Ethik in der Medizin: Literarische Texte für den neuen Querschnittsbereich GTE* (2013), co-authored and co-edited with Annette Kern-Stähler and Bettina Schöne Seifert, as well as several (forthcoming) articles about medicine and ethnicity, civil religion, and "9/11."

KIRSTEN TWELBECK is Assistant Professor of American Studies at the University of Hanover, Germany, with an interest in questions of identity formation and nation-building. Much of her scholarship analyzes intersections of gender, race, citizenship, and religion, focusing on cultural conflict as a driving force in American culture. She is the author of *No Korean Is Whole—Wherever He Or She May Be* (Peter Lang, 2002), that discusses Korean American literature in a transpacific context. Her current book project turns to Reconstruction-era literature and analyzes the struggle to define the meaning of democracy and citizenship during the "Second Founding." Her project centers on the Civil War hospital as an intercultural contact zone and a metaphorical site where healing was associated with national recovery. She has also lectured and taught courses on the cultural relationship between Germany and America, focusing on medicine, science, and education.